AF870213

Cataract Surgery Complications

Cataract Surgery Complications

Lucio Buratto, MD
Centro Ambrosiano Oftalmico
Milan, Italy

Stephen F. Brint, MD, FACS
Associate Clinical Professor of Ophthalmology
Tulane University School of Medicine
New Orleans, Louisiana

Mario R. Romano, MD, PhD
Department of Ophthalmology
Head of Vitreo-Retinal Service
Istituto Clinico e di Ricerca Humanitas, IRCSS
Rozzano (Milan), Italy

CRC Press
Taylor & Francis Group
Boca Raton London New York

CRC Press is an imprint of the
Taylor & Francis Group, an **informa** business

Illustrations courtesy of Massimiliano Crespi and Lucio Buratto.

First published 2013 by SLACK Incorporated

Published 2024 by CRC Press
2385 NW Executive Center Drive, Suite 320, Boca Raton FL 33431

and by CRC Press
4 Park Square, Milton Park, Abingdon, Oxon, OX14 4RN

CRC Press is an imprint of Taylor & Francis Group, LLC

© 2013 Taylor & Francis Group, LLC

This book contains information obtained from authentic and highly regarded sources. While all reasonable efforts have been made to publish reliable data and information, neither the author[s] nor the publisher can accept any legal responsibility or liability for any errors or omissions that may be made. The publishers wish to make clear that any views or opinions expressed in this book by individual editors, authors or contributors are personal to them and do not necessarily reflect the views/opinions of the publishers. The information or guidance contained in this book is intended for use by medical, scientific or health-care professionals and is provided strictly as a supplement to the medical or other professional's own judgement, their knowledge of the patient's medical history, relevant manufacturer's instructions and the appropriate best practice guidelines. Because of the rapid advances in medical science, any information or advice on dosages, procedures or diagnoses should be independently verified. The reader is strongly urged to consult the relevant national drug formulary and the drug companies' and device or material manufacturers' printed instructions, and their websites, before administering or utilizing any of the drugs, devices or materials mentioned in this book. This book does not indicate whether a particular treatment is appropriate or suitable for a particular individual. Ultimately it is the sole responsibility of the medical professional to make his or her own professional judgements, so as to advise and treat patients appropriately. The authors and publishers have also attempted to trace the copyright holders of all material reproduced in this publication and apologize to copyright holders if permission to publish in this form has not been obtained. If any copyright material has not been acknowledged please write and let us know so we may rectify in any future reprint.

Except as permitted under U.S. Copyright Law, no part of this book may be reprinted, reproduced, transmitted, or utilized in any form by any electronic, mechanical, or other means, now known or hereafter invented, including photocopying, microfilming, and recording, or in any information storage or retrieval system, without written permission from the publishers.

For permission to photocopy or use material electronically from this work, access www.copyright.com or contact the Copyright Clearance Center, Inc. (CCC), 222 Rosewood Drive, Danvers, MA 01923, 978-750-8400. For works that are not available on CCC please contact mpkbookspermissions@tandf.co.uk

Trademark notice: Product or corporate names may be trademarks or registered trademarks and are used only for identification and explanation without intent to infringe.

Library of Congress Cataloging-in-Publication Data

Buratto, Lucio.
Cataract surgery complications / Lucio Buratto, Stephen F. Brint, Mario R. Romano.
p. ; cm.
Includes bibliographical references and index.
ISBN 978-1-61711-608-7 (alk. paper)
I. Brint, Stephen F., 1946- II. Romano, Mario R. III. Title.
[DNLM: 1. Cataract Extraction--adverse effects. 2. Cataract Extraction--methods. WW 260]

617.7'4201--dc23

2012038582

ISBN: 9781617116087 (hbk)
ISBN: 9781003522881 (ebk)

DOI: 10.1201/9781003522881

Dedication

All surgeons have complications...we hope you only have a few and I hope that this book will help to resolve them very well.
Lucio Buratto, MD

I have been so fortunate to have great teachers and friends who have helped me though the management of the inevitable complications of cataract surgery, and have made me a better surgeon.
Stephen F. Brint, MD, FACS

To my father, the guide of my first steps in surgery and in life.
Mario R. Romano, MD, PhD

Contents

Acknowledgments

Publishing a book is a very exhausting task. There is an incredible amount of work involved. All of this would not have been possible without the smooth-running organization and help from a number of people that I would now like to thank personally:

I would like to thank Mario Romano for his active collaboration. His support has contributed greatly to the highly scientific content of this book.

My sincere appreciation to Stephen Brint for his invaluable contribution, his scientific skill, and for supervising the English translation of these books.

My sincere thanks goes to Massimiliano Crespi, the artist who created all of the magnificent drawings in this book, particularly for his ability to transfer the author's thoughts onto paper; also Salvatore Ferrandes, who was responsible for the clinical iconographic portions.

I would also like to thank the staff of Medicongress, in particular Monica Gingardi, for the organizational and operational support provided.

My translator Fiona Johnston for her precise and accurate translation of the Italian texts.

Many thanks also to Vittorio Picardo, a warm friend, for his supervision of the final text in Italian.

And AISO (Accademia Italiana di Scienze Oftalmologiche) for their scientific support and grant for the publication of this work.

And finally I would like to thank SLACK Incorporated, my publisher, for asking me to produce a new book on cataract surgery.

Lucio Buratto, MD

About the Editors

Lucio Buratto, MD is a leading international expert in cataract and myopia surgery, and a pioneer in the ocular techniques of intraocular lens (IOL) implantation, in the phacoemulsification procedure for the cataract, in the laser techniques for myopia, astigmatism and hyperopia. In 1978, Dr. Buratto began using the Kelman phacoemulsification technique, and in 1979 he started using posterior chamber intraocular lenses. Since 1980, he has organized and presided over 48 updating congresses on the surgery of cataract and glaucoma and on laser therapy, organized 54 practical courses for the teaching of eye surgery, and taken part as spokesman and teacher in more than 400 courses and congresses.

In 1989, Dr. Buratto became the world's first surgeon to use excimer laser intrastromal keratomileusis, and concurrently began to treat low myopia using PRK techniques. In 1995, he was appointed as Monitor of the United States Food and Drug Administration. In 1996, Dr. Buratto became the world's first surgeon to use a new technique called Down-Up LASIK, which improved the LASIK procedure for the correction of myopia; he holds a United States patent for this technique.

For teaching purposes, Dr. Buratto has performed surgical operations during live surgery sessions for more than 200 international and Italian congresses, performed surgery during satellite broadcasts to 54 countries on 4 different continents, and designed and produced 143 instruments for ocular surgery. In 2004, he was a speaker at the Binkhorst Medal Lecture during the XXII Annual Meeting of the European Society of Cataract and Refractive Surgeons (ESCRS) in Paris, and was the first European surgeon to use the new intralase laser for refractive surgery. In 2011, Dr. Buratto was the first West European surgeon to use the femtosecond laser for cataract surgery.

Dr. Buratto has published over 125 scientific publications and 59 monographs (of which 24 are on cataract surgery, 5 are on glaucoma surgery, and 11 are on myopia). His recent works include, *Phakic IOLs: State of the Art*, *LASIK: The Evolution of Refractive Surgery*, and *PRK: The Past, Present, and Future of Surface Ablation*.

If you would like to contact Dr. Buratto, you can email him at bookspublishing@wyanokegroup.com.

Stephen F. Brint, MD, FACS was the first physician in the United States to perform the LASIK procedure in June 1991, after working with Dr. Lucio Buratto in Milan to perfect the technique. He was the medical monitor for the first United States Food and Drug Administration LASIK study, Wavelight Allegretto study, Wavefront Optimized study, and custom studies and lead investigator for the Alcon Custom Cornea LASIK procedure. He graduated from Tulane University School of Medicine in New Orleans, Louisiana where he completed his residency in 1977, where he continues to serve as Associate Clinical Professor of Ophthalmology. In addition to his vast LASIK experience of over 30,000 LASIK procedures, many with the Intralase All Laser LASIK technique, he is a renowned cataract/lens surgeon, having participated in the Food and Drug Administration clinical trials of the new intraocular lenses including ReSTOR, ReZOOM, and toric IOLs.

He is board certified by the American Board of Ophthalmology and a Fellow of the American College of Surgeons. He has been recognized as "The Best Doctor in New Orleans" by *New Orleans Magazine* for the last 10 years and has been selected by his peers for the 2000-2012 editions of "The Best Doctors in America." Dr. Brint is a leading cataract surgeon and instructor, and the author of the 3 definitive textbooks on LASIK and cataract surgery including the most recent, *Custom LASIK*.

Dr. Brint performs surgery and lectures around the world, including Europe, Russia, China, Japan, Australia, Singapore, Africa, and South America.

Dr. Brint has a passion for education and research, and most recently has been involved with the refinement of the intraoperative aberrometer for selecting IOL power and femtosecond laser-assisted cataract surgery.

Mario R. Romano, MD, PhD enriched his training in vitreo-retinal surgery with clinical and research activities at the Massachusetts Eye & Ear Infirmary in Boston, Massachusetts and at the Royal Liverpool University Hospital in Liverpool, England. He also completed his PhD in Pharmacology and Molecular Oncology in 2009. His research projects account for endo-tamponade, intraocular temperature, vitreo-retinal disease, intraocular inflammation, and degenerative ocular disease. Dr. Romano is an active member of numerous scientific international societies, and he also serves as a referee for several peer-reviewed journals. Dr. Romano is in charge of the vitreo-retinal service of the Istituto Clinico e di Ricerca Humanitas in Milan, Italy.

Contributing Authors

Athiya Agarwal, MD, DO (Chapter 17)
Director
Dr. Agarwal's Eye Hospitals
Chennai, India

Jorge L. Alió, MD, PhD (Chapter 22)
Professor and Chairman
Vissum Corporacion
Instituto Oftalmologico De Alicante
Universidad Miguel Hernández
Alicante, Spain

Iva Dekaris, MD, PhD (Chapter 20)
Professor of Ophthalmology
University of Rijeka Medical School
Medical Director, Svjetlost Hospital
Head of Corneal and Refractive Surgery
University Eye Hospital Svjetlost
President, European Eye Bank Association
Zagreb, Croatia

Nikica Gabric, MD, PhD (Chapter 20)
Professor of Ophthalmology
University of Rijeka Medical School
Head of Eye Hospital Svjetlost
University Eye Hospital Svjetlost
Zagreb, Croatia

Tsutomu Hara, MD (Chapter 21)
Hara Eye Hospital
Utsunomiya, Japan

Ozana Moraru, MD (Chapter 15)
Medical Director
Oculus Eye Clinic
Bucharest, Romania

Mauricio A. Perez, MD (Chapter 14)
Cincinnati Eye Institute
University of Cincinnati
Cincinnati, Ohio

Šárka Pitrová, MD (Chapters 18, 19)
Assistant Professor of Ophthalmology
Private Eye Clinic
Prague, Czech Republic

Michael E. Snyder, MD (Chapter 14)
Consultant Surgeon and Board of Directors
Cincinnati Eye Institute
Volunteer Assistant Professor of Ophthalmology
University of Cincinnati
Cincinnati, Ohio

Felipe Soria, MD (Chapter 22)
Fellow, Cataract and Refractive Surgery
Vissum Corporacion
Alicante, Spain

Roger F. Steinert, MD (Chapter 16)
Irving H. Leopold Professor of Ophthalmology
Professor of Biomedical Engineering
Chair of Ophthalmology
Director, Gavin Herbert Eye Institute
University of California, Irvine
Irvine, California

Eva Vlková, MD (Chapters 18, 19)
Professor of Ophthalmology
Department of Ophthalmology
University Hospital of Masaryk University
Brno, Czech Republic

Introduction

During my professional life, I have published various books on cataract surgery; 24 in total, in all different languages.

Atlas of Intraocular Lenses published in 1984 was the first Italian work to introduce Italian ophthalmologists to the world of modern intraocular lenses; and the last *Phacoemulsification: Principles and Techniques* published by my American publisher, SLACK Incorporated in 2003, was a work with international acclaim that has provided important information covering the entire operative procedure; this work is still utilized today.

Now, almost 10 years later, I introduce 5 new works to the world of cataract surgery with 5 big promises of eye surgery.

The first of this series to be published with Mario Romano is about the difficult subject of intra- and postoperative complications and their prevention and treatment.

Volume 2, with Luigi Caretti, covers the surgery of complicated cases, another topic of great interest.

Finally, the last 3 books are on routine cataract surgery with a book dedicated to the preparation of the patient and the first operating steps with Laura Sacchi, one on the topic of phacoemulsification with Rosalia Sorce, and the last is dedicated to intraocular lenses with Domenico Boccuzzi.

With all those books there is the invaluable contribution of Stephen Brint, a very renowned cataract surgeon and a very good friend of mine.

I hope that these books are useful and will constitute a basis lasting many years for teaching and consulting for all eye surgeons searching for continuous improvements.

Lucio Buratto, MD

Section I

1

Anesthesia by Injection

Lucio Buratto, MD; Stephen F. Brint, MD, FACS; and Mario R. Romano, MD, PhD

Introduction of minimally invasive techniques, better control during intraoperative procedures, and more rapid postoperative recovery are just some of the factors driving the cataract surgeon to use safer and less invasive anesthesia techniques that ensure intraoperative analgesia without resorting to akinesia of the extraocular muscles.

Peri- or retrobulbar infiltration of anesthetic agents has the objective of inducing akinesia and analgesia in order to prevent contraction of the extraocular muscles. This contraction can result in expulsion of the globe contents through larger incisions, which are necessary for extra- or intracapsular surgery.

The commonly used terms *peribulbar* and *retrobulbar* do not adequately describe the technique and are ambiguous. It would be more appropriate to define the retrobulbar injection technique as *intraconical*, as described by Atkinson in 1936, and *extraconical*, the technique of peribulbar injection described later by Hamilton[1,2] (Figure 1-1).

The original description by Atkinson was an injection of approximately 3 mL of local anesthetic through the medial third and the lateral third of the lower edge of the orbit to reach the apex of the muscular cone. This maneuver requires patient cooperation, as the patient is asked to look upwards in a superior-nasal direction.[1]

Iatrogenic Damage and Axial Length

Complications with local/regional injection anesthesia for cataract surgery are estimated to be between 0.009% and 0.13% for globe perforation and between 0.09% and 0.79% with involvement of the encephalic trunk.[3-5] These occur because of lack of knowledge of anatomical relationships within the orbit and anatomical abnormalities of the globe or orbit.

A detailed clinical history prior to performing the injection can raise alarms. The patient should be questioned about previous eye surgeries (episcleral surgery for retinal detachment) or myopic refractive errors. The myopic eye has a different relationship to the orbit as opposed to the emmetropic eye. In particular, the equator of the globe in an emmetropic eye is located approximately 12.5 mm posterior to the limbus; it is located more posteriorly in the myopic eye, creating a different anatomical relationship with the margin of the orbit, used as the reference point for the insertion of the needle.

Myopic eyes with posterior staphylomas have a mean axial length of 27.5 mm, compared to 9% of cases without staphyloma having an axial length greater than 25 mm. The literature also reports eyes having an axial length of 32.5 mm without posterior staphylomas.[6] Moreover, scleral ectasia may not be symmetrical at the posterior pole making it difficult to define a scleral profile and a margin of safety. The morphological profile of the staphyloma is most dangerous in Type I (single scleral ectasia at the posterior pole), Type VI (double ectasia at the posterior pole and the macula), and Type IX (staphyloma is split into compartments by thin folds). Compared to the other types described, these have a longer axial length and a greater degree of asymmetry[7] (Figure 1-2). The incidence of staphyloma tends to increase with age and increases in axial length.[8]

Buratto L, Brint SF, Romano MR.
Cataract Surgery Complications (pp 3-10).
© 2013 Taylor & Francis Group.

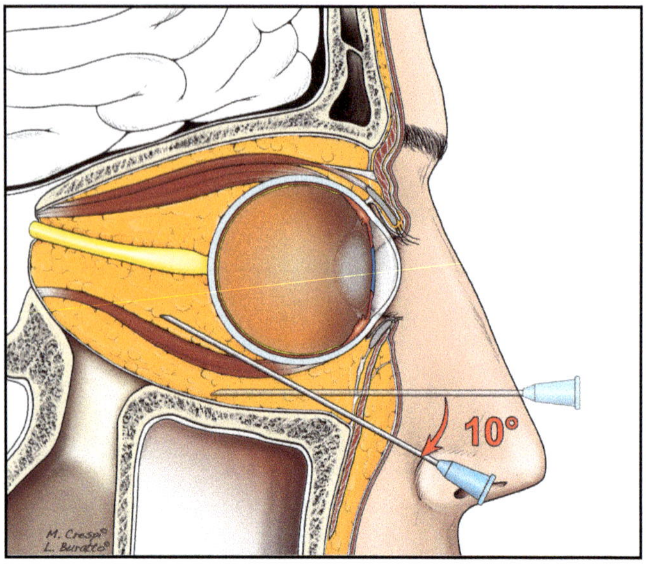

Figure 1-1. Intraconical and extraconical local/regional anesthetic. The image shows the position of the needle tip insertion, in the inferotemporal quadrant (between the lateral and medial rectus muscles) with the bevel of the needle toward the globe. The needle is inserted through the eyelid (transpalpebral) and is inserted parallel to the floor of the orbit in the extraconical technique. In the intraconical technique, once the needle has passed the equator of the globe, the needle is tilted approximately 10 degrees upward and medially to reach the intraconical space.

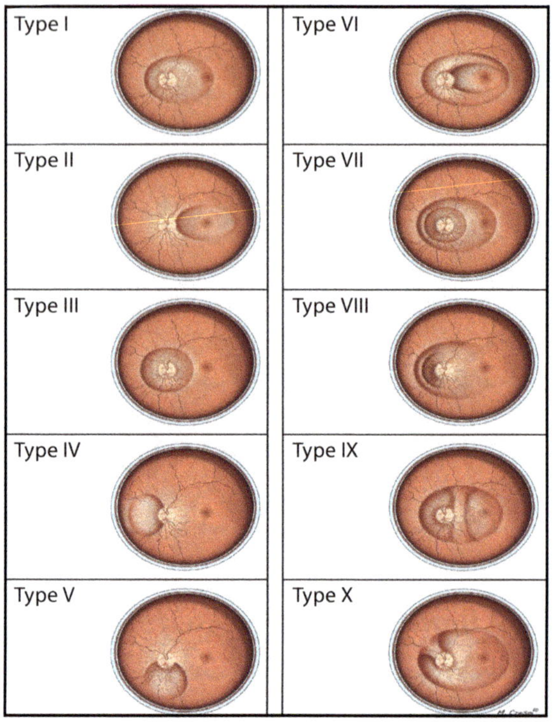

Figure 1-2. Classification of staphylomas. One should immediately remove the needle as the injection of even a few milliliters of anesthetic can lead to central retinal vein occlusion or necrotizing retinal phenomena. Other direct signs include loss of the red reflex of the fundus caused by vitreous hemorrhage, retinal detachment, and choroidal hemorrhage.

Injection Techniques

Intraconical Injection

The patient is supine with the eye in the primary position. Introduce the needle (25 to 27 gauge) in the inferotemporal quadrant (between the lateral and medial rectus muscles) with the bevel of the needle toward the globe. The needle is introduced through the eyelid and moved posteriorly, parallel to the floor of the orbit. The surgeon's finger, positioned between the edge of the orbit and the globe, can facilitate the introduction of the needle (Figure 1-3). Once the needle has passed the equator of the globe, it is tilted upwards and medially to reach the intraconical space (see Figure 1-3). Following aspiration to exclude penetration of a blood vessel, 3.5 to 5 mL of anesthetic solution is slowly injected over a period of 60 to 90 seconds to prevent sudden increase in the intraorbital pressure. At the end of the procedure, the surgeon should gently compress the eye for approximately 20 minutes to allow the anesthetic agent to diffuse and to reduce the intraocular pressure.

Extraconical Injection

The patient is again in a supine position with the eye in the primary position. The injection is performed with a 25- to 27-gauge needle and involves administration of 7 to 10 mL of anesthetic agent in 2 places (Figure 1-4). The first injection is performed in the inferotemporal quadrant (between the lateral and medial rectus muscles) introducing the needle parallel to the floor of the orbit, at a depth of 2.5 mm from the lower edge of the orbit. The second injection is performed in the superonasal quadrant at the margin of the superior rectus muscle (see Figure 1-4). The eye is again gently compressed for approximately 20 minutes.

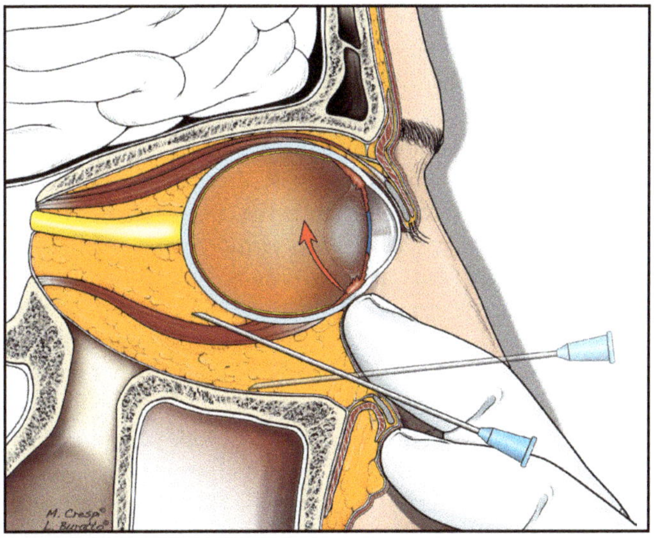

Figure 1-3. Intraconical injection. The surgeon's finger is placed between the orbital rim and the globe to move the globe upward and facilitate introduction of the needle into the extraconical space. The needle is tilted about 10 degrees with respect to the corneal plane, advancing, and eventually tilting, the tip of the needle toward the apex of the cone once the needle has passed the equator. Once the intraconical position is achieved, 3.5 to 5 mL of anesthetic should be injected.

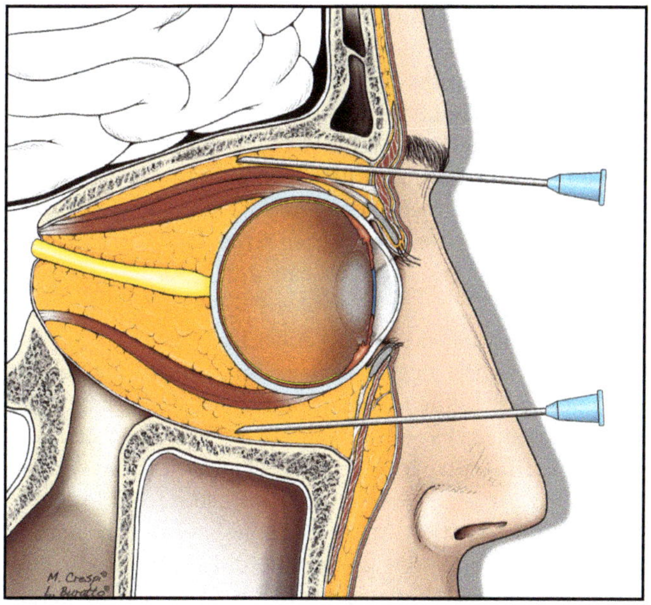

Figure 1-4. Extraconical injection. This involves an injection of 7 to 10 mL of anesthetic administered in 2 locations: The first injection is performed in the inferotemporal quadrant (between the medial and lateral rectus muscles) placing the needle parallel to the floor of the orbit about 2.5 mm from the inferior orbital margin. The second injection is performed in the superonasal quadrant near the margin of the superior rectus muscle.

A similar anatomical situation is seen in an emmetropic eye with a small orbit. Here, the equator of the globe is more posterior with respect to the orbital rim (Figure 1-5). Under these conditions, the space available for needle placement is reduced with increased risk of iatrogenic damage.

Complications

Perforation of the Globe

Perforation of the globe and even more so, intraocular injection of anesthetic, are the most feared complications associated with retrobulbar injections. Trauma induced by the needle may be penetrating or perforating. Penetrating the globe can result in the injection of anesthetic agent into the vitreous cavity with a corresponding increase in intraocular pressure (IOP), with the risk of rupture of the globe.[9] Consequently, the surgeon must recognize perforation of the globe before the damage can be aggravated by the intraocular injection.

From the literature, it is clear that it is difficult to describe the sensations perceived when the globe is perforated during administration of the anesthesia. The pressure required to inject anesthetic into the sheath of the optic nerve or into the sclera is approximately 138 mm Hg, 4 times the resistance encountered by injection into the retrobulbar adipose tissue (approximately 35 mm Hg).[10] Resistance to intraocular perforation has been described as being very low and can often be confused with the needle passing through a layer of orbital connective tissue.

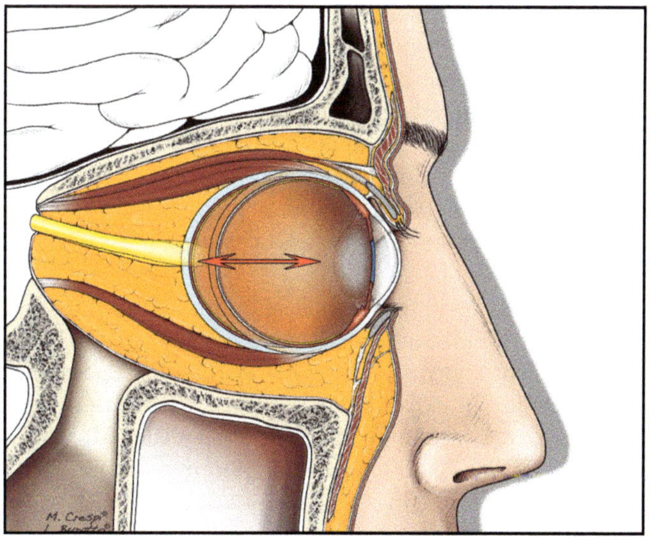

Figure 1-5. Posterior staphyloma. The presence of staphylomas or small orbits are risk factors that should be considered if the surgeon uses an intraconical or extraconical local/regional block. The equator of an emmetropic eye is located approximately 12.5 mm behind the limbus. It lies more posteriorly in a myopic eye. The equator of the globe will therefore be more posterior when used as a reference point for insertion of the needle. Consequently, working space is reduced with an increased risk of damage.

An important warning sign is localized pain reported by the patient when the anesthetic agent has been injected; this is caused by an immediate increase in IOP. If the surgeon has any doubt about the occurrence of penetration, he or she should immediately remove the needle as the injection of even a few mL of anesthetic can lead to central retinal vein occlusion or necrotizing retinal phenomena. Other direct signs include loss of the red reflex caused by vitreous hemorrhage, retinal detachment, and choroidal hemorrhage.

Perforating trauma, on the other hand, is characterized by the exit of the needle passing through the globe in a position closer to the posterior pole. In this case, iatrogenic damage is caused by the needle pass. Retinal tears can result with direct macular involvement. The block in these cases will be perfect with total akinesia resulting from localized intraconical injection of the anesthetic. For this reason, perforating trauma may go unnoticed during the administration of the anesthetic agent. IOP is the most important parameter. If penetrating trauma with intraocular injection of the anesthetic and increased IOP occurs, the surgeon must immediately begin pharmacological management (with mannitol) or a surgical intervention to lower the increased pressure. In this case, emergency vitrectomy is recommended.

Retrobulbar Hemorrhage

The needle movement through the orbit can damage venous or arterial blood vessels, leading to an accumulation of retrobulbar blood with dangerous compression. Retrobulbar hemorrhage is a rare complication; however, the consequences are potentially irreversible because of the increased pressure on the optic nerve. The symptoms include eye pain, vomiting, proptosis, and vision loss. Adequate decompression will ensure good functional recovery.

In order to avoid this complication, the surgeon should inject into the inferotemporal quadrant for an intraconical approach, and in the inferotemporal and superonasal quadrants for an extraconical approach, as these are relatively avascularized sites in the anterior orbit. Moreover, the use of a needle no longer than 30 mm will reduce the probability of damaging large blood vessels located at the apex of the orbit.

The rupture of a vein will lead to a slow accumulation of blood and is often self-limiting; however, penetration of a retrobulbar artery will lead to a much more rapid accumulation of blood. In this case, the appearance of symptoms is much more rapid and clearly visible, characterized by marked proptosis and immobility of the globe.

The incidence of retrobulbar hemorrhage varies between 0.44% and 3% and is more frequent in patients who are using anticoagulant drugs.

When retrobulbar compression of the central retinal artery is seen with the ophthalmoscope, the surgeon must immediately decompress the anterior orbit. The most common methods are incision of the inferior fornix and lateral canthotomy. It may be possible to manage the IOP by massaging the area with the fingers and injecting mannitol directly into the vessel.

The surgeon should also remember that increased IOP, caused by orbital hemorrhage, will affect ocular perfusion even when there is no occlusion of the central retinal artery. Diabetic patients, patients with hemorrhagic tendencies, and glaucoma patients also have more sensitivity to small changes in perfusion pressure; these may sometimes be irreversible and cannot be explained. The situation is very different from a complication-free surgery with excellent postoperative outcomes.[11]

The difficulty of surgery performed following retrobulbar hemorrhage is associated with the intraocular pressure induced. With good IOP, it is possible to proceed with surgery; if the IOP is excessive, surgery should be postponed 3 to 5 days to avoid intraoperative difficulties associated with posterior vitreous pressure.

In the differential diagnosis of retrobulbar hemorrhage, the surgeon should remember that hyaluronidase can induce formation of an orbital pseudotumor as a reaction to hypersensitivity to hyaluronidase, with subsequent compression.[12]

Palsy of the Extraocular Muscles

The cataract surgeon requires complete akinesia of the extraocular muscles when dealing with extremely complex cases. Rarely, there may be persistent palsy of the extraocular muscles (the inferior rectus muscles in particular). This damage may be caused by myotoxicity of the anesthetic agent from hypoperfusion of the muscle due to laceration of the anterior ciliary arteries following incorrect movements, or direct injection of anesthetic deep into the muscle, inducing mechanical damage of the muscle. The use of hyaluronidase, in addition to anesthetic, can create localized periocular areas of accumulated anesthetic that can induce potential toxicity in the muscle. The inferior rectus muscle is often involved in these cases, presumably because of the injection from the inferotemporal quadrant.[13]

Palsy may be due to strabismus camouflaged by the cataract or anisometropia. After the cataract surgery, this may result in a lack of central fusion of the image, frequently resulting in diplopia.

Lesion of the Optic Nerve

Another dreaded complication is injection of anesthetic into the optic nerve sheath (Figure 1-6). The direct connection between the optic nerve sheath and the subarachnoid and subdural spaces allows direct involvement of the central nervous system, potential respiratory arrest, arrhythmias, cardiopulmonary arrest, and involvement of the cranial nerves. Subarachnoid injection of local anesthesia reaches the sheaths of the contralateral optic nerve through the nerve sheaths. Patients report bilateral reduction in visual acuity and ophthalmoplegia, with variable central nervous system symptoms.[14]

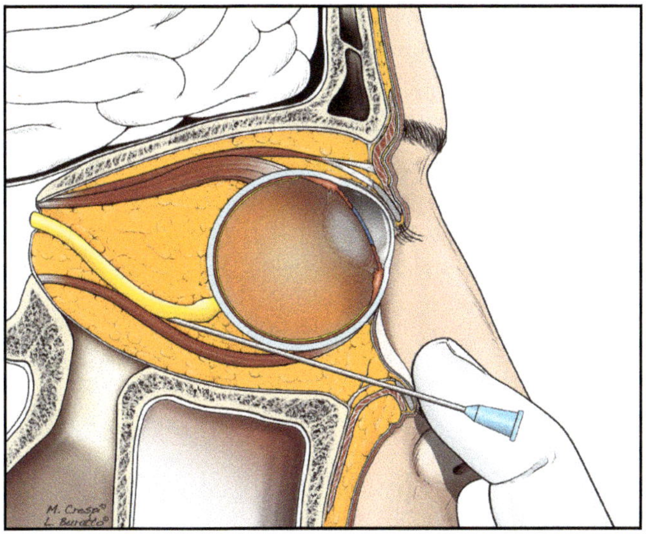

Figure 1-6. Damage to the optic nerve. The patient should not be asked to look up and in as this will tend to bring the sclera and/or the optic nerve sheath closer to the needle inserted in the inferotemporal quadrant.

Injection of the anesthetic into the cerebrospinal fluid can also induce a vagal stimulus up to 15 minutes after the injection. This complication requires immediate diagnosis and support from a medical team specialized in resuscitation.[15]

Oculocardiac Reflex

Described in 1908 by Aschner, the oculocardiac reflex, also known as the phenomenon of Aschner, involves a decreased pulse rate following traction on the extraocular muscles and/or compression of the globe. The reflex is mediated through connections of the trigeminal nerve and parasympathetic system mediated by the vagus nerve. This can lead to bradycardia, asystole, and death on rare occasions.

The oculocardiac stimulation is therefore due to an arc reflex with the afferent branch of the trigeminal nerve starting from the orbit. The orbit, when rapidly filled with anesthetic through a large bore needle, stimulates the trigeminal nerve before the transmission has been blocked by the anesthetic itself. The oculocardiac reflex may be minimized by a slow gradual injection of anesthetic through a small bore needle; this will achieve the nerve block before the stimulation of the arc reflex.

Block of the Facial Nerve

Injection of anesthetic close to the stylomastoid opening is an invasive procedure not free from complications. Currently, this technique is almost obsolete. Paralysis of the facial nerve and the large pharyngeal nerve can cause breathing difficulties that are sometimes complicated by vagal nerve involvement. Many surgeons are of the opinion that the block of the VII cranial nerve for cataract surgery should be avoided even in complicated cases.

Exposure Keratitis

Exposure keratitis is a result of eyelid akinesia. When this occurs, it is necessary to close the eyelid with a pressure patch in order to avoid keratitis due to the lack of blinking.

Atonic Pupil

Another complication that has been described is an atonic pupil following cataract surgery. The reasons for this have not been well defined. Damage to the ciliary ganglion or direct alteration of the iris sphincter are considered to be the most probable causes.

Modified Injection Technique

The classic retrobulbar injection has been replaced by a modified peribulbar approach that can minimize complications and ensure adequate anesthesia and akinesia.[16] A short, sharp needle (25 to 30 mm) is preferable, with a lateral approach and an injection of larger volumes of anesthetic (7 to 10 mL). Clinically, we would suggest approaching the inferotemporal quadrant, displacing the globe from the orbital rim using a finger, with the objective of creating space and reaching the equator of the globe more easily.

One important consideration is the length and gauge of the needle used; the ciliary ganglion lies approximately 35 mm from the inferior orbital rim. A needle 25 to 30 mm in length can reach the extraconical and intraconical space with excellent results in terms of anesthesia and akinesia. The smaller gauge of the needle creates less stress through the orbital structure, and at the same time, a slower, more gradual injection of anesthetic, in order to avoid stimulating the trigeminal reflexes with vagal effects. Finally, the use of sharp (as opposed to blunt) needles facilitates penetration of the tissues, reducing discomfort for the patient. This approach carries the risk of inducing penetrating damage as blunt needles induce greater tissue trauma, but with a lower incidence of direct penetration.

An injection in the extreme inferotemporal angle (less medial than the technique described by Atkinson) is far away from the globe and maintains a fixed angle with respect to the orbital rim that should not be altered during the injection to allow an increase in the intraconical space. When the needle direction is changed beyond the equator, retrobulbar damage may occur.

If the surgeon wishes to increase the depth of anesthesia, he or she should insert the needle at the caruncle with the bevel facing away from the globe (medial block) to a depth of 20 mm, injecting approximately 3 mL of anesthetic to combine intraconical and extraconical anesthesia.

There are multiple openings between the intraconical and extraconical space, so a greater amount of peribulbar anesthetic injected (5 to 10 mL) can induce adequate akinesia.

Hyaluronidase (3.5 units/mL) contributes to the induction of anesthesia, improving the quality of the block and assisting diffusion. Researchers have described a hypothetical mechanism of toxicity induced by localization of the anesthetic agent enhanced by hyaluronidase.[13] Clinically, an excellent block can be achieved without using hyaluronidase.

Modified Injection Technique

Patient in a Supine Position
With the Eye in a Primary Position

An injection of approximately 10 mL of anesthetic using a needle measuring 25 to 30 mm in length. Approaching the inferotemporal quadrant, displacing the globe from the orbital rim with fingers is recommended in order to create space and pass the equator more easily. The surgeon proceeds with introduction of the needle at an angle of approximately 10 degrees with respect to the corneal plane. The surgeon proceeds progressively, with the tip of the needle facing toward the apex of the cone once it has passed the equator of the globe.

Tips and Tricks

The axial length of the eye is an important consideration when injecting. Clinically, the following may prove useful:

- Discuss the surgery with the patient and ask for assistance by staring in the primary position. In the event that cooperation is poor, the patient should be sedated prior to proceeding.
- Use needles no longer than 30 mm.
- Inject the anesthetic slowly as the needle progresses in the orbit. The objective is to displace blood vessels; if the surgeon perceives resistance to the injection syringe because of hitting the sclera, he or she should stop.
- Pay great attention to the angle of incline of the needle with respect to the globe in eyes with an axial length greater than 26 mm.
- Do not ask the patient to look in a superonasal position as this could bring the sclera and/or the sheath of the optic nerve closer to the needle inserted in the inferotemporal quadrant (see Figure 1-6).
- Avoid a second injection of anesthetic unless absolutely necessary.
- Judge whether the analgesia is adequate by gently pinching the conjunctiva.
- Do not always attempt to achieve akinesia of the extraocular muscles and amaurosis.
- It should be remembered that a retrobulbar injection of just 3 mL of anesthetic causes an increase in intraocular pressure of approximately 12% to 80%, reaching a mean value of approximately 37 mm Hg.[17] Finger massage of the globe (or use of the Honan balloon) for 3 to 5 minutes after the injection of anesthetic is always recommended, as it can reduce the IOP to baseline in 60% to 80% of cases.

Other Injection Techniques

The retrobulbar or intraconical injection can also be done with a transconjunctival injection of 2% lidocaine to anesthetize the conjunctiva. A good tip is to displace the conjunctiva, better exposing the equator of the globe prior to introducing the needle through the conjunctiva, and directly reaching the intraconical space with a needle no longer than 20 mm.

Retrobulbar Injection With a Transconjunctival Approach

Patient in a Supine Position
With the Eye in a Primary Position

Conjunctival anesthesia is induced with 2 to 3 drops of topical anesthesia (2% lidocaine). The bulbar conjunctiva is displaced to expose the equator of the globe, allowing introduction of the needle (25 to 27 gauge, no longer than 20 mm) through the conjunctiva of the inferotemporal quadrant with an inclination of approximately 10 degrees (Figure 1-7).

The surgeon continues in this direction, tilting the tip toward the apex of the cone while injecting 4 to 5 mL of anesthetic.

Another injection technique is sub-Tenon's infiltration of anesthetic as described by Stevens in 1993. It is used primarily in patients having phacoemulsification.[18] Akinesia is not complete but can be achieved with additional infiltrations of anesthetic in other quadrants.

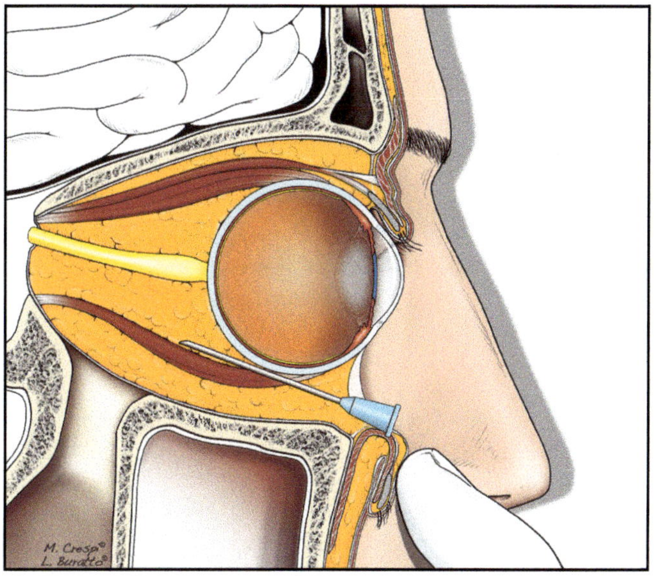

Figure 1-7. Transconjunctival injection. The conjunctiva is displaced to expose the equator of the globe; the surgeon then proceeds with needle insertion (25 to 27 gauge, length no greater than 20 mm) into the conjunctiva in the inferotemporal quadrant with an inclination of approximately 10 degrees with respect to the corneal plane. The needle continues in this direction, tilting the tip toward the apex of the cone, and injecting 4 to 5 mL.

Technique of Sub-Tenon's Injection

Patient in a Supine Position With the Eye in a Primary Position

The technique is straightforward direct transconjunctival infiltration (following conjunctival peritomy in the inferonasal quadrant or cauterization of the conjunctiva[19]) of local anesthesia directly into sub-Tenon's space with a blunt 19-gauge Southampton cannula.[20] The use of a blunt cannula reduces the risk of perforating any retrobulbar structures but does not alter the risk of infection (orbital cellulitis).[21]

References

1. Atkinson WS. Local anesthesia in ophthalmology. *Am J Ophthalmol.* 1946;29(11):1451.
2. Hamilton RC. A discourse on the complications of retrobulbar and peribulbar blockade. *Can J Ophthalmol.* 2000;35(7):363-372.
3. Edge R, Navon S. Scleral perforation during retrobulbar and peribulbar anesthesia: risk factors and outcome in 50,000 consecutive injections. *J Cataract Refract Surg.* 1999;25(9):1237-1244.
4. Schrader WF, Schargus M, Schneider E, Josifova T. Risks and sequelae of scleral perforation during peribulbar or retrobulbar anesthesia. *J Cataract Refract Surg.* 2010;36(6):885-889.
5. Hay A, Flynn HW Jr, Hoffman JI, Rivera AH. Needle penetration of the globe during retrobulbar and peribulbar injections. *Ophthalmology.* 1991;98(7):1017-1024.
6. Edge R, Navon S. Axial length and posterior staphyloma in Saudi Arabian cataract patients. *J Cataract Refract Surg.* 1999;25(1):91-95.
7. Curtin BJ. The posterior staphyloma of pathologic myopia. *Trans Am Ophthalmol Soc.* 1977;75:67-86.
8. Saka N, Ohno-Matsui K, Shimada N, et al. Long-term changes in axial length in adult eyes with pathologic myopia. *Am J Ophthalmol.* 2010;150(4):562-568.
9. Bullock JD, Warwar RE, Green WR. Ocular explosion during cataract surgery: a clinical, histopathological, experimental, and biophysical study. *Trans Am Ophthalmol Soc.* 1998;96:243-276; discussion 76-81.
10. Wang BC, Bogart B, Hillman DE, Turndorf H. Subarachnoid injection—a potential complication of retrobulbar block. *Anesthesiology.* 1989;71(6):845-847.
11. Munteanu G, Munteanu M. Anterior ischemic optic neuropathy secondary to retrobulbar hematoma. *Oftalmologia.* 2000;52(3):49-52.
12. Kempeneers A, Dralands L, Ceuppens J. Hyaluronidase induced orbital pseudotumor as complication of retrobulbar anesthesia. *Bull Soc Belge Ophtalmol.* 1992;243:159-166.
13. Brown SM, Brooks SE, Mazow ML, et al. Cluster of diplopia cases after periocular anesthesia without hyaluronidase. *J Cataract Refract Surg.* 1999;25(9):1245-1249.
14. Ahn JC, Stanley JA. Subarachnoid injection as a complication of retrobulbar anesthesia. *Am J Ophthalmol.* 1987;103(2):225-230.
15. Brookshire GL, Gleitsmann KY, Schenk EC. Life-threatening complication of retrobulbar block. A hypothesis. *Ophthalmology.* 1986;93(11):1476-1478.
16. Kumar CM. Needle-based blocks for the 21st century ophthalmology. *Acta Ophthalmol.* 2011;89(1):5-9.
17. Nwosu SN, Apakama AI, Ochiogu BC, et al. Intraocular pressure, retrobulbar anaesthesia and digital ocular massage. *Niger J Clin Pract.* 2010;13(2):125-127.
18. Stevens JD, Foss AJ, Hamilton AM. No-needle one-quadrant sub-Tenon anaesthesia for panretinal photocoagulation. *Eye (Lond).* 1993;7 (pt 6):768-771.
19. Gauba V, Saleh GM, Watson K, Chung A. Sub-Tenon anaesthesia: reduction in subconjunctival haemorrhage with controlled bipolar conjunctival cautery. *Eye (Lond).* 2007;21(11):1387-1390.
20. Kumar CM, Williamson S, Chabria R. A simple method of sub-Tenon anaesthesia delivery. *Anaesthesia.* 2000;55(6):612-613.
21. Liang SY, Moloney G, O'Donnell BA, Fernando G. Orbital cellulitis as a postoperative complication of sub-Tenon anaesthesia in cataract surgery. *Clin Experiment Ophthalmol.* 2006;34(9):897-899.

2

The Corneal Incision

Lucio Buratto, MD; Stephen F. Brint, MD, FACS; and Mario R. Romano, MD, PhD

The surgeon decides on the size and shape of the corneal incision prior to phacoemulsification and it is important in the surgical outcome. The incision should provide easy access for the instruments, provide stable fluidics, allow sutureless closure of the incision, and induce astigmatism. The width, location, and shape of the corneal incision depends on various parameters that we will analyze later; the determining features are the planned surgical technique and the intraocular lens (IOL) implantation.

Phaco incisions began in 1972 as limbal incisions that were large and straight.[1] Subsequently in 1977, Kratz introduced a scleral tunnel approach. This induced less astigmatism as opposed to corneal incisions.[2] This has evolved into clear corneal incisions as described by Fine in 1991 with external and internal incisions of 4 mm or less, and tunnels 1.75 mm long.[3] Initially, a single corneal suture was used as described by Shepherd.[4]

The development of foldable IOLs that can be injected through corneal incisions now down to 1.7 mm allow sutureless and astigmatic neutral surgery. A proper corneal tunnel that sustains the surgical stress induced by phacoemulsification and can be made watertight with incision hydration is required.[5,6] The astigmatic advantages are statistically significant for sutureless incisions less than 3.2 mm.[5]

Recently the introduction of gluing with liquid hydrogel applied to the incision and a protective collagen shell is felt to have significant advantages in terms of closure of the incision and improvement in postoperative comfort.[7,8]

Traumatic dehiscence post "small sutureless water tight incisions" is seen less frequently than with larger incisions, but is still occasionally reported.[9,10]

Clear Corneal Incisions

There are 3 steps recommended in clear cornea: external incision, the tunnel, and internal incision. Each has to support a different degree of mechanical stress induced by surgery and allow a watertight corneal incision at the end.[11]

The Anatomy of the Limbus

Knowledge of the limbal anatomy is required for the creation of a good corneal tunnel. The limbus has a width of 2 mm. The anterior margin is delineated by the conjunctival capillaries extending into clear cornea (corresponding to the external margin of Bowman's); the posterior margin of the limbus merges with the scleral spur. Between the anterior and the posterior margins of the limbus, an area of blue reflex is seen corresponding to the termination of Descemet's membrane ending in Schwalbe's line (Figure 2-1).

Buratto L, Brint SF, Romano MR.
Cataract Surgery Complications (pp 11-18).
© 2013 Taylor & Francis Group.

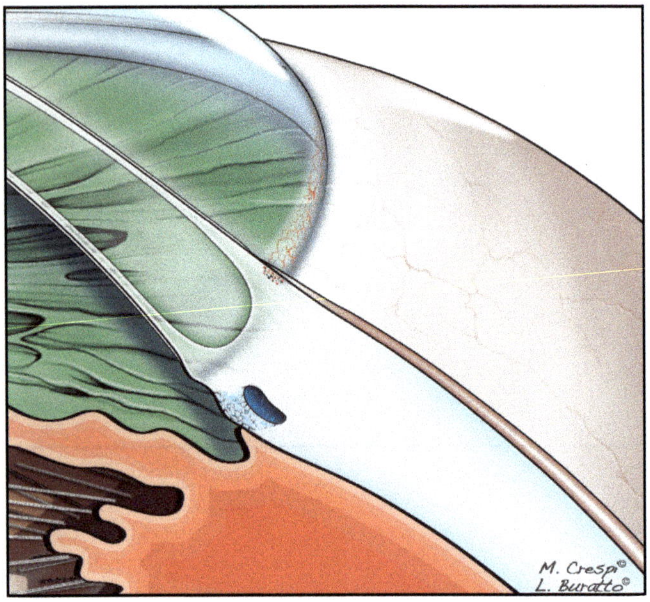

Figure 2-1. Limbal anatomy. The limbus measures 2 mm in width, and the anterior limit is defined by the conjunctival capillary vessels extending into clear cornea (corresponding to the outer limit of Bowman's membrane). The peripheral limit of the limbus merges into the scleral spur between the anterior and posterior margins of the limbus for approximately 1 mm starting at the anterior margin. One can see an area with a blue reflex defining the end of Descemet's membrane, ending with Schwalbe's line.

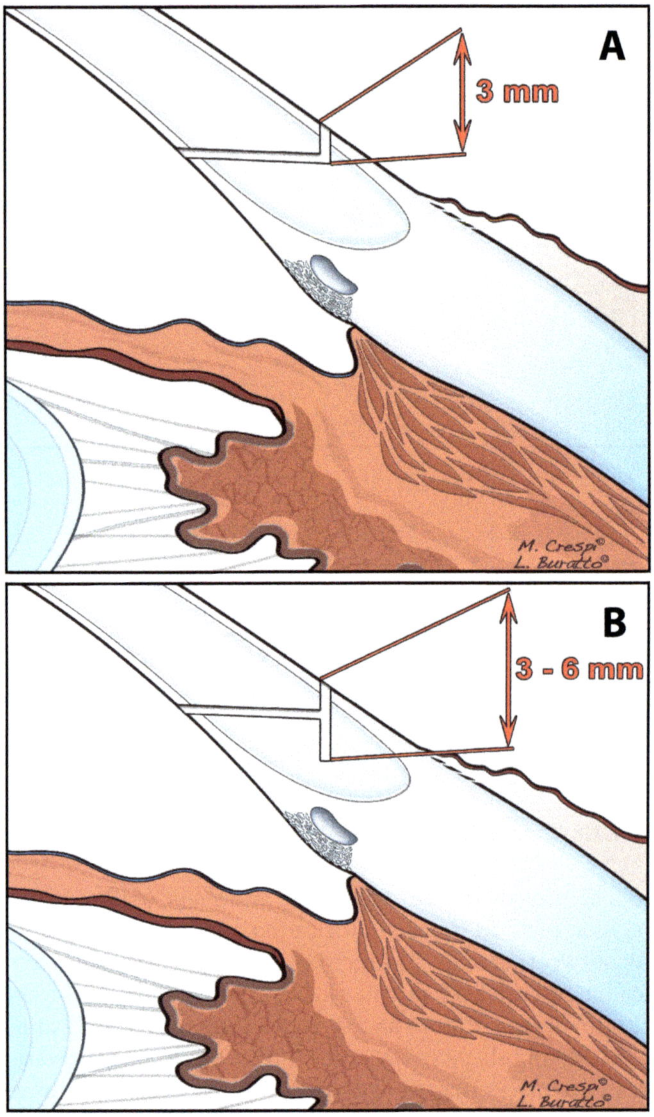

Figure 2-3. Grooved incisions. (A) A groove approximately 3 mm long allows the incision to be initiated at a deeper plane, producing a tunnel roof with greater thickness that will resist the pressure and stress from surgical instrumentation. (B) Creation of a groove 3- to 6-mm long is also an option, entering the AC with the blade and creating a tunnel 3 mm in length to ensure a better valve effect.

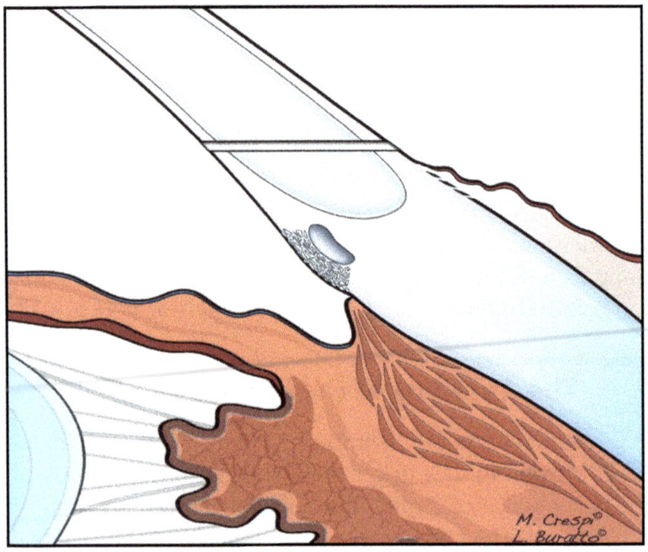

Figure 2-2. Clear corneal incisions. Clear corneal incisions create an external layer that may be thin and fragile. It may tear with excessive surgical trauma.

The external corneal incision is initiated at the anterior margin of the limbus, just in front of the conjunctival arcades, to the anterior edge of the blue limbal reflex, as it relates to the external margin of Bowman's membrane. Some recommend the "near clear" corneal incision using a slightly more peripheral approach, avoiding excessively long tunnels potentially impinging on the visual axis. The external incision may be straight or initiated with a groove the same width as the corneal incision, usually 1.7 to 3.0 mm in width (Figure 2-2).

A groove approximately 3 mm in length allows the tunnel incision to be deeper, with a thicker tunnel roof that will resist stress and pressure from the phaco and other instruments (Figure 2-3A). A groove longer than 3 mm (between 3 and 6 mm) can be made; the surgeon then uses a metal or diamond blade with a width of up to 3 mm to create a better valve effect (Figure 2-3B). Very deep grooves cause instability in the corneal incision and may be perceived postoperatively as a foreign body sensation lasting several months after the surgery.

The corneal tunnel is created along the stromal plane from the external scleral incision for a length of 2 mm (see Figure 2-3B). Different thicknesses of the roof may lead to incorrect margins of the incision, making it less watertight.

The ideal tunnel is square shaped, equally wide and long to create a watertight corneal incision.

The internal corneal incision requires cutting Descemet's membrane and corneal endothelium. In the last step of corneal tunnel creation, the blade angle is turned toward the anterior chamber (AC). At this point, the incision of Descemet's membrane should have smooth edges. If not, the fluid entering and leaving the AC may create a Descemet's detachment during phacoemulsification or cortical aspiration. This complication is normally easy to manage by injecting an air bubble into the AC at the end of surgery. Sometimes the damage may be irreversible if the flap of Descemet's membrane is accidentally removed during aspiration with phaco or irrigation/aspiration (I/A).

Blades play an essential role in the correct creation of the corneal incision and tunnel. Diamond blades usually produce cleaner cuts in the stroma and endothelium with better apposition of the corneal layers after surgery.

Moreover, there is less of a chance of an incomplete cut into Descemet's membrane that may result in its detachment. Incisions with diamond blades, though more expensive, provide less resistance to corneal penetration. Recently, blades for microincisional surgery were introduced with options of a bevel on the anterior and posterior portions of the blade, with a cutting edge at the tip (as opposed to the edge of the blade), optimizing creation of the tunnel, and avoiding wound stress from movements of the phaco tip.

Complications of the External Incision

An excessively peripheral incision may create an excessively long tunnel, leading to intraoperative problems with corneal distortion and wound burn (Figure 2-4). Moreover, long tunnels restrict movement of the phaco, causing corneal distortion with poor visualization. Lifting the phaco tip vertically becomes difficult, but necessary for good sculpting. This may lead to a tear of the tunnel or corneal distortion, creating corneal edema or Descemet's folds postoperatively. A long tunnel also decreases the flow of fluid leaving the AC and cooling the phaco tip. Edema of the corneal incision is induced by localized increase in temperature with the incision becoming less watertight.

The surgeon should create the external incision carefully in previous laser in situ keratomileusis (LASIK) patients. The risk is associated with the corneal LASIK flap and epithelial ingrowth.[12]

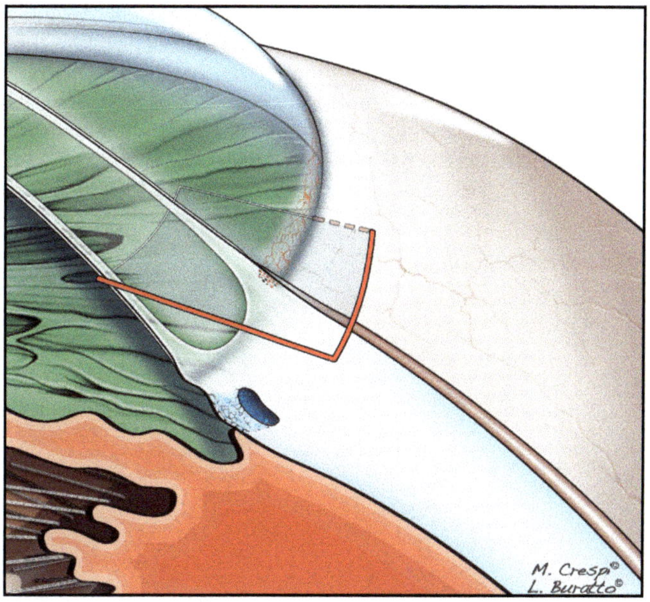

Figure 2-4. External incision that is too peripheral. An external incision that is too peripheral may create an excessively long tunnel. The tunnel may overheat and corneal distortion can occur from maneuvers of the phaco tip. The surgeon may not be able to tilt the phaco tip enough for good sculpting.

Deep external incisions may allow premature entrance of the blade into the AC with creation of an excessively short tunnel, sometimes associated with a Descemet's detachment.

Superficial external incisions may create a very thin tunnel roof that may tear during phacoemulsification.

Long external incisions may result in excessive wound leak during phaco with a shallow AC. Increasing flow does not always increase chamber depth and may create instability of the AC.

Short external incisions: Excessive stress on the tunnel may occur along with sleeve compression, reduction of flow from the chamber, and lack of cooling of the tip. Descemet's detachment may also occur. Moreover, moving the phaco tip may displace the eye, making phacoemulsification and IOL implantation more difficult.[13]

Complications From the Internal Incision

An incision that is excessively peripheral may permit premature entry into the AC with formation of an excessively short tunnel (Figure 2-5). Also, the incision of Descemet's membrane may be incomplete because it is posterior to Schwalbe's line, leading to a Descemet's detachment. Moreover, a short tunnel may not be watertight.

Finally, it predisposes the wound to iris prolapse with its associated intraoperative complications (see Figures A1 and A2).

Shallow chamber depth, postoperative hypotony, and wound leak/gape may allow passage of bacteria into the AC, leading to endophthalmitis.[14,15]

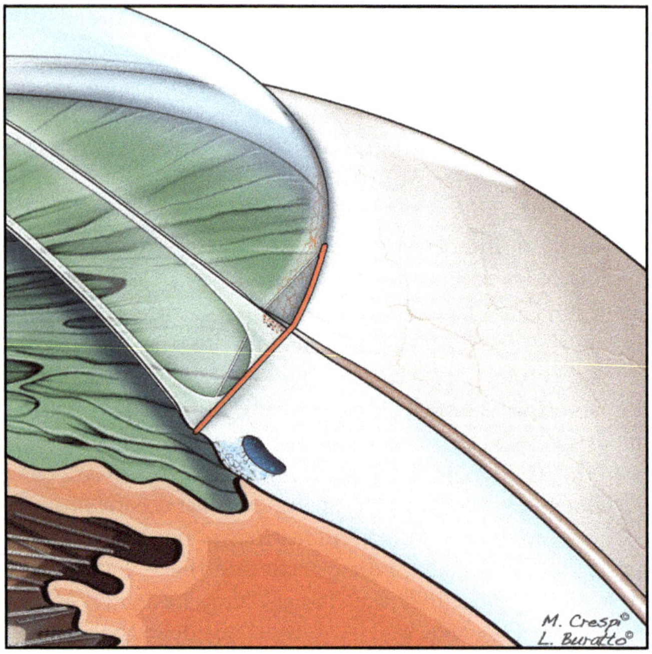

Figure 2-5. Internal incision that is too peripheral. An internal incision that is too peripheral allows premature entry into the AC with the creation of a short tunnel. The incision of Descemet's membrane may not be complete because it is partially behind Schwalbe's line, allowing detachment of Descemet's membrane. This also increases the risk of iris prolapse.

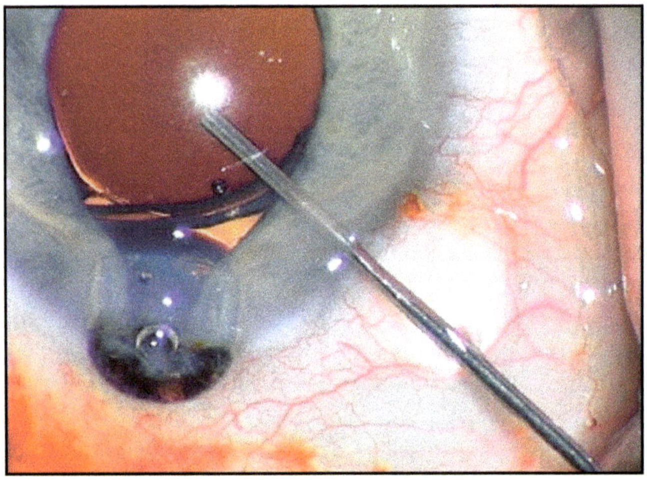

Figure A1. At the end of surgery, OVD is injected in order to correctly position the IOL that was not been properly inserted into the bag. This causes iris prolapse through the corneal incision.

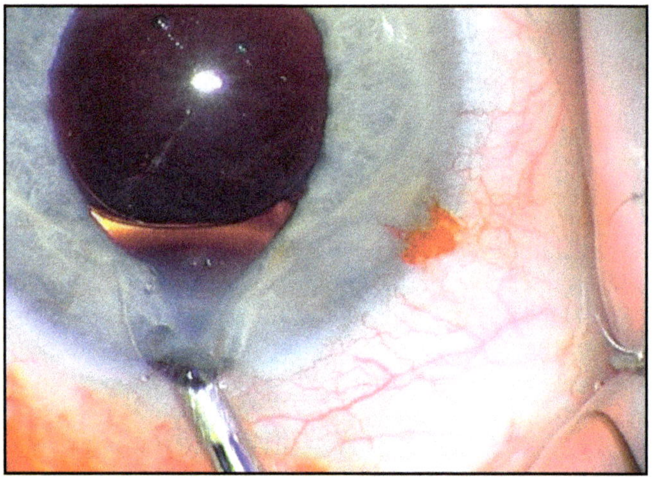

Figure A2. OVD is aspirated through the corneal paracentesis and the iris is repositary.

Management of Complications From a Poorly Constructed Incision

In these cases, the surgeon should suture the corneal incision at the end of surgery or abandon the poorly constructed incision, creating a new one to avoid potential intra- and postoperative complications.

Previous or combined vitreo-retinal surgery does not affect the stability of the sutureless incision.[16]

Sclerocorneal Incisions

Initially, sutureless cataract surgery involved a tangential sclerocorneal incision as described by McFarland in 1990.[17] Evolution of the technique included curved external incisions (frown incision) enlarged prior to lens implantation that are concave, fornix-based, 2 mm posterior to the limbus, varying in length from 2.8 to 3.4 mm with a depth of 0.3 mm. At this plane, the surgeon extends beyond Schwalbe's line, entering the AC with an internal incision approximately 1 mm from the external one, creating a valve to prevent iris prolapse.

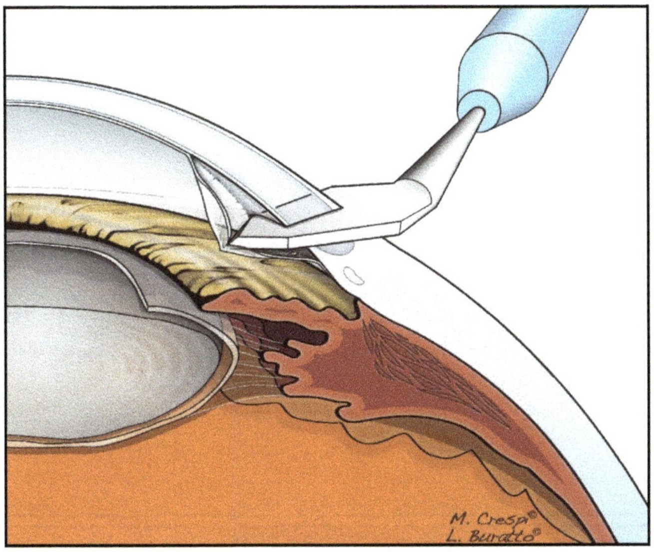

Figure 2-6. Cutting Descemet's membrane. The blade entering the AC should smoothly incise Descemet's membrane. An excessively posterior incision intersecting Schwalbe's line or an excessively anterior one can create a tear in Descemet's membrane. This tear may extend, resulting in detachment.

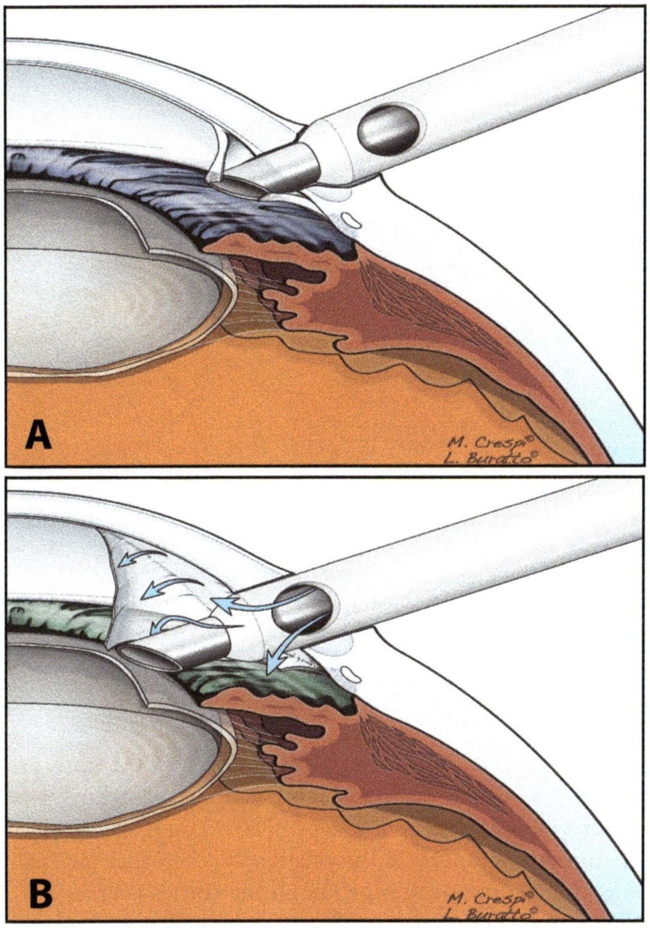

Figure 2-7. Descemet's membrane detachment. Detachment of Descemet's membrane is common. (A) It may be caused by insertion of the phaco tip, (B) turbulence of fluid in the AC, and aspiration maneuvers of the tip and IOL injection.

Excessively central external incisions and/or premature internal incisions will create a tunnel that is too short to seal and may require a suture. This also may lead to intra- and postoperative iris prolapse.

Excessively deep external incisions may expose the ciliary body. The surgeon should suture the incision and create another incision in another location.

A superficial external incision may create instability of the tunnel roof with possible tears or buttonholes.

Descemet's Membrane Detachment

Descemet's membrane tears may create detachment of the membrane and corneal endothelium, allowing corneal decompensation. The blade entering the AC should cut Descemet's cleanly without causing damage. A cut that is excessively peripheral, crossing Schwalbe's line, or excessively central and parallel to the pre-Descemet's plane, may cause a tear extending detachment of the membrane (Figure 2-6).

The surgeon should not ignore even small tears of Descemet's membrane. Progression of the detachment is a common problem due to turbulence from fluid flow in the AC, manipulation of the aspiration tip, and maneuvers associated with IOL injection (Figures 2-7).

A number of different solutions have been recommended for this complication: full-thickness sutures involving stroma, endothelium, and Descemet's membrane; injection of OVD into the AC; and injection of gas into the AC.[18]

In our experience, placing an air bubble into the AC with the patient in a supine position for 24 hours is adequate to ensure adhesion between the membrane and the stroma, assisted by good endothelial pump function. Only suturing the stroma, endothelium, and Descemet's can manage larger tears, as injection of OVD can create an interface between the membrane and the stroma, actually preventing adhesion. The use of 20% sulfur hexafluoride in a nonexpandable dilution can create excessive filling of the AC and pupillary block.

Avoiding Descemet's Membrane Detachment

In order to avoid Descemet's membrane detachment, the surgeon should do the following:

- Use sharp blades to enter the AC
- Introduce the phaco tip in a direction parallel to the corneal tunnel
- Avoid stress to the anterior edge of the incision when entering the AC
- Not proceed with surgery if the tunnel is too short
- Not force the IOL through a small corneal tunnel

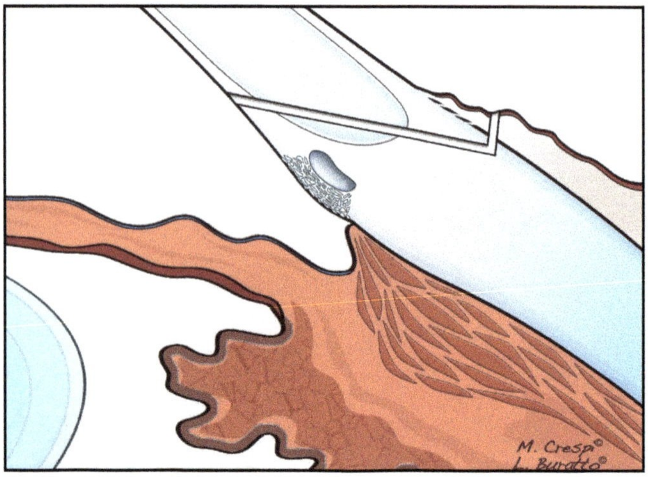

Figure 2-8. Conjunctival chemosis. Chemosis of the conjunctiva is caused by incisions that are too peripheral. It is not just the position of the incision, but may also depend on the location of the conjunctival insertion on the cornea when an incision is created peripheral to the limbal attachment of Tenon's capsule.

Conjunctival Chemosis

Conjunctival chemosis is common when the external incision is created peripheral to the limbal attachment of Tenon's capsule. It does not depend solely on the location of the incision but also on the relationship between the incision and conjunctival insertion on the cornea (Figure 2-8). This complication results from incising Tenon's capsule leading to escape of the fluid leaving the AC under Tenon's capsule. Chemosis of the conjunctiva results with a ballooning effect allowing pooling of fluid on the cornea resulting in poor visualization during phacoemulsification and cortical aspiration. This complication also results from poor placement of the side port incision. The surgeon should identify this problem early on, performing a peritomy to ensure that fluid leaving the AC does not reach the sub-Tenon's space.

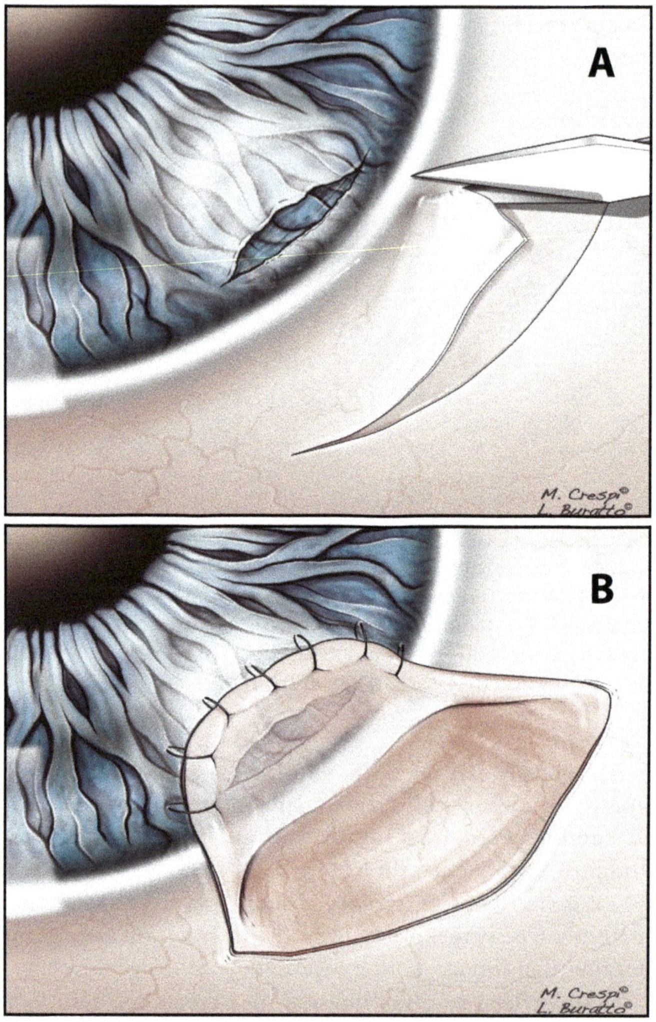

Figure 2-9. Conjunctival patching. Heating of the corneal tunnel may cause wound burn with scleral necrosis. In these cases, covering the wound with conjunctiva may prove useful, creating a conjunctival flap with a limbal base (A) large enough to cover the corneal incision and sutured to the cornea using a 10-0 nylon suture far from the damaged area (B).

Wound Burn

Corneal damage from localized wound heating can create damage based on the degree of burn. Modern phaco equipment software controls the duty cycle of ultrasound, spacing the effective stroke of the phaco tip with micropulsations that cool the tip and increase ultrasound efficiency.[19] With burns of the corneal incision, the surgeon should suture and avoid further damaging the swollen incision.

The most common causes of this problem include the following:

- An incision that is excessively small or long, as this will not permit adequate passage of fluid through the sleeve necessary to cool the phaco tip.
- Prolonged surgical time; the high frequency of the ultrasound creates heat.
- Blockage of flow by OVD in the AC. This appears when ultrasound is used in an AC that has been over-filled with OVD, preventing both fluid aspiration by the phaco tip and fluid outflow from the cooling sleeve. The surgeon should aspirate some of the OVD prior to initiating ultrasound. Sometimes heating can lead to sclerocorneal necrosis (melting) that may require a conjunctival flap to cover the corneal wound or a scleral graft to cover both cornea and sclera, sutured into place with individual sutures (Figure 2-9).

References

1. Parkash O. A new technique of wound closure in cataract surgery. *Indian J Ophthalmol.* 1972;20(3):113-119.
2. Kratz RP. Intraocular lens complications and how to avoid them. *Trans Pac Coast Otoophthalmol Soc Annu Meet.* 1977;58:211-216.
3. Fine IH. Architecture and construction of a self-sealing incision for cataract surgery. *J Cataract Refract Surg.* 1991;17(suppl): 672-676.
4. Shepherd JR. Induced astigmatism in small incision cataract surgery. *J Cataract Refract Surg.* 1989;15(1):85-88.
5. Martin RG, Sanders DR, Miller JD, Cox CC III, Ballew C. Effect of cataract wound incision size on acute changes in corneal topography. *J Cataract Refract Surg.* 1993;19(suppl):170-177.
6. Steinert RF, Brint SF, White SM, Fine IH. Astigmatism after small incision cataract surgery. A prospective, randomized, multicenter comparison of 4- and 6.5-mm incisions. *Ophthalmology.* 1991;98(4):417-423; discussion 423-414.
7. Dell SJ, Hovanesian JA, Raizman MB, et al. Randomized comparison of postoperative use of hydrogel ocular bandage and collagen corneal shield for wound protection and patient tolerability after cataract surgery. *J Cataract Refract Surg.* 2011;37(1):113-121.
8. Hovanesian JA. Cataract wound closure with a polymerizing liquid hydrogel ocular bandage. *J Cataract Refract Surg.* 2009;35(5):912-916.
9. Ball JL, McLeod BK. Traumatic wound dehiscence following cataract surgery: a thing of the past? *Eye (Lond).* 2001;15(pt 1):42-44.
10. Chowers I, Anteby I, Ever-Hadani P, Frucht-Pery J. Traumatic wound dehiscence after cataract extraction. *J Cataract Refract Surg.* 2001;27(8):1238-1242.
11. Masket S, Belani S. Proper wound construction to prevent short-term ocular hypotony after clear corneal incision cataract surgery. *J Cataract Refract Surg.* 2007;33(3):383-386.
12. Cheng CJ, Stark WJ. Wound instability and management after cataract surgery in a patient with prior laser in situ keratomileusis. *J Cataract Refract Surg.* 2007;33(7):1315-1317.
13. Kumar R, Reeves DL, Olson RJ. Wound complications associated with incision enlargement for foldable intraocular lens implantation during cataract surgery. *J Cataract Refract Surg.* 2001;27(2):224-226.
14. Francis IC, Roufas A, Figueira EC, Pandya VB, Bhardwaj G, Chui J. Endophthalmitis following cataract surgery: the sucking corneal wound. *J Cataract Refract Surg.* 2009;35(9):1643-1645.
15. Kehdi EE, Watson SL, Francis IC, et al. Spectrum of clear corneal incision cataract wound infection. *J Cataract Refract Surg.* 2005;31(9):1702-1706.
16. Wyszynski RE, Khosrof S, Shands P, Kalski RS, Bruner WE. Effect of scleral buckling on unsutured cataract wound strength. *Ophthalmic Surg Lasers.* 1996;27(9):787-789.
17. McFarland M. Surgeon undertakes phaco, foldable IOL series sans sutures. *Ocular Surg News.* 1990;8.
18. Assia EI, Levkovich-Verbin H, Blumenthal M. Management of Descemet's membrane detachment. *J Cataract Refract Surg.* 1995;21(6):714-717.
19. Wahab S, Faiz-ur-Rub K, Hargun LD. Comparison of conventional phacoemulsification technique vs cool phacoemulsification technique with the importance of phacoemulsification variables. *J Coll Physicians Surg Pak.* 2010;20(7):449-453.

3

Capsulorrhexis

Lucio Buratto, MD; Stephen F. Brint, MD, FACS; and Mario R. Romano, MD, PhD

Anterior Capsulorrhexis

Anterior capsulorrhexis (ACR) remains a critical step in surgery due to aging fragility of the capsular bag, secondary to degeneration and ocular trauma.

The capsular bag is an elastic basement membrane of Type IV collagen approximately 20 microns thick, with zonule attachment approximately 2.5 mm anterior to the equator. The thickness of the anterior chamber (AC) is approximately 14 microns, and the thickness of the posterior capsule (PC) varies between 2 to 4 microns. Capsulorrhexis provides the surgeon with access to the lens, allowing straightforward in the bag phacoemulsification, which allows stress induced by surgical manipulations.[1]

In 1990, Gimbel and colleagues proposed continuous curvilinear capsulorrhexis (CCC), which provides excellent resistance to the outward forces required in surgery, which tend to create radial tears of the rhexis with potential zonule and PC disruption.[2]

CCC allows better control of forces, avoiding radial tears that can compromise the integrity of the capsular bag (see Figures A1 to A6).[1]

Outward Forces and Positive Pressure

Cataract development induces progressive increase in lens thickness with an increase in capsular bag tension (Figure 3-1).

Surgical incision of the capsule tends to generate a centrifugal vector force that may lead to extension of the rhexis. The surgeon should always fill the AC with a cohesive ophthalmic viscoelastic device (OVD), particularly in cases with increased risk factors like intumescent lenses or posterior pressure[1] (see Figure 3-1). Positive pressure can be induced by the speculum, lid squeezing, excess peribulbar injection, and suprachoroidal hemorrhage. Following incision of the capsule with a cystotome or rhexis forceps, the surgeon proceeds by creating a vector tangential to the desired opening. The surgeon should maintain the capsular tear with anterior and centripetal tension, anticipating the direction of the CCC as the forceps move.

If the rhexis tries to escape, additional OVD should be injected to reduce centrifugal forces.

The flap is then grasped near its edge, moving in a centripetal manner. This maneuver will not be successful if the rhexis has extended to the zonules. In this case, the surgeon should stop, as his or her actions could extend the tear to the PC. One suggestion is to begin a new tear at a different point. The AC may be cut tangentially using Gills Walsh Vannas scissors, and the rhexis is completed continuing in the opposite direction (Figure 3-2).

Size of the Anterior Capsulorrhexis

When planning the size of the CCC, the surgeon should consider the anatomy. The lens has a mean diameter of 10.5 mm. The zonules extend approximately 2.5 mm

Buratto L, Brint SF, Romano MR.
Cataract Surgery Complications (pp 19-28).
© 2013 Taylor & Francis Group.

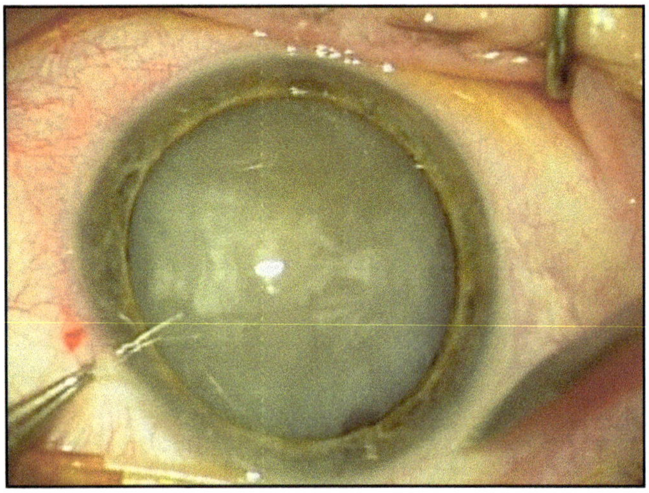

Figure A1. Hard intumescent cataract.

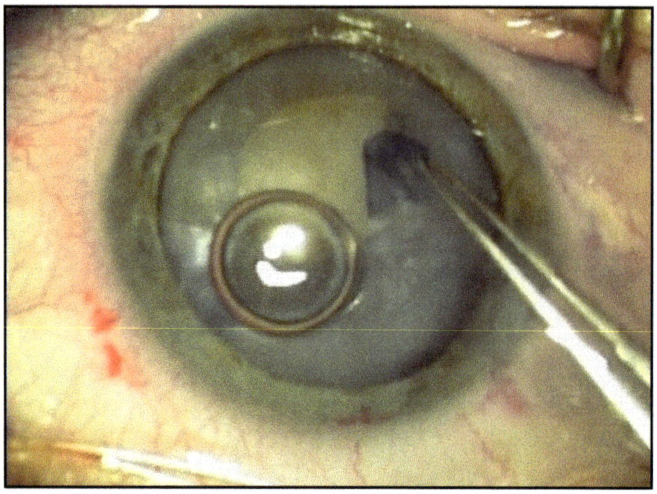

Figure A2. After staining of anterior capsulorrhexis with trypan blue and injection of OVD, the surgeon starts to perform the capsulorrhexis.

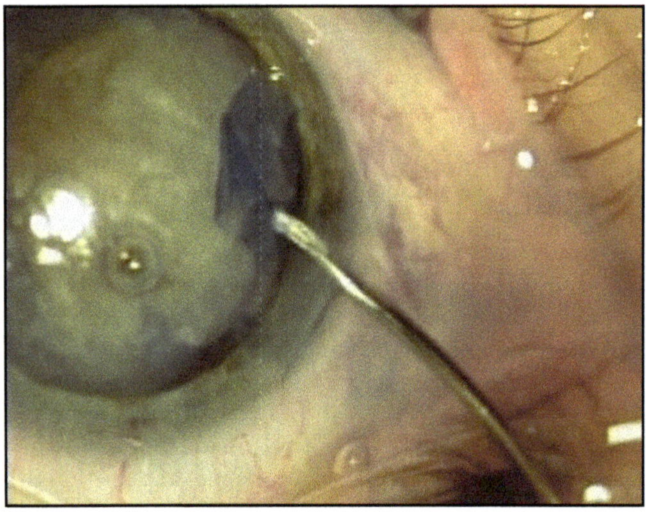

Figure A3. The anterior capsulorrhexis is escaping. It is grasped from another location but is still escaping.

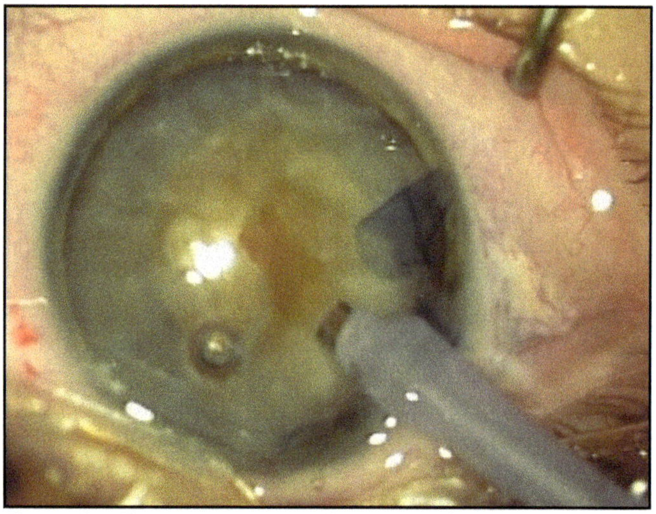

Figure A4. The surgeon starts phacoemulsification.

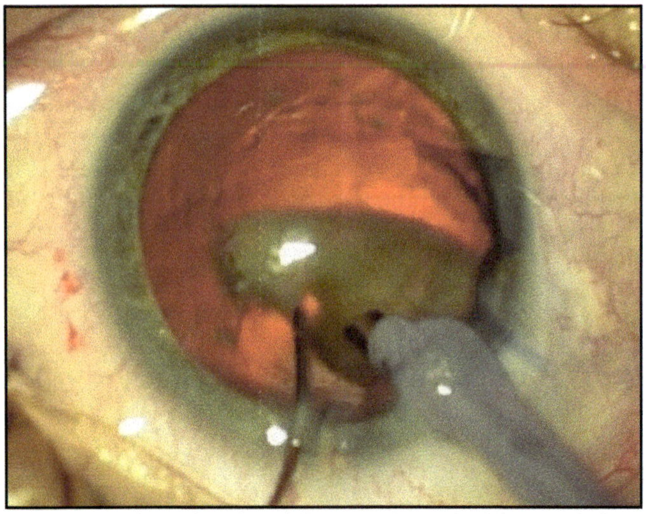

Figure A5. Three-fourths of the way through phacoemulsification procedures, the surgeon realizes that the posterior capsule is opened.

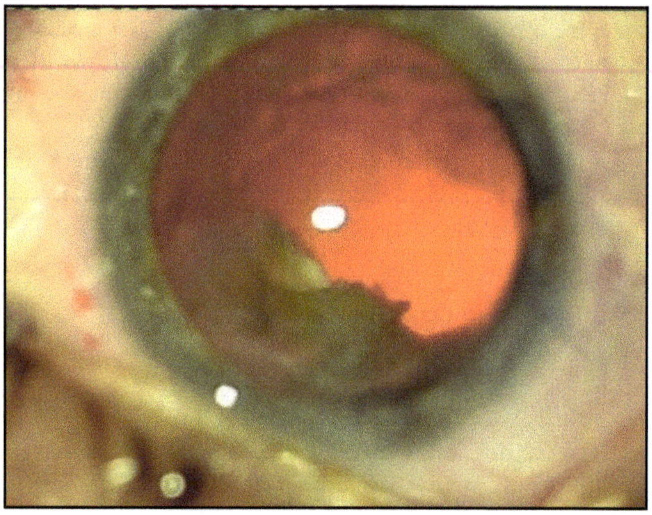

Figure A6. Part of the nucleus falls into the vitreous; posterior vitrectomy is required.

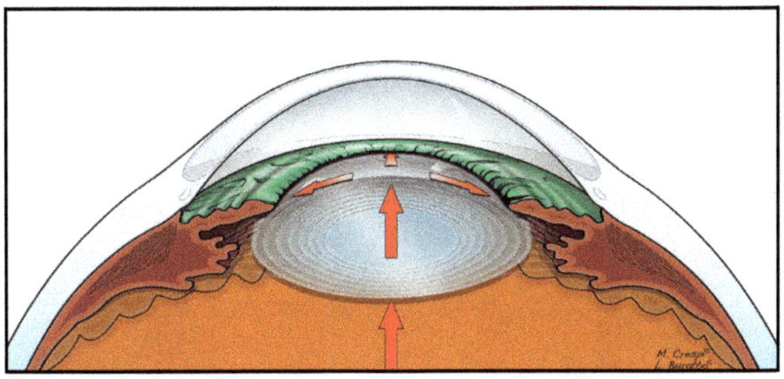

Figure 3-1. Centrifugal force and positive pressure. Increase in volume and curvature of the lens caused by intumescent cataracts induces increased pressure in the capsular bag. This force may be associated with posterior vitreous force increasing capsular pressure. Incision of the anterior capsule may initiate a centrifugal force, allowing escape of the tear of the anterior capsule. The surgeon should always fill the AC with cohesive OVD, particularly in eyes with increased risk factors.

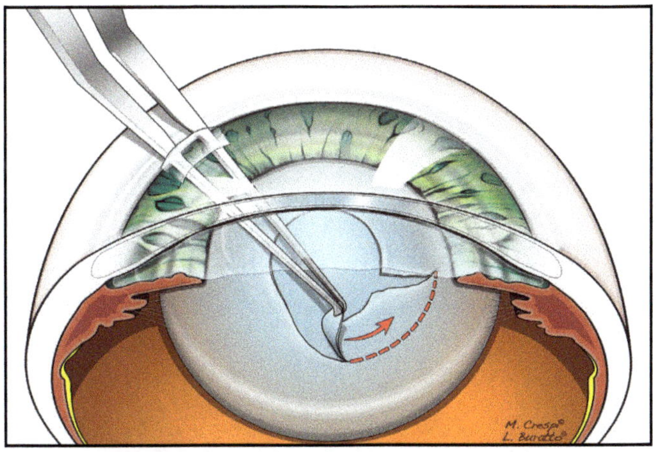

Figure 3-2. Escape of the anterior capsulorrhexis. If the margin of the rhexis escapes before reaching the zonules, the surgeon should make a cut in the opposite direction and initiate a new CCC. This may create an eccentric, asymmetric, noncontinuous CCC allowing poor IOL centration, but is preferable to PC rupture.

anterior to the equator. A rhexis larger than 5.5 mm will cut some of the zonules, affecting stability of the bag and continuity of the CCC.[3]

With a mature nuclear cataract, the surgeon should create a larger CCC to facilitate manipulation of the enlarged nucleus. Conversely, with a mature cortical cataract, even when it is white, the surgeon does not necessarily need to create a large rhexis. If the rhexis is less than 4.0 mm, the surgeon should enlarge it (Figure 3-3). The dimensions of the CCC also vary based on the size of the intraocular lens (IOL).

Dimensions of the Continuous Curvilinear Capsulorrhexis

The diameter of the CCC should be 0.5 mm smaller than the diameter of the optic of the IOL for the following reasons:

- There will be greater stability of the implant in the capsular bag, avoiding lens tilt, induced by asymmetric contraction of the bag after adhesion of the AC to the PC, possible decentration induced by Nd:YAG capsulotomy.
- It creates a barrier to epithelial cell migration across the PC because of adhesion between the AC, the "square edge" of the IOL, and the PC.
- It creates compartmentalization from the vitreous cavity and posterior chamber, even following capsulotomy, to prevent anterior migration of vitreous with subsequent retinal traction.
- With PC rupture, a rhexis that is smaller than the diameter of the optic provides excellent support for an implant in the sulcus and allows the IOL optic to be placed posterior to the CCC.

Finally, it is important to remember that the CCC should be concentric with the optic. If the CCC is not continuous or is decentered over the IOL, or if it is asymmetric, there will be asymmetric adhesion between the AC, IOL, and PC, resulting in constriction of the capsular bag, not concentric with the lens. There is increased risk of epithelial cell migration, dislocation, and tilt of the IOL[4] (Figure 3-4). With bag implantation of silicone lenses, dislocation of the IOL may occur after Nd:YAG posterior capsulotomy, even years after the cataract surgery.[5]

Intraocular inflammation, pseudoexfoliation, and weak zonules may make it difficult to perform a CCC because of capsular fibrosis. In some cases, it is possible to initiate the rhexis using scissors to avoid stress the zonule.

The most frequent complications of a CCC less than 4.5 mm include the following:

- PC rupture during hydrodissection due to a lack of fluid escape as the balanced saline solution (BSS) is trapped between the lens and PC (Figure 3-5).
- Tear of the CCC during phacoemulsification or hydrodissection if the CCC is not continuous, with potential risk of extension to a PC rupture (Figure 3-6).
- Contraction of the bag with decentration of the lens and possible haptic deformation.[6]
- Capsular phymosis.
- Myopic shift induced by accumulation of material between the IOL and PC (capsular block syndrome, frequent with silicone or acrylic IOLs),[7] normally treated by Nd:YAG capsulotomy.

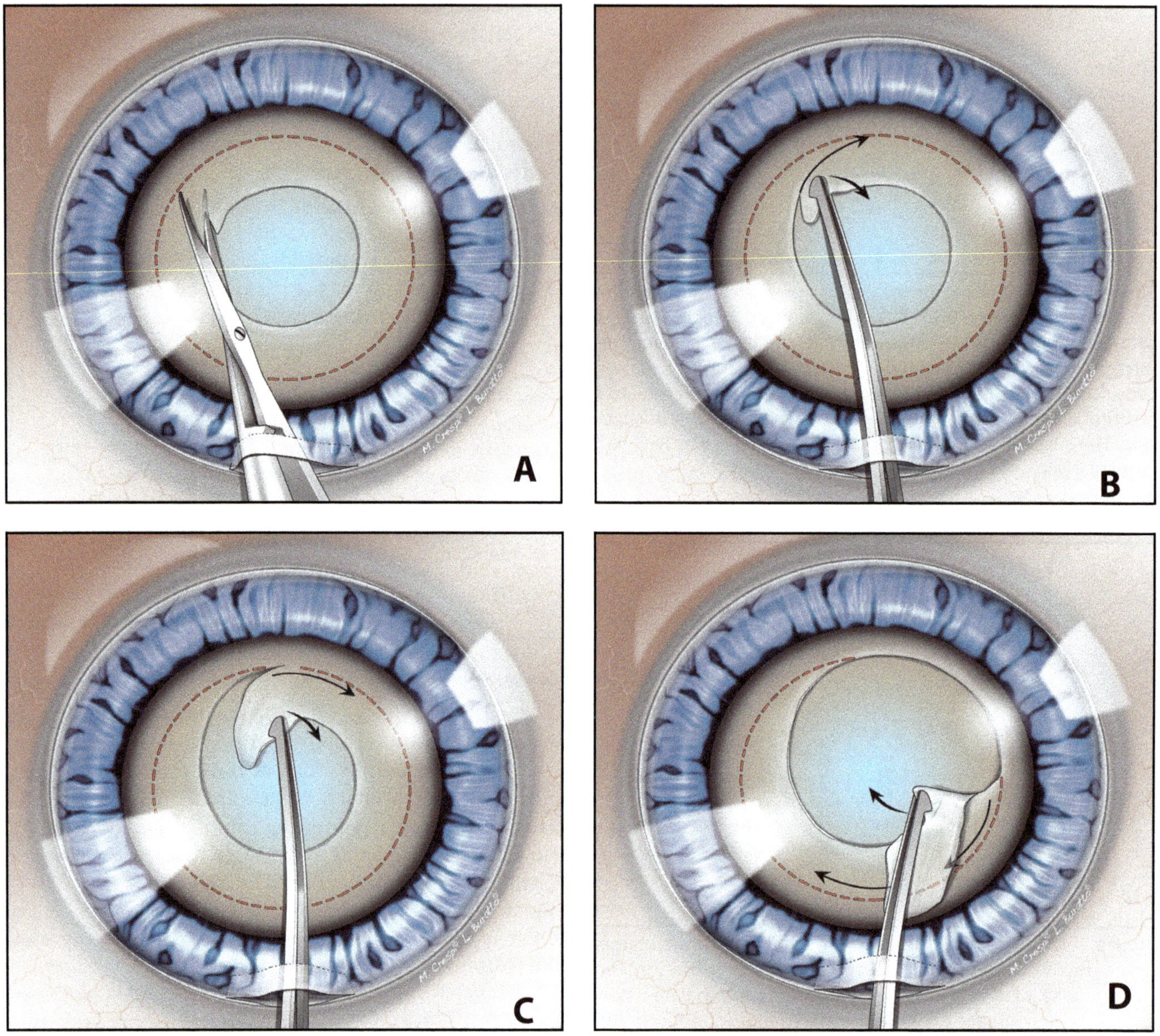

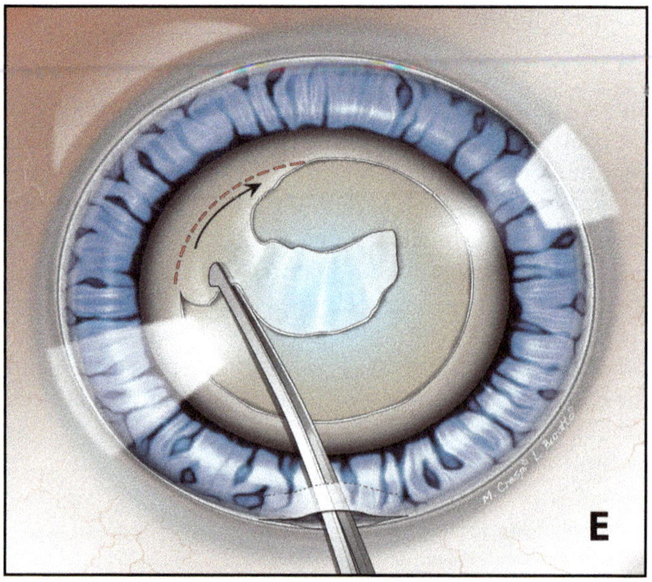

Figure 3-3. Enlargement of the rhexis. With a rhexis smaller than 4.0 mm, the surgeon should enlarge the rhexis during surgery. He or she should use microscissors to create a small radial enlargement of the existing rhexis, then, with the AC filled with OVD (A), he or she should use capsulorrhexis forceps carefully to tear a new, larger rhexis concentric and slightly larger than the previous one (B to E).

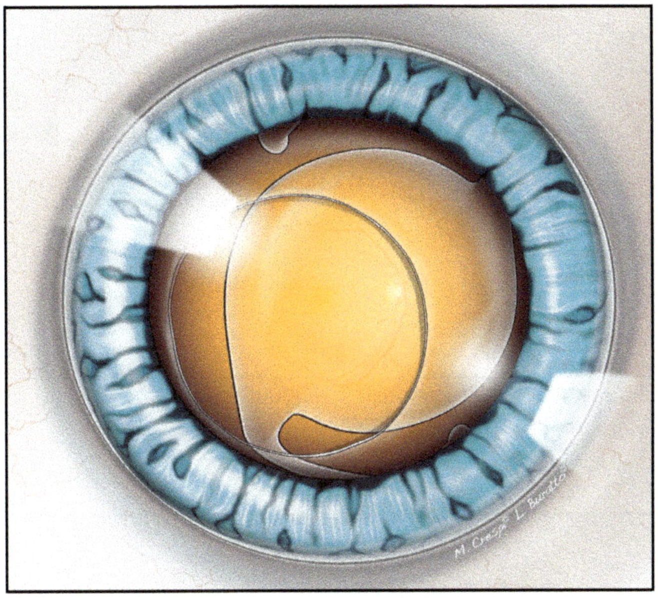

Figure 3-4. Symmetry of the ACR. The ACR should be concentric with the IOL optic. If the ACR is not continuous, decentered, or asymmetric to the optic, asymmetric adhesion will develop between the ACR, IOL, and PC, allowing asymmetric contraction of the bag with IOL decentration.

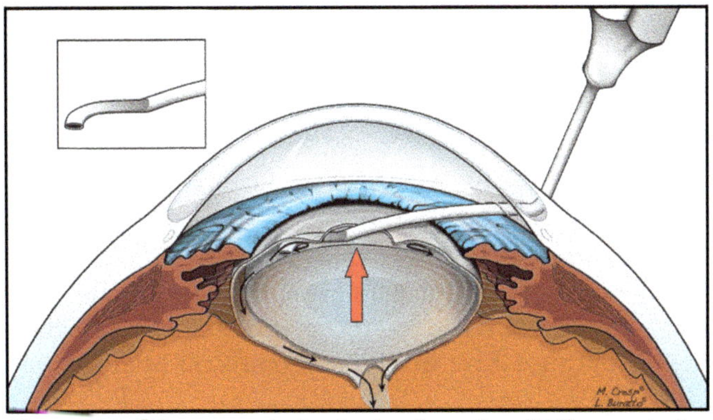

Figure 3-5. PC rupture during hydrodissection. With an anterior capsulorrhexis smaller than 4.5 mm, the fluid from hydrodissection may be trapped between the lens and the PC, leading to increased pressure on the capsule with subsequent rupture.

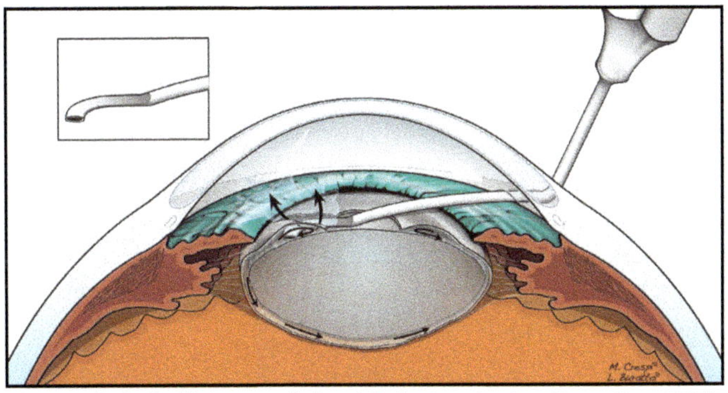

Figure 3-6. Radial tear of the AC during hydrodissection. With a noncontinuous ACR, hydrodissection increases the pressure inside the capsular bag with potential risk of anterior radial tear extension leading to PC rupture.

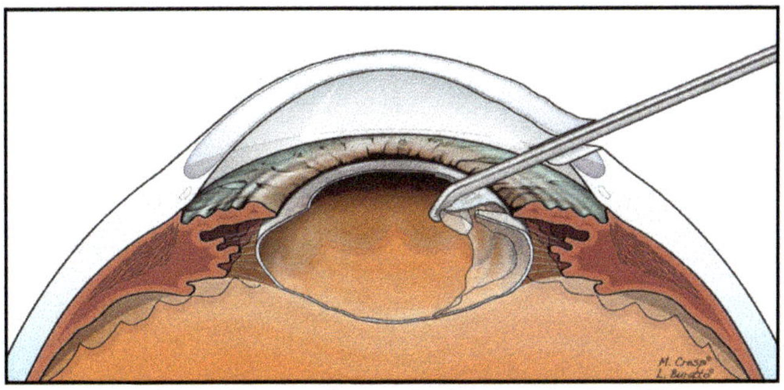

Figure 3-7. AC radial tear during cortical aspiration. This occurs more frequently when coaxial I/A is used to reach subincisional cortex. This may be complicated further by shallowing of the AC caused by incomplete placement of the I/A tip into the AC. Here, a bimanual I/A approach is recommended.

Anterior Capsule Tears

A tear of the CCC has an incidence of 0.7%; it may occur during phacoemulsification, with contact of the phaco tip or second instrument to the CCC and in cracking or chopping maneuvers.

In these cases, the surgeon should inject an OVD above and below the capsular tear to counteract centripetal forces, allowing complete escape of the rhexis. The surgeon should perform a centripetal maneuver with AC forceps to prevent extension of the rhexis before it reaches the zonules (see Figure 3-2). The CCC that results is eccentric and asymmetric but can still resist phacoemulsification forces.[3]

If the CCC has extended to the equator of the lens, the surgeon should continue very cautiously with hydrodissection and delicate manipulation of the nucleus to avoid induced surgical stress to the posterior zonules and PC rupture (which may jeopardize implantation of the IOL in the sulcus). If the surgeon anticipates PC rupture secondary to rhexis extension, the CCC should be enlarged as much as possible using a low molecular weight OVD injected underneath the nucleus to allow expression of the lens. Introducing a phaco tip into the AC is not recommended, as the infusion fluid pressure could induce dislocation of the lens into the vitreous. If the surgeon is ready to insert the phaco tip, he or she should aspirate some of the OVD from the AC; the phaco tip can then be introduced and the infusion bottle lowered to 30 to 40 cm above the patient's head. The capsule may also tear during cortical aspiration (Figure 3-7). This occurs more frequently with subincisional cortical aspiration. If aspiration is performed coaxially, there are often problems with distortion of the cornea. This can be further complicated by shallow AC depth due to incomplete insertion of the irrigation/aspiration (I/A) tip. Angled I/A tips are better with a coaxial approach. We recommend a bimanual approach with infusion separate from aspiration; a Buratto style bimanual I/A cannula can be used to easily engage the cortex without corneal distortion and stress to the corneal incisions (see Figures B1 to B4).

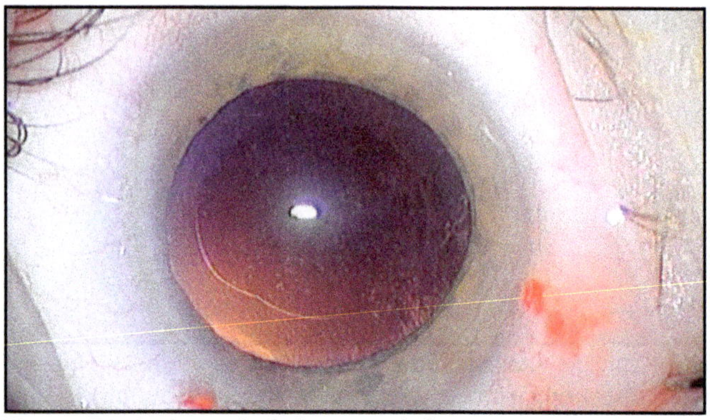

Figure B1. At the end of phacoemulsification and I/A, the anterior capsulorrhexis is intact.

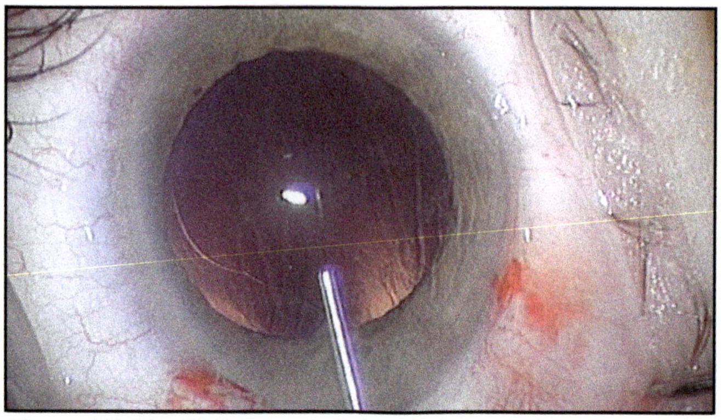

Figure B2. The OVD cannula is inserted.

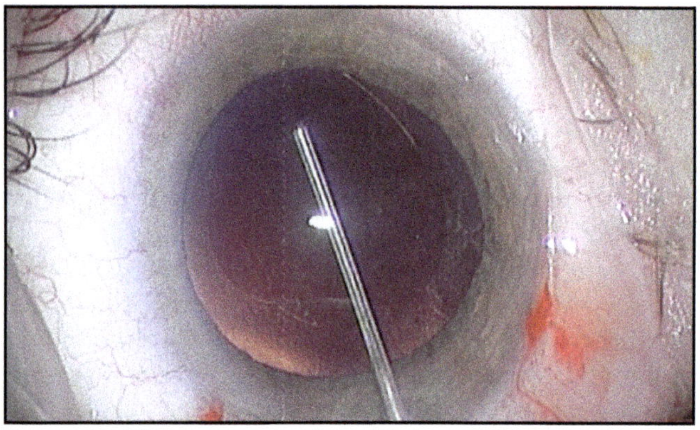

Figure B3. The surgeon begins injection of OVD.

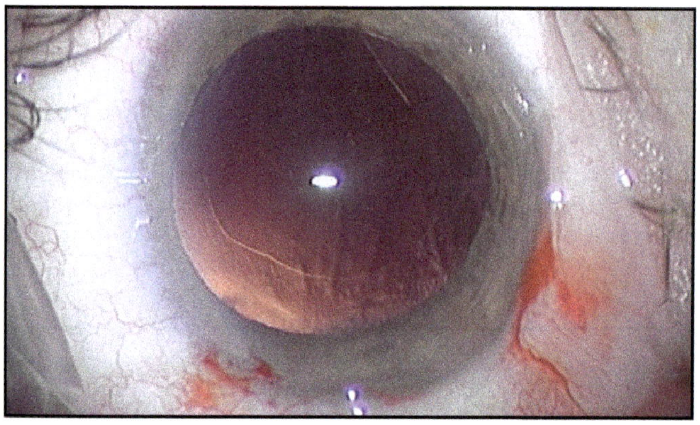

Figure B4. The capsulorrhexis is opened as the OVD is injected.

Implantation in the Bag Following Tear of the Anterior Capsule

A lens can be implanted in the capsular bag even with an AC tear. Here, the surgeon should implant a 3-piece IOL no shorter than 13.0 mm. The haptics should be positioned in the capsular bag, avoiding rotation, in a direction perpendicular to the tear. Sometimes the surgeon will create opposite cuts in the capsular bag to prevent asymmetric contraction forces on the bag.

Anterior Capsulorrhexis With Intumescent Cataracts

The first problem is visualization of the CCC due to decreased contrast, poor red reflex, and presence of lens milk once the anterior capsule has been opened. First, the surgeon should stain the capsule with dye (0.1% trypan blue).[9] Previously to improve the reflex, Gills proposed a retroillumination technique using an external light with scleral contact to increase the reflex.

The surgeon should also use a high molecular weight OVD (eg, Healon 5 [Abbott Laboratories Inc, Abbott Park, IL] or Viscoat [Alcon Laboratories Inc, Fort Worth, TX]) that can decrease the anterior curvature of the lens, reducing the outward force from the intumescent cataract[9] (see Figure 3-1).

Despite these attempts to control the CCC, positive pressure from an intumescent lens may lead to rhexis escape.

The surgeon can decompress the capsular bag by aspirating liquefied cortex prior to completing the anterior CCC. Recently, preoperative treatment using a YAG laser was proposed to create an anterior CCC in intumescent cataracts. There were no reports of complications in the 11 patients treated in this study.[10] Encouraging results have been seen with a femtosecond laser CCC in high-risk cases.[11]

The same applies to the results of the microincisional approach (MICS) with intumescent cataracts. Complications associated with a discontinuous CCC occurred in 4% of cases, and corneal edema was reported in 7% of cases (see Figures C1 to C6).[12]

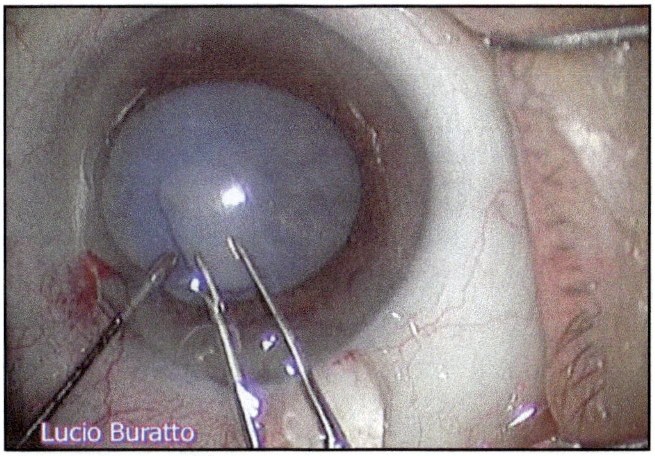

Figure C1. The capsule has been stained with trypan blue. The chamber is formed with high molecular weight ophthalmic viscoelastic device (OVD) and the capsulorrhexis has been started. Abundant milky fluid flows through the anterior capsule opening.

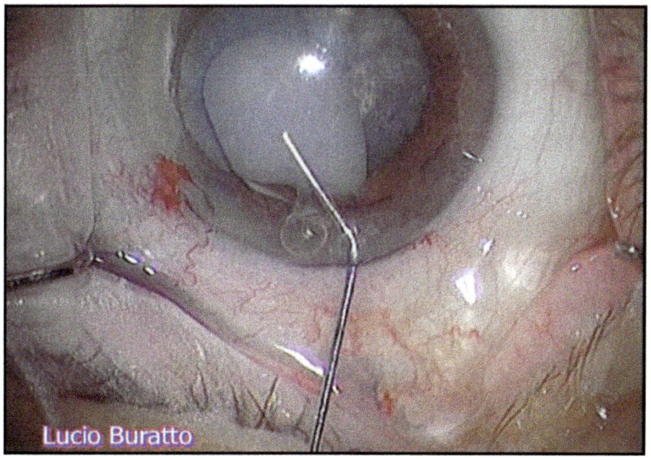

Figure C2. The liquid is aspirated using a cannula.

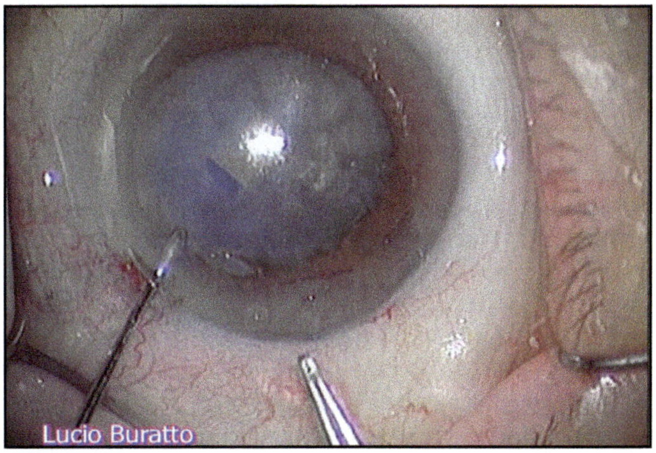

Figure C3. The capsular bag is decompressed and more OVD is injected.

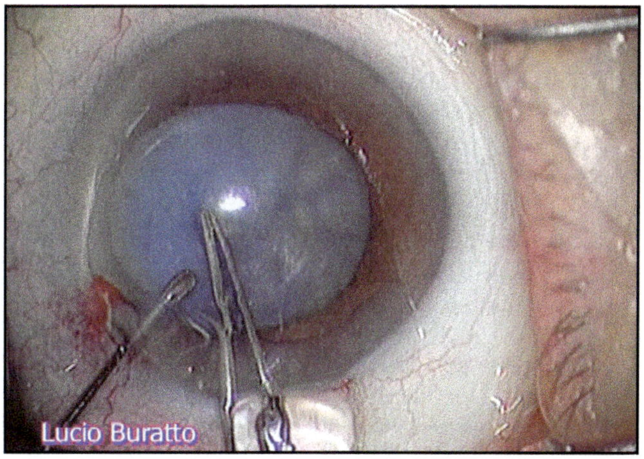

Figure C4. Capsulotomy restarts.

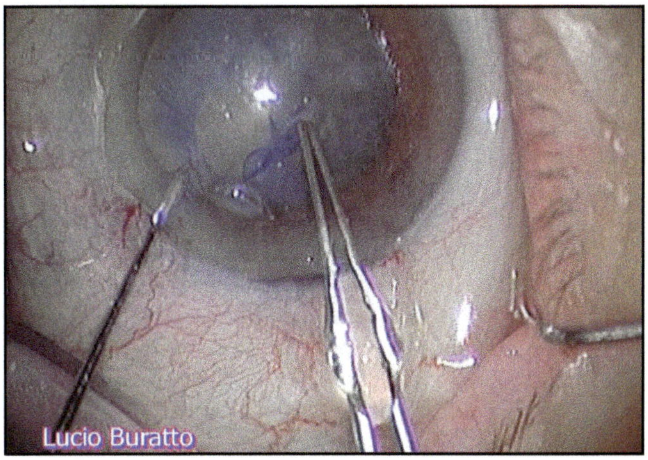

Figure C5. The capsulorrhexis is completed using forceps.

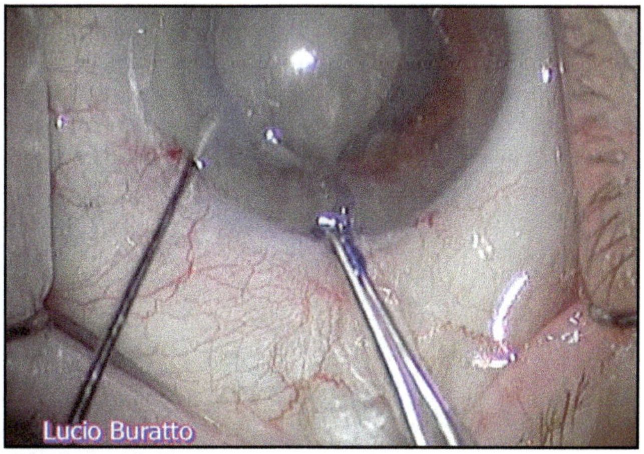

Figure C6. The large anterior capsulorrhexis is completed and the capsule removed.

Anterior Capsulorrhexis in Small Pupils

CCC is more difficult with pupils smaller than 4.5 mm. Here, the surgeon should ensure the CCC is intact prior to proceeding with other maneuvers.[13]

Vasavada reported good results with phacoemulsification performed in the central 4 mm, creating a deep central approach in the lens. A chop technique with low flow and high aspiration is recommended and is performed with a small pupil to create separation of the nucleus peripherally, which is otherwise difficult to access.[13]

If a CCC larger than the pupil diameter is needed, the surgeon should carefully control the tear. Occasionally, the surgeon may need iris retractors or pupil enlargement devices (Malyugin ring).[14]

Coaxial Forceps for Anterior Capsulorrhexis

Current microincision techniques use a primary corneal incision of 1.8 to 2.00 mm. The creation of a CCC through this small incision is more difficult using traditional forceps, as they are difficult to maneuver when the arms are open inside the small corneal tunnel. Corneal distortion with poor visualization of the rhexis results.

Coaxial forceps are useful in microincision techniques as they are easier to maneuver inside the AC (Figure 3-8). The main advantage is that the joint between the arms of the forceps is actually within the AC; this does not exert any pressure on the edges of the incision, making it easier to reach every point in the AC.[15]

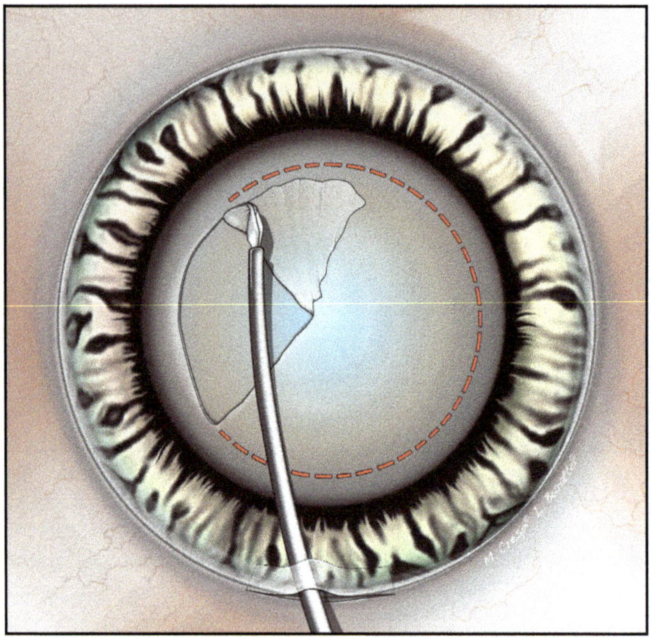

Figure 3-8. Coaxial forceps for ACR. The main advantage is that the hinge of the forceps is inside the AC and is smaller than the incision; therefore, the incision doesn't stretch, and it is easily maneuverable inside the AC.

Anterior Capsulorrhexis With Loose Zonules

With loose zonules or zonular dialysis, the surgeon must carefully perform the CCC, trying to avoid further stress to the zonules. The surgeon should initiate the incision of the capsule perpendicular to the zonules suspected of being loose. A sharp cystotome should be used to reduce stress on the zonules. Insertion of a capsular tension ring prior to phacoemulsification is recommended to more evenly distend the bag.[16]

Posterior Capsulorrhexis

Posterior capsulorrhexis (PCR) is a technique for PC opacity in children, rupture of the PC with an intact hyaloid face, or posterior fibrosis. The PCR technique is similar to the ACR technique.

The main difference is in the thinness of the PC (2 to 4 microns), adhesion of the ligament between the PC and the anterior hyaloid (Wieger's ligament), and the vitreous being closer to the PCR.[17] The surgeon should attempt to create a posterior CCC avoiding potential of escape or asymmetry, common with ACR.[18]

Prior to initiating PCR, the surgeon should puncture the PC and inject low molecular weight OVD to overcome the resistance of the capsule hyaloid ligament and displace the vitreous face away from the PC (Figure 3-9A). The capsular bag is stabilized with high molecular weight cohesive viscoelastic. The surgeon should create a posterior CCC approximately 3.5 to 4 mm in diameter; he or she should remember that escape of the ACR may lead to loss of capsular support for the IOL (Figure 3-9B).

The PCR is primarily used to capture the IOL optic in children[19] and to prevent PC opacity and capsular contraction with subsequent decentration. Recent studies recommend posterior CCC with optic capture as a routine approach in adult patients, along with decreasing inflammation, refractive variations, IOP increases, and accumulation of OVD underneath the IOL.[20-22] Menapace and colleagues recommended the use of this technique particularly in patients with pseudoexfoliation, severe myopia, peripheral retinal degeneration, and implantation of toric and multifocal lenses.[23]

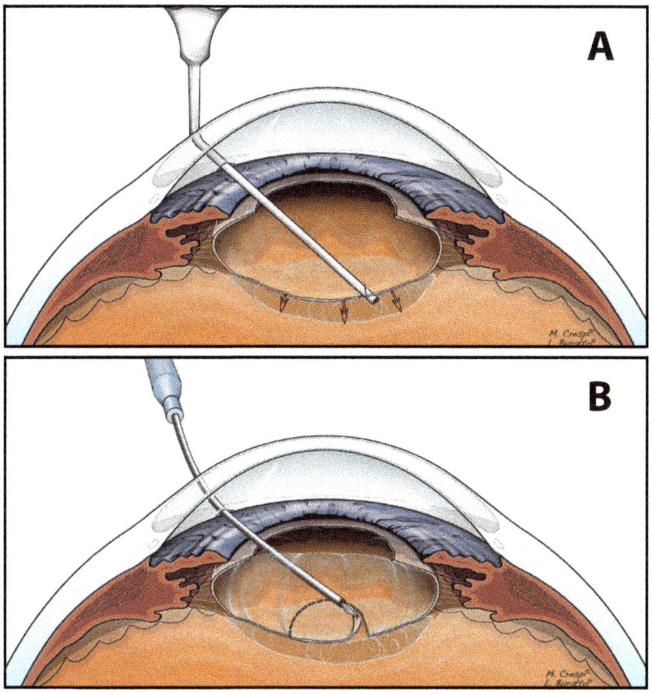

Figure 3-9. PCR. (A) Prior to performing PCR, the surgeon should puncture the PC, injecting low molecular weight OVD to break the resistance of the capsular hyaloid ligament and push the anterior hyaloid face away from the PC. The bag is then filled with high molecular weight cohesive OVD. (B) The surgeon creates a continuous PCR with a diameter approximately 3.5 to 4 mm.

References

1. Arshinoff S. Mechanics of capsulorrhexis. *J Cataract Refract Surg.* 1992;18(6):623-662.
2. Gimbel HV, Neuhann T. Development, advantages, and methods of the continuous circular capsulorrhexis technique. *J Cataract Refract Surg.* 1990;16(1):31-37.
3. Arshinoff S. Classifying capsulorrhexis complications. *J Cataract Refract Surg.* 1994;20:475.
4. Tappin MJ, Larkin DF. Factors leading to lens implant decentration and exchange. *Eye (Lond).* 2000;14(pt 5):773-776.
5. Petersen AM, Bluth LL, Campion M. Delayed posterior dislocation of silicone plate-haptic lenses after neodymium:yag capsulotomy. *J Cataract Refract Surg.* 2000;26(12):1827-1829.
6. Michael K, O'Colmain U, Vallance JH, Cormack TG. Capsule contraction syndrome with haptic deformation and flexion. *J Cataract Refract Surg.* 2010;36(4):686-689.
7. Namba H, Namba R, Sugiura T, Miyauchi S. Accumulation of milky fluid: a late complication of cataract surgery. *J Cataract Refract Surg.* 1999;25(7):1019-1023.
8. Miyake K, Ota I, Ichihashi S, Miyake S, Tanaka Y, Terasaki H. New classification of capsular block syndrome. *J Cataract Refract Surg.* 1998;24(9):1230-1234.
9. Goldman JM, Karp CL. Adjunct devices for managing challenging cases in cataract surgery: capsular staining and ophthalmic viscosurgical devices. *Curr Opin Ophthalmol.* 2007;18(1):52-57.
10. Coelho RP, Paula JS, Silva RN, Garcia TV, Martin LF. Preoperative Nd:YAG laser anterior capsulotomy in white intumescent cataracts: report of 11 cases. *Arq Bras Oftalmol.* 2009;72(1):113-115.
11. Friedman NJ, Palanker DV, Schuele G, et al. Femtosecond laser capsulotomy. *J Cataract Refract Surg.* 2011;37:1189-1198.
12. Venkatesh R, Das M, Prashanth S, Muralikrishnan R. Manual small incision cataract surgery in eyes with white cataracts. *Indian J Ophthalmol.* 2005;53(3):173-176.
13. Vasavada A, Singh R. Phacoemulsification in eyes with a small pupil. *J Cataract Refract Surg.* 2000;26:1210-1218.
14. Santoro S, Sannace C, Cascella MC, Lavermicocca N. Subluxated lens: phacoemulsification with iris hooks. *J Cataract Refract Surg.* 2003;29(12):2269-2273.
15. Ratnarajan G, Calladine D, Watson SL. Cross-action capsulorrhexis forceps for coaxial microincision cataract surgery. *J Cataract Refract Surg.* 2011;37(8):1559-1560.
16. Bayraktar S, Altan T, Kucuksumer Y, Yilmaz OF. Capsular tension ring implantation after capsulorrhexis in phacoemulsification of cataracts associated with pseudoexfoliation syndrome. Intraoperative complications and early postoperative findings. *J Cataract Refract Surg.* 2001;27(10):1620-1628.
17. Sun R. Advantage and disadvantage of posterior continuous curvilinear capsulorrhexis. *J Cataract Refract Surg.* 2007;33(12):2004-2005; author reply 2005-2007.
18. Fan H, Wing Lee VY, Li Liu DT, Chiu Lam DS. Clinical effects of primary posterior continuous curvilinear capsulorrhexis. *J Cataract Refract Surg.* 2007;33(12):2002; author reply 2002-2004.
19. Dadeya S. Posterior continuous curvilinear capsulorrhexis with and without optic capture of the posterior chamber intraocular lens in the absence of vitrectomy. *J Pediatr Ophthalmol Strabismus.* 2003;40(3):130-131; author reply 131.
20. Stifter E, Menapace R, Kriechbaum K, Vock L, Luksch A. Effect of primary posterior continuous curvilinear capsulorrhexis with and without posterior optic buttonholing on postoperative anterior chamber flare. *J Cataract Refract Surg.* 2009;35(3):480-484.
21. Stifter E, Menapace R, Kriechbaum K, Luksch A. Posterior optic buttonholing prevents intraocular pressure peaks after cataract surgery with primary posterior capsulorrhexis. *Graefes Arch Clin Exp Ophthalmol.* 2010;248(11):1595-1600.
22. Stifter E, Menapace R, Luksch A, Neumayer T, Sacu S. Anterior chamber depth and change in axial intraocular lens position after cataract surgery with primary posterior capsulorrhexis and posterior optic buttonholing. *J Cataract Refract Surg.* 2008;34(5):749-754.
23. Menapace R. Posterior capsulorrhexis combined with optic buttonholing: an alternative to standard in-the-bag implantation of sharp-edged intraocular lenses? A critical analysis of 1000 consecutive cases. *Graefes Arch Clin Exp Ophthalmol.* 2008;246(6):787-801.

4

Hydroseparation Maneuvers

Lucio Buratto, MD; Stephen F. Brint, MD, FACS; and Mario R. Romano, MD, PhD

Hydrodissection and hydrodelineation are techniques to free the lens from the capsule by using an injection of balanced saline solution (BSS). With hydrodissection, the cortex is separated from the capsular bag; with hydrodelineation, the nucleus is separated from the epinucleus.

With loose zonules and capsule weakness, hydroseparation can cause posterior capsule rupture or lack of loosening of the lens and its adhesions from the capsular bag.[1]

The lens has an average thickness of 10 mm and a diameter of approximately 4.5 mm. The capsular bag is approximately 20 microns thick at its equator. It thickens near the zonular attachment (that extend anteriorly for approximately 2.5 mm and 1 mm posterior to the equator), having a thickness of approximately 14 microns anteriorly and 3 microns at its posterior pole. Development of the lens leads to formation of new lens fibers that tend to compress and dehydrate older fibers. This leads to an increase in density and size of the lens with an increase in capsular pressure.

Hydrodissection Maneuvers

With hydrodissection, a 27-gauge cannula with a flat tip is used, creating laminar flow. The cannula may be straight or curved and should reach the edge of the anterior capsule and the equator of the capsular bag easily.[2] The flow should be directed just under the anterior capsule. With infusion of BSS into the bag, the surgeon lifts the cannula upward against the posterior surface of the anterior capsule to create a better flow just within the capsular bag. This should be forceful enough to separate the adhesions between the cortical fibers and the bag (cortical cleaving hydrodissection[3] [Figure 4-1]).

At the same time, the surgeon should exert mild pressure on the posterior lip of the corneal tunnel to allow the exit of fluid, avoiding increased intracapsular pressure (see Figure 4-1).

The BSS flows along the bag, eventually reaching the capsule equator distal to the cannula, then the posterior capsule, the distal capsular equator, and finally the proximal anterior capsule.

If performed correctly, the surgeon sees progression of fluid flow that progressively surrounds the lens. If hydrodissection is performed with the cannula placed into the cortex, a cleavage plane within the cortex remains partly adhered to the capsular bag. Now, more irrigation/aspiration (I/A) will be necessary with the associated risks of capsular rupture.

Hydrodelineation

Hydrodelineation separates the nucleus from the epinucleus. It uses an infusion of a lamellar flow of BSS. The

Buratto L, Brint SF, Romano MR.
Cataract Surgery Complications (pp 29-34).
© 2013 Taylor & Francis Group.

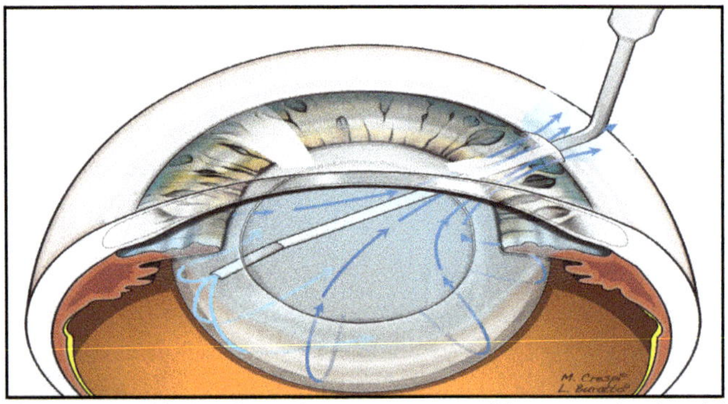

Figure 4-1. Hydrodissection maneuvers. The cannula should exert mild upward pressure on the posterior surface of the anterior capsule parallel to the anterior capsule, creating a flow just inside the capsular bag. At the same time, the surgeon exerts mild pressure on the posterior lip of the corneal incision to encourage escape of fluid, avoiding increased pressure on the capsule.

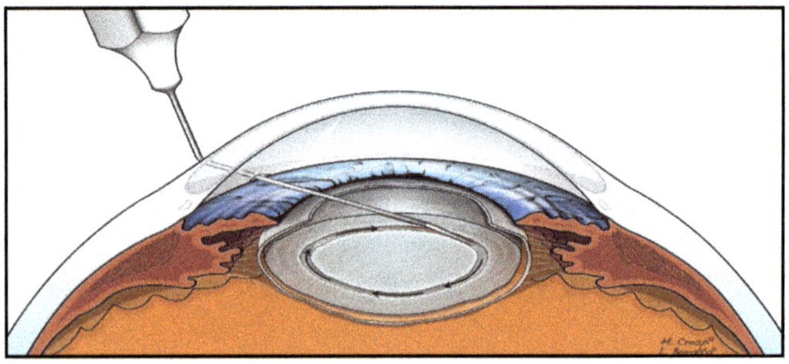

Figure 4-2. Hydrodelineation maneuvers. Hydrodelineation is performed by injecting BSS into the paracentral area of the nucleus to separate the nucleus from the epinucleus with a laminar flow of BSS. This should be performed following hydrodissection. If hydrodelineation is the only procedure performed, strong adhesion persists between the capsular bag, the epinucleus, and the cortex, making it more difficult to remove the cortex with I/A.

separation is achieved by injecting BSS into the paracentral zone of the nucleus (Figure 4-2). It should be performed following hydrodissection as it mobilizes the central nucleus. In cases in which hydrodelineation alone is performed, strong adhesion between the capsular bag and epinucleus/cortex of the lens persists, making it more difficult to remove cortex with I/A. Rarely, only hydrodelineation should be performed (see posterior polar cataract on page 32) as the cortex protects the posterior capsule during phacoemulsification.

Complications Associated With Hydroseparation

Complications associated with hydroseparation occur from excessive injection of fluid, inappropriate use of hydrodissection, or problems associated with the capsule or zonules.

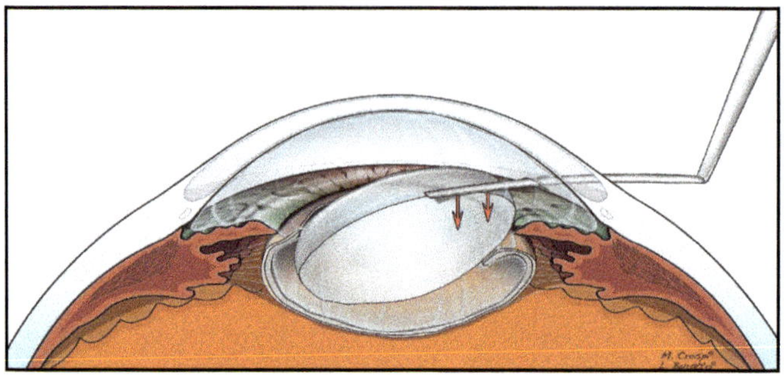

Figure 4-3. Prolapse of the nucleus during hydrodissection. The nucleus shifts anteriorly following hydrodissection, indicating complete mobilization. Here, the size of the nucleus must be reduced in the bag; it is pushed back into the bag to facilitate successive steps of phacoemulsification.

Maneuvers of Hydroseparation

Hydroseparation must be performed carefully with equal amounts of fluid entering and leaving the eye. The volume of BSS injected must be equal to the volume leaving the anterior chamber (AC) through the main corneal incision.

Prior to hydrodissection, a portion of the cohesive ophthalmic viscoelastic device (OVD) should be aspirated from the AC to facilitate internal flow of BSS, avoiding blockage of fluid egress. The maneuvers of hydrodissection should include slight posterior wound pressure as this will open the incision, allowing some of the OVD and fluid to escape from the AC.

During hydrodissection, the surgeon perceives an increase in AC depth (as the flow passes around the lens) and subsequent reduction in depth (when the flow reaches the AC and leaves the eye). Sometimes the nucleus or the combined nucleus cortex shifts forward during this maneuver. This indicates complete mobilization. The nucleus must be reposited into the bag to facilitate subsequent phacoemulsification in the posterior chamber (Figure 4-3).

Excessive Fluid Injection

A rapid increase in the volume of the bag due to injecting too much or too rapidly may result in capsular rupture jeopardizing subsequent phacoemulsification. Rupture of the posterior capsule can occur because of excessive fluid pressure on the posterior capsule; there is no good exit for the amount and force of the fluid (the situation is often aggravated by a small anterior capsulorrhexis). This can result in a localized pressure increase on the posterior capsule (Figure 4-4). Rupture of the posterior capsule may not be noticed during hydrodissection. The surgeon becomes aware of the situation when the phaco tip with infusion is placed into the eye. The surgeon sees posterior dislocation of the nucleus under pressure from the infusion fluid.

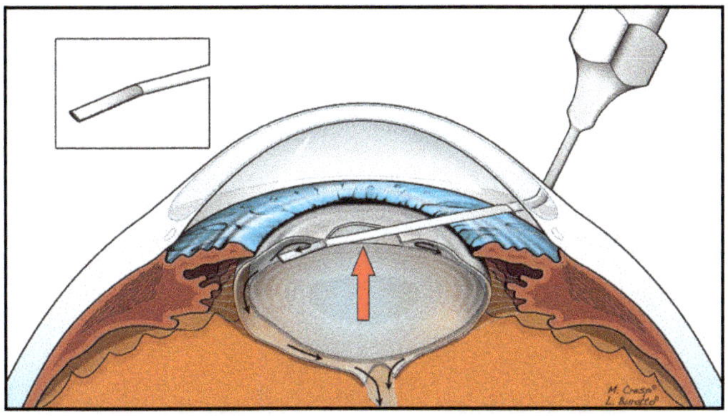

Figure 4-4. Rupture of the posterior capsule caused by excessive fluid pressure. Rupture of the posterior capsule occurs because of excessive fluid pressure on the posterior capsule. The fluid injected does not have an adequate exit (a situation sometimes caused by a small anterior capsulorrhexis), generating increased pressure localized to the posterior capsule.

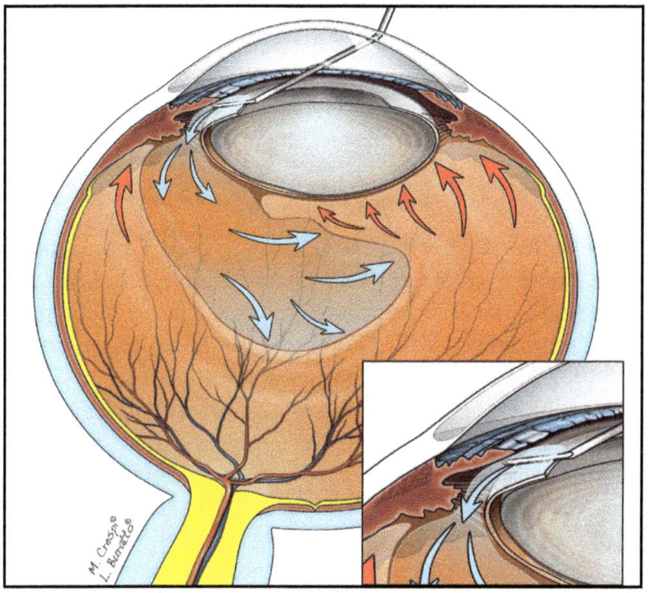

Figure 4-5. Fluid misdirection. If the hydrodissection cannula is placed between the iris and the anterior capsule, a flow will be generated that reaches the vitreous through the zonules, resulting in increased hydrostatic pressure inside the vitreous chamber with subsequent anterior displacement of the bag, and potential dehiscence of the zonules.

Complications Resulting From Incorrect Hydrodissection Maneuvers

Incorrect Direction of the Flow

Hydrodissection with small pupils and poor visibility of the margin of the anterior rhexis can be performed incorrectly in a different plane than desired. If the cannula is positioned between the iris and anterior capsule, flow will be generated reaching the vitreous through the zonules. This leads to an increase in pressure in the vitreous with subsequent anterior displacement of the bag, and possibly dehiscence of the zonules (Figure 4-5). In more serious cases, the surgeon may see luxation of the entire lens into the AC and sometimes into the vitreous because of zonule rupture, due to inward flow of BSS directed through the zonules and positive posterior pressure resulting from the passage of BSS into the vitreous.

The surgeon should proceed with rapid 20% IV mannitol infusion to dehydrate the vitreous. If the zonule damage is minimal and vitreous is absent from the AC, the surgeon should inject high molecular weight OVD into the AC and infusion fluid to maintain appropriate depth of the AC for successful completion of the surgery. With prolapse of the lens with vitreous into the AC, the surgeon should perform a total vitrectomy (see Chapters 10 and 11).

Management of soft cataracts has also been described.[13] Once the central nucleus has been removed, viscoelastic is injected between the cortex and the epinucleus (viscodissection) to elevate it. The epinucleus and cortex are then removed using low aspiration.

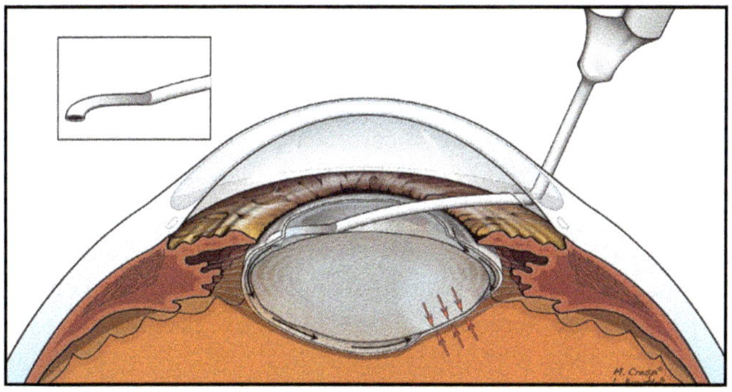

Figure 4-6. Incomplete hydrodissection. Incomplete hydrodissection will result in poor separation of the cortical adhesions with the bag. It will not be easy for the surgeon to rotate the nucleus during successive phacoemulsification. This leads to excessive stress on the zonules induced by additional rotational maneuvers.

Inadequate Hydrodissection

The complications from hydrodissection come from inadequate cleaving of cortical adhesions from the bag. In this case, successive rotation of the nucleus during phacoemulsification will not be easy. Excessive stress of the zonules is induced by forceful rotation of the nucleus (Figure 4-6). With persistent posterior adhesions, phaco must be interrupted. The surgeon should inject a small amount of OVD and cautiously perform 360 degrees of hydrodissection. Alternatively, the surgeon can perform nuclear cracking without rotation. This will allow fluid to flow underneath the nucleus without involving the zonules.

Complications Associated With Abnormalities of the Bag

A Too Small Anterior Capsulorrhexis

An anterior capsulorrhexis smaller than 5 mm with a large, dense nucleus can block the outward hydrodissection from under the anterior capsulorrhexis. There will be posterior segregation of the fluid between the posterior cortex and the posterior capsule (see Figure 4-4).

This block may also occur with anterior prolapse of a soft nucleus following excessive and rapid fluid injection into the capsular bag regardless of the capsulorrhexis diameter. Prior to additional maneuvers, the surgeon should push the nucleus back into the bag to allow fluid to flow into the AC and decompress the capsular bag. Rupture of the posterior capsule with an intact anterior capsule is rare with an incidence of 0.04%, but may lead to complete dislocation of the lens into the vitreous.[4]

Tear of the Anterior Capsulorrhexis

With a tear and/or escape of the anterior capsulorrhexis, hydrodissection generates centrifugal forces that tend to further open the anterior capsule as far as the equator (Figure 4-7). Discontinuity or tear of the anterior capsulorrhexis has an incidence of 0.79%.[5] Most anterior capsulorrhexis tears (if the surgeon carefully performs hydrodissection) can be stopped by the zonules prior to reaching the equator.

However, if the rhexis escape reaches the equator of the bag, the posterior capsule opens with a difficult procedure required (see Chapter 10). With anterior escape, the surgeon proceeds with hydrodissection with great caution, working with low infusion pressure and using phacoemulsification techniques that will not increase stress to the bag and zonules.

Pseudoexfoliation

The incidence of pseudoexfoliation (PXF) varies from 0.2% to 20%. It is unilateral in 50% of cases and associated with glaucoma in 20% of patients. There are associated complications during cataract surgery, primarily associated with zonular lysis (13% to 18% of cases), lens subluxation (10.6%), and capsular rupture (2%).[6] Hydrodissection is extremely important with PXF. Adequate hydrodissection allows good rotation of the nucleus in the bag, avoiding further stress to the already compromised zonules during phacoemulsification. The surgeon should perform multiple small amounts of hydrodissection in the 4 quadrants, avoiding sudden changes in AC depth that can increase stress on the zonules. Hydrodelineation of the nucleus is not recommended as increased amounts of cortex remain and more aspiration will be required. In cases of PXF with loose zonules, the surgeon should insert a capsular tension ring immediately after completion of the capsulorrhexis.[7] The tension ring stabilizes the equator of the bag during cortical aspiration with the stress distributed 360 degrees from the zonules. The tension ring may complicate cortical removal with its inevitable cortical obstruction. Alternately, the ring may be inserted following complete cortical removal to resist bag contraction postoperatively by metaplasia and fibrosis.

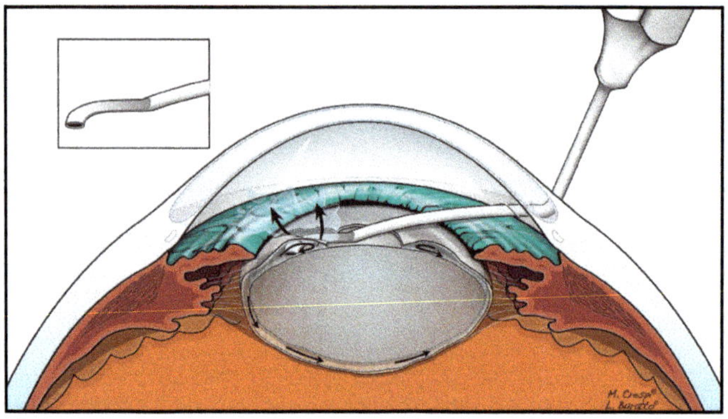

Figure 4-7. Escape of the anterior capsulorrhexis during hydrodissection. Hydrodissection generates centrifugal forces that, with a tear or escape of the anterior capsulorrhexis, tend to extend the tear until it reaches the equator of the bag.

Posterior Polar Cataract

The posterior polar cataract (PPC) is a white circular opacity occupying the posterior cortical and subcapsular region of the lens.

The incidence of posterior capsule rupture with PPC varies from 26% to 36%.[8,9]

Adjacent to the PPC, the posterior capsule is thin and fragile, having marked adherence with capsular connective tissue. It has been hypothesized that the posterior capsule can actually be absent in the area of the PPC.

Cortical cleaving hydrodissection is contraindicated in these cases: When flow from hydrodissection meets the point where the PPC is adhered to the posterior capsule, hydraulic rupture of the posterior capsule tends to extend toward the equator[3] with dislocation of the entire lens. Instead, hydrodelineation should be performed gently in all 4 quadrants with the fluid wave being contained within the proximal margin of the PPC[10] (Figure 4-8).

Hydrodelineation of the nucleus preserves the cortex and protects the posterior capsule during phacoemulsification. Once the nucleus has been freed, the surgeon proceeds with aspiration of the nucleus and cortex using I/A. He or she should attempt to leave a central zone of cortex as protection until the final steps. The PPC should be managed with low levels of aspiration in a centripetal direction. A more prudent approach has also been proposed using the YAG laser later for subsequent posterior capsulotomy.[11]

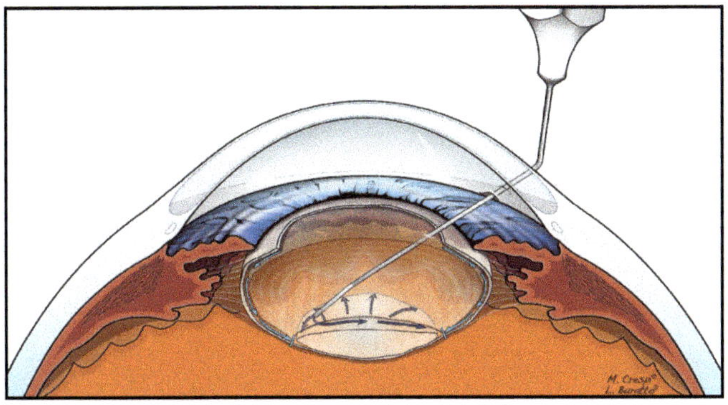

Figure 4-8. Hydrodissection and hydrodelineation of a posterior polar cataract. With a posterior polar cataract (PPC), if hydrodissection is performed it must be minimal, ensuring that the wave does not extend far beyond the margin of the CCC, and it should be sequentially performed in all 4 quadrants. Hydrodelineation of the nucleus is preferred in order to preserve the cortex to protect the posterior capsule during phacoemulsification.

Recently, Salahuddin proposed a technique of hydrodelineation followed by viscodelineation and viscodissection in cases of PPC. Posterior capsular rupture was reported in 7% of cases.[12] The technique first described hydrodelamination of the nucleus. Then, low molecular weight OVD was injected below the central nucleus (viscodelineation) with the intention of separating it totally from the epinucleus, creating a shell of viscoelastic to protect the epinucleus.[12] The surgeon continues with minimal hydrodissection, followed by sculpting. Fracture of the nucleus induced by injection of OVD deep into the nucleus of soft cataracts has also been described.[13] Once the central nucleus has been removed, viscoelastic is injected between the cortex and the epinucleus (viscodissection) to elevate it. The epinucleus and the cortex are then removed using low aspiration.

References

1. Dooley IJ, O'Brien PD. Subjective difficulty of each stage of phacoemulsification cataract surgery performed by basic surgical trainees. *J Cataract Refract Surg.* 2006;32(4):604-608.
2. Levy JH, Pisacano AM, Yalon M. New and efficient hydrodissection cannula to enhance fluid distribution around the nucleus. *J Cataract Refract Surg.* 1994;20(4):478-479.
3. Fine IH. Cortical cleaving hydrodissection. *J Cataract Refract Surg.* 1992;18(5):508-512.
4. Ota I, Miyake S, Miyake K. Dislocation of the lens nucleus into the vitreous cavity after standard hydrodissection. *Am J Ophthalmol.* 1996;121(6):706-708.
5. Marques FF, Marques DM, Osher RH, Osher JM. Fate of anterior capsule tears during cataract surgery. *J Cataract Refract Surg.* 2006;32(10):1638-1642.
6. Kuchle M, Viestenz A, Martus P, Handel A, Junemann A, Naumann GO. Anterior chamber depth and complications during cataract surgery in eyes with pseudoexfoliation syndrome. *Am J Ophthalmol.* 2000;129(3):281-285.
7. Fine IH, Hoffman RS. Phacoemulsification in the presence of pseudoexfoliation: challenges and options. *J Cataract Refract Surg.* 1997;23(2):160-165.
8. Vasavada A, Singh R. Phacoemulsification in eyes with posterior polar cataract. *J Cataract Refract Surg.* 1999;25(2):238-245.
9. Osher RH, Yu BC, Koch DD. Posterior polar cataracts: a predisposition to intraoperative posterior capsular rupture. *J Cataract Refract Surg.* 1990;16(2):157-162.
10. Vasavada AR, Dholakia SA, Raj SM, Singh R. Effect of cortical cleaving hydrodissection on posterior capsule opacification in age-related nuclear cataract. *J Cataract Refract Surg.* 2006;32(7):1196-1200.
11. Siatiri H, Moghimi S. Posterior polar cataract: minimizing risk of posterior capsule rupture. *Eye (Lond).* 2006;20(7):814-816.
12. Salahuddin A. Inverse horseshoe technique for phacoemulsification of posterior polar cataract. *Can J Ophthalmol.* 2010;45(2):154-156.
13. Malavazzi GR, Nery RG. Viscofracture technique for soft lens cataract removal. *J Cataract Refract Surg.* 2011;37(1):11-12.

5

Complications of Phacoemulsification

Lucio Buratto, MD; Stephen F. Brint, MD, FACS; and Mario R. Romano, MD, PhD

Phacoemulsification techniques should minimize the use of ultrasound and optimize efficiency of lens removal without causing damage. It is well known that the longitudinal motion of phaco creates a double disadvantage: localized increase in temperature at the incision and repulsion of lens fragments.

The adjustment of aspiration parameters keeps the lens material as close as possible to the tip and reduces the temperature of the tip. With increased ultrasound power, the surgeon should increase aspiration flow, while increasing infusion flow by raising the balanced saline solution (BSS) bottle (Table 5-1). Recent developments in energy management of ultrasound have minimized thermal burns and optimized nuclear removal (see Figures A1 to A2 and B1 to B6).

Recent Developments

Recently, torsional movement (Ozil) allows an oscillating movement of the tip, reducing repulsion and decreasing thermal phenomena. The advantage is better efficiency of phacoemulsification, with decreased infusion and aspiration. The newest phacoemulsification equipment also minimizes post-occlusion surge. The surge is much less to a reduction in compliance and internal diameter of the aspiration tubing. Also some systems utilize an Aspiration Bypass System (ABS) port on one side of the phaco tip, devised to maintain aspiration flow even when the tip is completely occluded. This ensures constant cooling of the tip and reduced vacuum levels. The new software can also monitor infusion pressure, vacuum, and aspiration flow to modulate the speed of the pump and ultrasound power and change the vacuum (dynamic rise). When the predetermined values of the vacuum are reached, the system releases a small burst of longitudinal ultrasound to break the occlusion then draws new lens material to the tip. Other systems regulate the duty cycle of the phaco device modulating the on/off cycles of ultrasound (8 to 16 ms). Some software updates can regulate the duty cycle in relation to the stroke of the phaco tip; that is modified based of the density of the lens.

Buratto L, Brint SF, Romano MR.
Cataract Surgery Complications (pp 35-46).
© 2013 Taylor & Francis Group.

Table 5-1

Suggested Parameters for Phacoemulsification

	Ultrasound %*	Torsional %**	Aspiration (cc/min)	Vacuum (mm Hg)	Irrigation (cm H_2O)
Pre-phaco	10	20	20 to 25	140 to 180	80 to 100
Sculpting	30 to 70	80	28 to 32	80 to 100	80 to 100
Quadrant	10 to 50	60	32 to 40	300 to 400***	110 to 120
Cortex			32 to 35	500	110 to 120

*The ultrasound energy is kept at low values if the torsional function is active on the phaco device.

**When Ozil used may be zero.

***Values at higher limits if a chop technique is used.

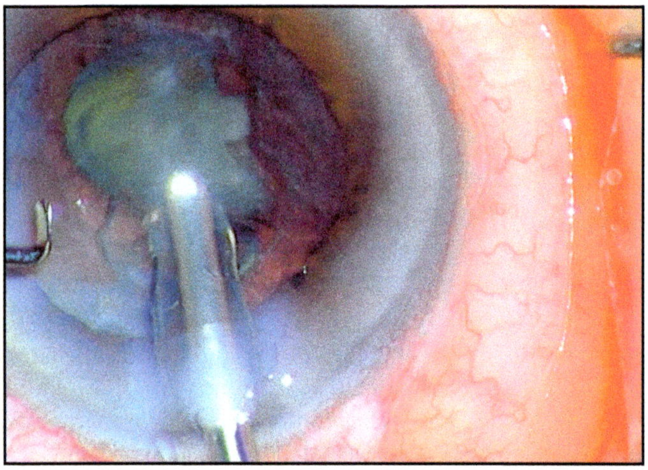

Figure A1. Phacoemulsification may result in a wound burn using high power U/S with a chamber filled with viscous adhesive substance.

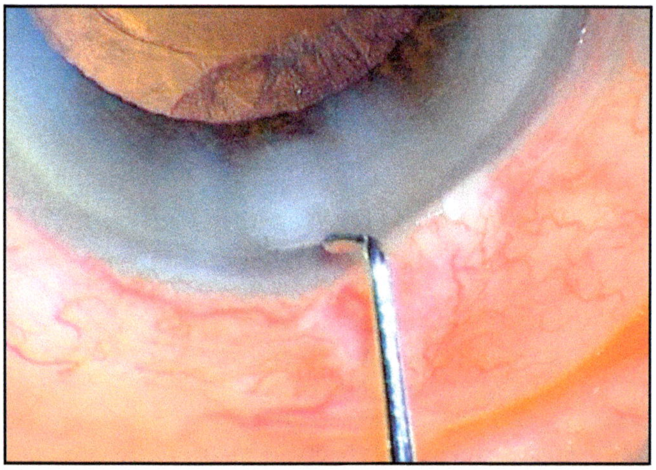

Figure A2. To prevent burns, it is necessary to aspirate some OVD first and then use low ultrasound energy at the beginning of phacoemulsification.

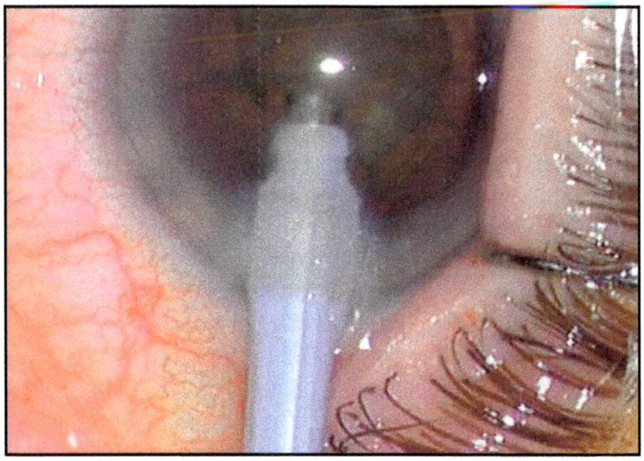

Figure B1. The AC is formed by OVD and the surgeon has set high ultrasound power. He is using an older generation phaco.

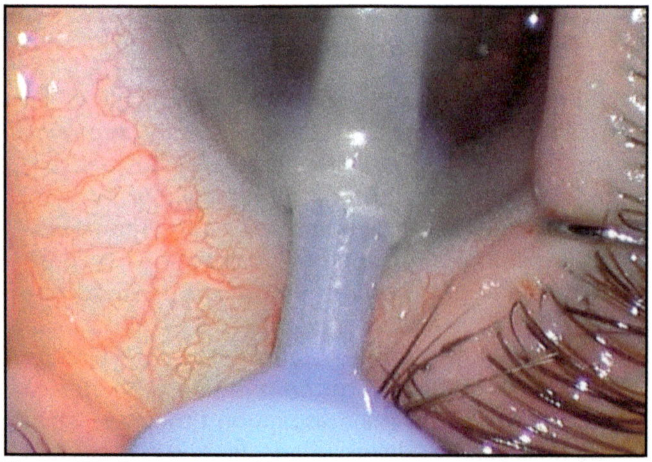

Figure B2. Severe wound burn.

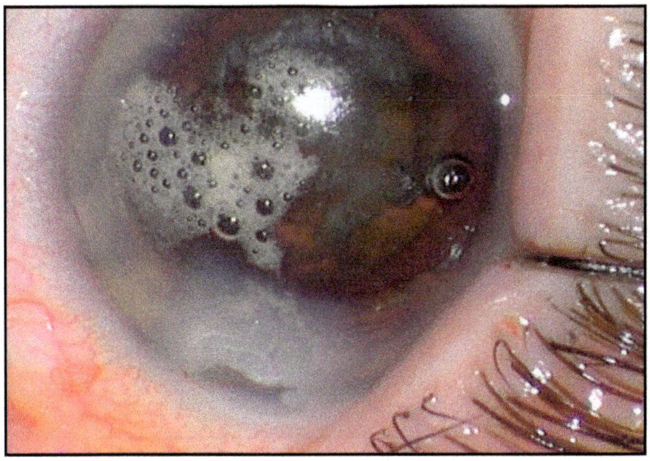

Figure B3. The edges of the incision are elevated.

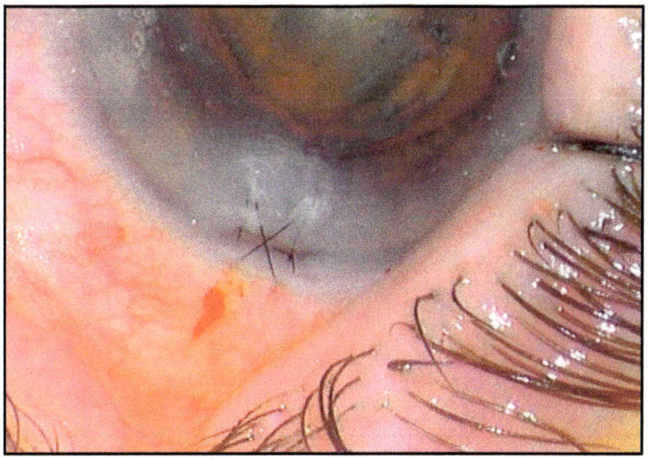

Figure B4. Suture of the wound burn.

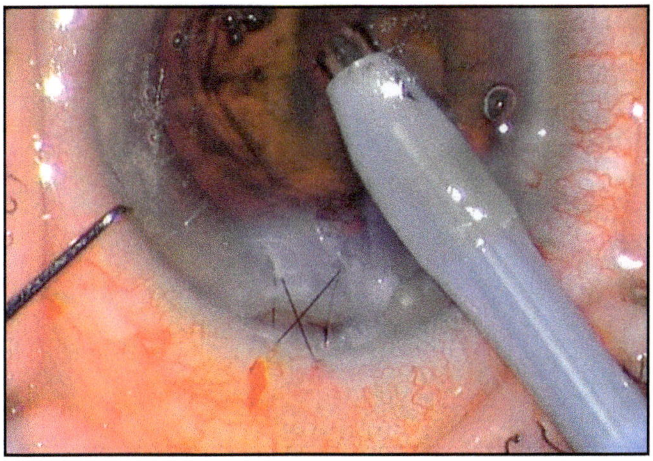

Figure B5. Make a new corneal incision and continue the operation.

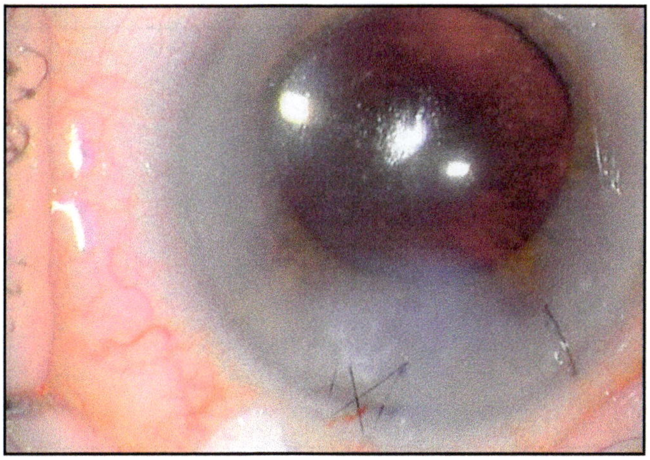

Figure B6. Operation completed.

Complications of Phacoemulsification

The surgeon must adapt his or her surgical technique to the type of cataract to be removed, taking into consideration the potential complications associated with each technique.[1] We will now take a look at the complications associated with the various phacoemulsification techniques (see Figures C1 to C6).

Technique Using Four Quadrant Divide and Conquer

This technique can be used by all surgeons, even the inexperienced, and it can be used with nuclei of almost all densities. However, it is not free from complications.[2,3]

Sculpting

If the nucleus is soft, peripheral lens material may be unexpectedly aspirated during sculpting. With a soft nucleus, aspiration settings should be kept low and the tip should not approach the equator. The problem comes from exposure of the posterior capsule to aspiration and direct ultrasound. The surgeon should create a deep, short groove to allow adequate cracking of the soft nucleus, or modify the technique to expression of the nuclei into the anterior chamber (AC) and perform supracapsular phaco.

If the nucleus is very hard, this method will require more ultrasound energy than other techniques with potential thermal damage to the incision and endothelium.[4,5] A hard nucleus can cause greater stress to the zonules compared to the "chop" techniques. The stress on the zonules comes from movement of the lens created by excessive force during sculpting of the 4 quadrants in a hard nucleus. The surgeon should increase ultrasound power, proceed with short ultrasound bursts, and create a long groove, approaching the equator of the lens in a dense nucleus. In these cases,

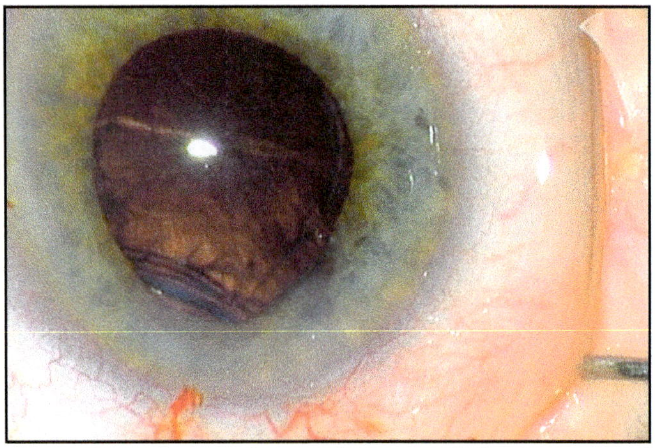

Figure C1. At the completion of phacoemulsification, a part of the capsular bag is clearly dislocated.

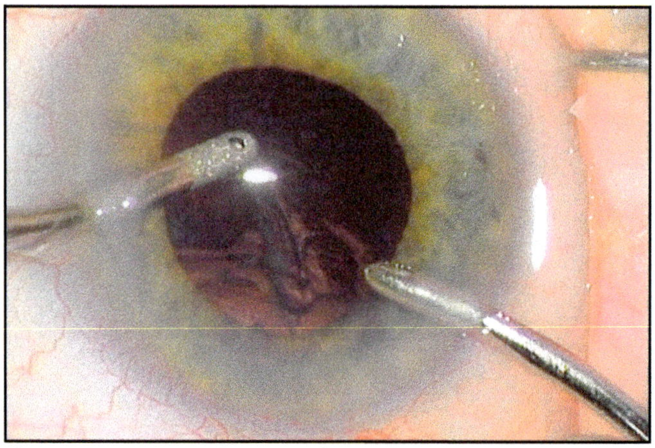

Figure C2. I/A procedure is performed with 2 hands and special care is used to not exert traction on the bag.

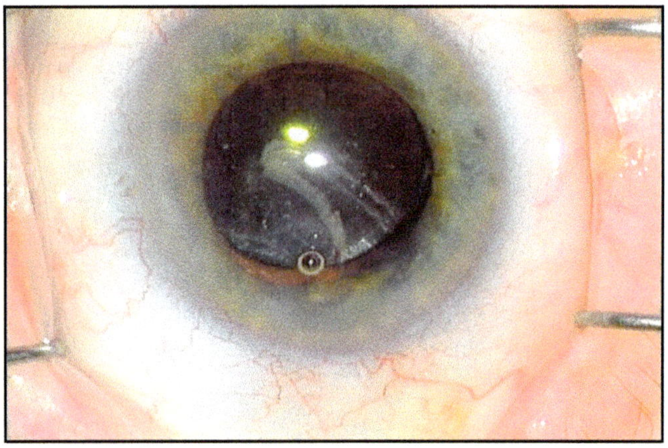

Figure C3. After the IOL implant, vitreous is seen in the AC.

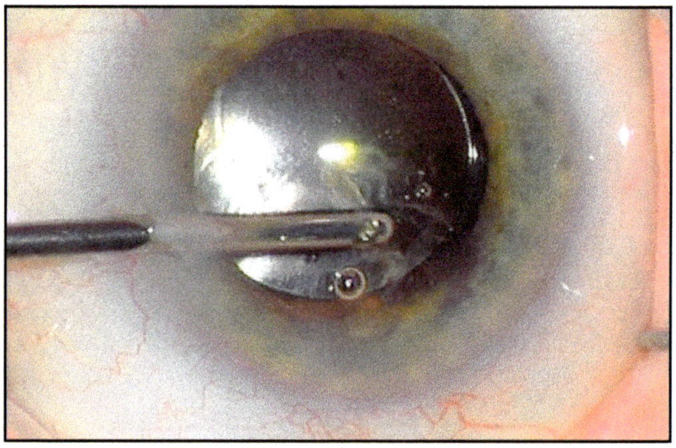

Figure C4. Anterior vitrectomy is performed.

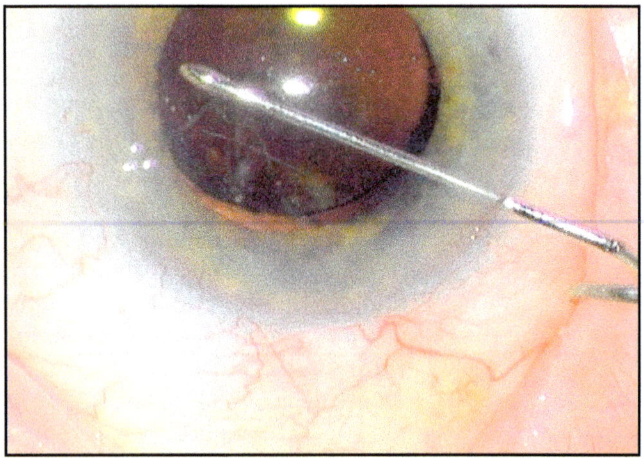

Figure C5. Using the spatula, vitreous strands are highlighted in the AC.

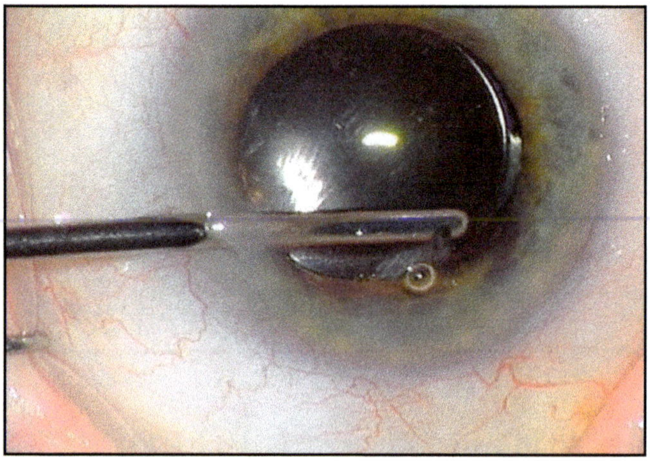

Figure C6. Additional anterior vitrectomy is then performed in order to remove all vitreous strands.

sculpting is facilitated by greater cavitation from angled tips (see Chapter 7). It is recommended to keep aspiration low to avoid additional stress on the zonules or accidental damage to the iris. However, minimal aspiration is necessary to prevent the tip from overheating as this may cause thermal burns. Prior to phacoemulsification of the quadrants, the surgeon should ensure that the quadrants are completely separated.

Very dense nuclei may contain residual posterior nuclear fibers that may prevent good cracking of the lens, increasing the complication potential associated with quadrant removal.

Quadrant Cracking

Potential complications are primarily associated with poor positioning of instruments within the groove or a too shallow groove. The instruments (spatula, nucleus manipulator, or forceps for nuclear cracking) are positioned just peripheral to the center of the nucleus to have good lens density to facilitate separation. If the instruments are positioned too peripherally, it is more difficult to completely separate the nucleus, and there is increased risk of iatrogenic damage to the posterior capsule. If the groove is not adequately deep, cracking maneuvers are less likely to be successful. In these cases, the surgeon should carefully deepen the groove in the posterior central part of the lens (see Figures D1 to D6).

Phaco Chop

The phaco chop technique, introduced by Nagahara in 1993, completely revolutionized the approach to cataract surgery, particularly when the cataract is very dense. This technique involves mechanical use of intraocular maneuvers as opposed to ultrasound, which may cause endothelial and capsule damage. The principle is based on separation of the quadrants using combined "phaco" and "chop" action. The lens is sculpted from the hydrodelineation line centrally, along the direction of its fibers. Along these lines, the resistance of the lens is lower and more easily split (Figure 5-1). If the maneuvers are performed correctly, this technique is extremely safe even in the initial phases of chopping.[6] The length of the tip of the various choppers is approximately 1.5 mm; the mean thickness of the lens is approximately 4.5 mm. The phaco chop technique has an enormous advantage of reducing the amount of energy necessary for phacoemulsification of dense nuclei, thus limiting endothelial damage.[7,8] Moreover, when performed correctly, it reduces stress on the zonules. With hard nuclei, there is considerable stress during sculpting.[4] The technique is also recommended in postvitrectomy eyes to minimize stress to the zonules without vitreous support.[9]

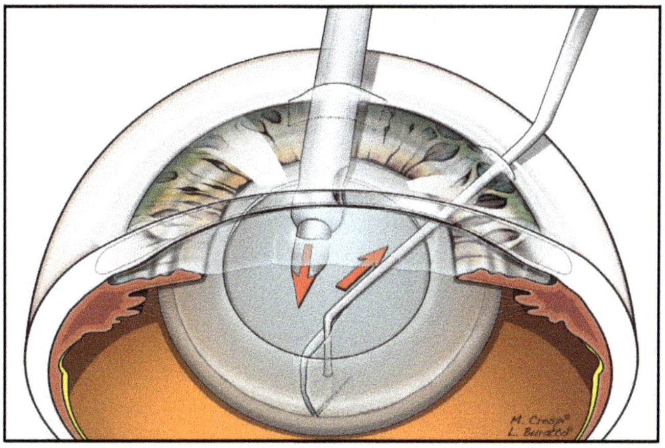

Figure 5-1. Combined phaco chopper action. This principle is based on opposite movements of the phaco tip and chopper to split the lens along the direction of its fibers. The lens has less resistance along these lines and splits more easily. This technique opts for mechanical action of intracapsular maneuvers as opposed to the use of ultrasound, which is associated with endothelial and capsule damage.

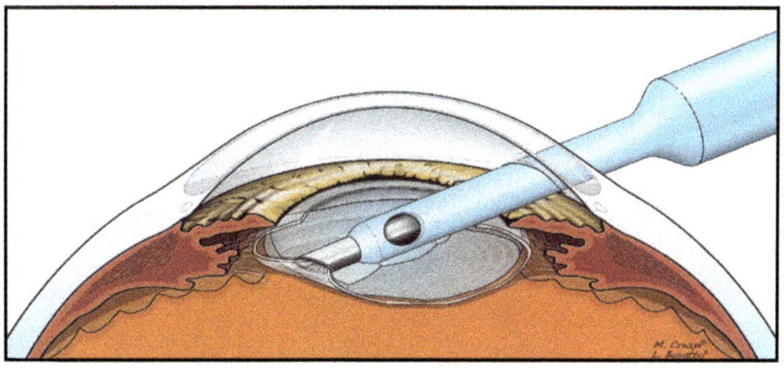

Figure 5-2. Aspiration of the posterior capsule. During chopping, the nucleus is engaged using constant aspiration. If the phaco tip is placed peripherally in a cataract that is not very dense, the surgeon runs the risk of aspirating epinucleus, touching the posterior capsule with consequent iatrogenic damage. In the chopping steps, the nucleus is held firmly using constant aspiration. This complication is more frequent with 0 degree or angled tips in the bevel-down position, as these lead to potential rapid aspiration of the epinucleus.

Sculpting

The phaco tip should proceed as far as the center of the nucleus, prior to initiating chopping. A more peripheral position of the tip will have a weaker grasp during the chopping as it will be unable to occlude the nucleus. During chopping, the surgeon must maintain a stable nucleus with constant aspiration; if the phaco tip is peripheral and next to the epinucleus, there is a risk of aspirating the nucleus and rapidly damaging the posterior capsule (Figure 5-2). Complete occlusion with 0 degree tips or angled tips in a bevel-down position increases the risk of rapid aspiration of the epinucleus. The same problem occurs if the technique is used with nuclei that are soft and do not provide resistance

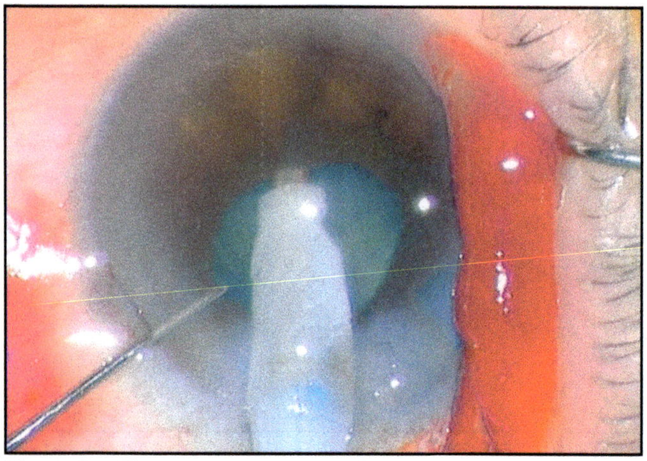

Figure D1. The operation starts with a poorly dilated pupil with hard cataracts; the tip of the U/S probe comes into contact with the iris.

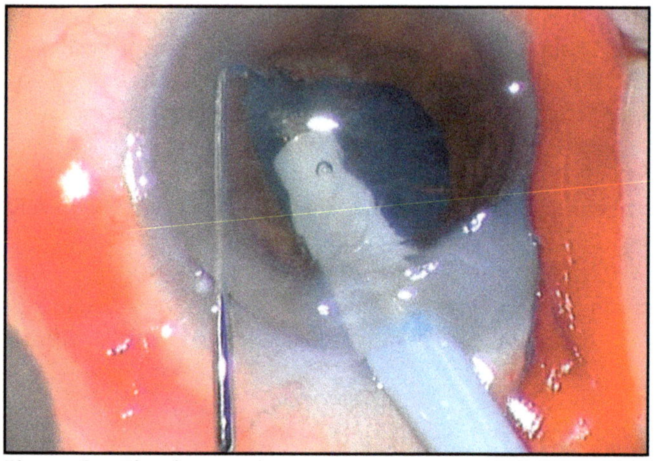

Figure D2. The damaged iris is retracted with a spatula. During fragmentation, the posterior capsule is broken.

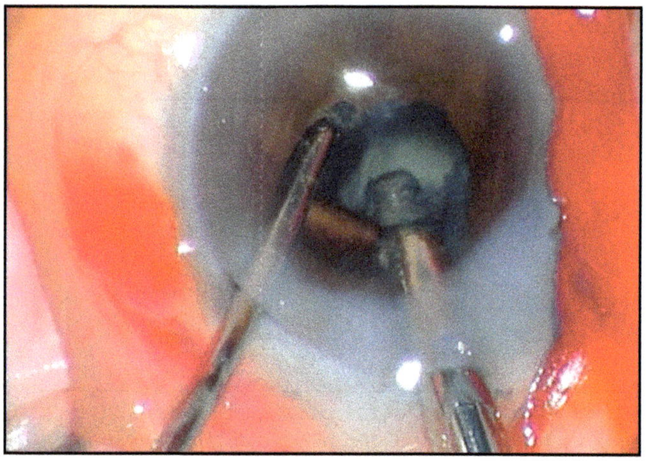

Figure D3. Bimanual anterior vitrectomy.

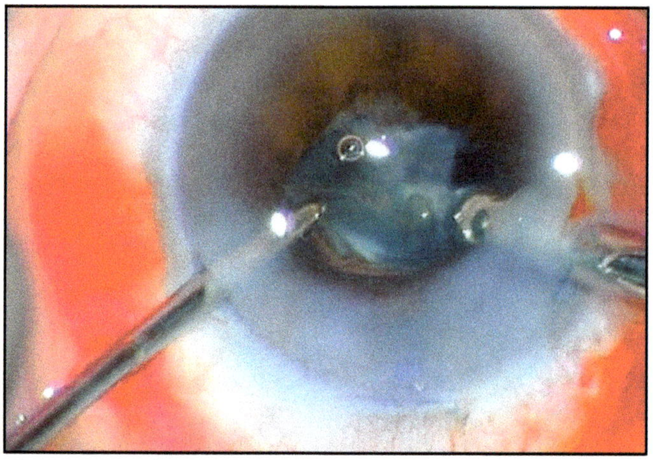

Figure D4. The operation continues with vitrectomy and removal of nuclear pieces.

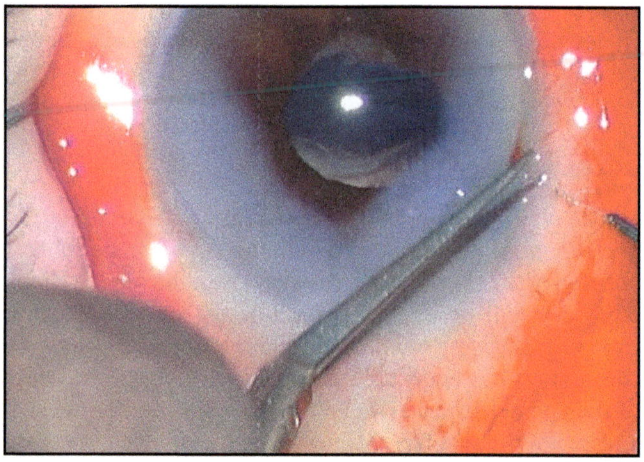

Figure D5. In the corneal incision, a vitreous strand is visible that is then cut.

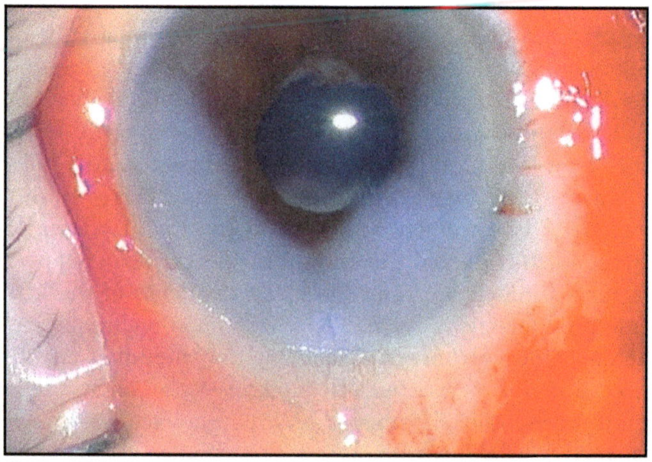

Figure D6. Extensive corneal edema induced by overhydration of the tunnel. In addition, an extensive hemorrhage caused by subconjunctival sub-Tenon's injection of anesthetic is visible.

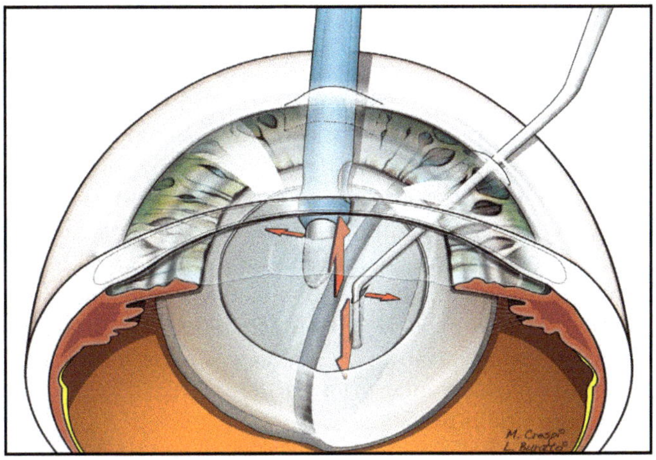

Figure 5-3. Vertical chopping or karate chop technique. The vertical or karate chop technique is recommended in eyes with small pupils and poor visibility of the lens. The lens is held firmly by the phaco tip and maneuvers are performed only in the central part of the nucleus with a slight vertical movement, pulling the nucleus upwards and simultaneously moving the chopper downwards. Both instruments must also move sideways to allow the division of the nucleus.

to aspiration (see Figure 5-2). Values of aspiration/vacuum of 150 to 350 mm Hg are used with a low flow rate (20 to 24 mL/min) and 70% ultrasound power.

Another potential complication is zonular dialysis from horizontal or vertical movements of the phaco tip once it has occluded the nucleus. If hydrodissection is incomplete, even successive rotation of the nucleus can induce varying amounts of zonular dialysis. Movement of the phaco tip must be minimal and separation of the quadrants must be performed with the chopper. Zonular dialysis can also occur with accidental contact between the chopper and the margin of the capsulorrhexis; this complication occurs more frequently when the capsulorrhexis has a diameter less than 5 mm. In these cases, the surgeon should prolapse the lens into the AC and proceed with phacoemulsification under protection of dispersive OVD, both above and below the nucleus.

If the pupil or the capsulorrhexis is small, the vertical chopping technique or karate chop may be useful. Once the lens has been engaged with the phaco tip, the surgeon chops only centrally in the nucleus with a slight vertical movement, bringing the nucleus upwards and simultaneously moving the chopper downwards (Figure 5-3). The phaco tip and chopper both penetrate at least as far as the center of the nucleus; here, the surgeon separates the quadrants of the nucleus with a horizontal movement. The maneuver is repeated by continually rotating the nucleus 180 degrees and subsequently repeated in the 2 heminuclei. The advantage of this technique is staying central in the nucleus and avoiding the periphery, which is difficult to see. The karate chop technique is also recommended in eyes with dense nuclei with a small amount of epinucleus.

Steps of Freeing and Phacoemulsification of Lens Fragments

The technique of phaco chop as described makes phacoemulsification of the fragments more difficult. When the fragments are separated they cannot be mobilized inside the capsular bag. The space required for mobilization comes from sculpting of the nucleus, which does not occur with this technique. Here, the surgeon should use a bimanual (spatula chopper) technique to ensure that all of the quadrants are completely separated. The surgeon should proceed by lifting the internal central apex of the nucleus to facilitate removal of the section from the bag.

Once the first quadrant or section is removed, the remaining fragments can be removed much more easily. With a large nucleus and a capsulorrhexis less than 5 mm, the anterior capsule margin may tear with potential extension into the zonules.

Stop and Chop Technique

The stop and chop technique involves a first step of sculpting then separation of the 2 hemiquadrants, then a second chopping step of the nucleus into smaller fragments.

Sculpting

The width of the groove must be larger as related to the hardness of the nucleus (approximately 3.5 mm). The objective is to create space for successive chopping maneuvers and mobilization of the fragments. The length of the groove must be longer with hard nuclei, and extend close to the periphery; the nucleus must be rotated 180 degrees to allow exposure of the opposite part of the groove.

The surgeon must always consider that, during sculpting, progressive peripheral movement of the phaco tip risks engaging an epinucleus that is less dense. Therefore, there is greater risk of sudden aspiration of softer lens material and hitting the posterior capsule (Figure 5-4).

The central depth of the groove is the essential determinant for good cracking ability. Things that can help the surgeon identify the correct plane include the color of the material in the deepest part of the groove (gray-orange) and the depth. Both are described in text books, but surgeon experience is necessary to evaluate each individual cataract on the basis of its size and density. Incorrect creation of the width and depth of the groove will lead to incomplete separation of the hemiquadrants, compromising the following steps.

The phaco tip should always be kept in a bevel-up position during sculpting as this ensures good control of the groove depth and avoids occlusion of the tip during sculpting. Occlusion of the tip during sculpting may lead to rapid aspiration of the lens material, even the posterior capsule (Figure 5-5).

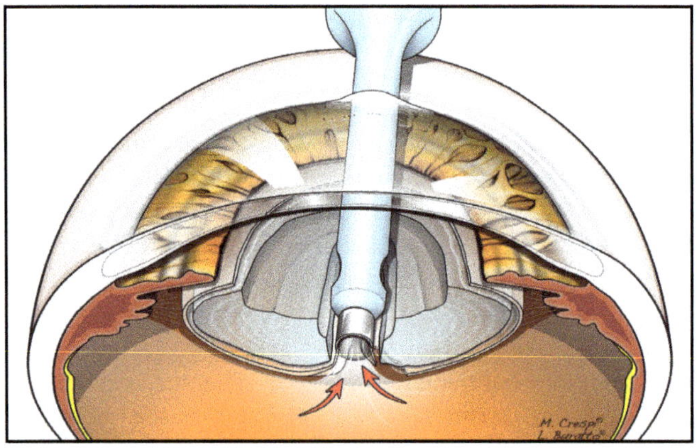

Figure 5-4. Contact between the phaco tip and posterior capsule. The phaco tip should always be in the bevel-up position during sculpting as this allows better control of the depth of the groove. Occlusion of the phaco tip in the bevel-down position will lead to more rapid aspiration of the lens material with potential contact with the posterior capsule.

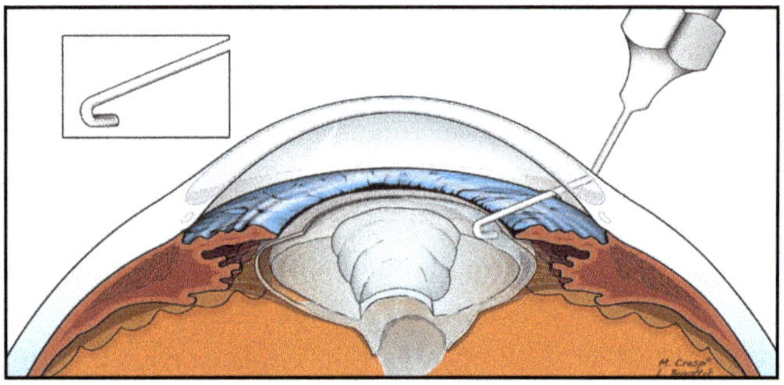

Figure 5-5. Deep sculpting. During sculpting, the phaco tip must be in the bevel-up position as this allows better control of groove depth, avoiding complete occlusion of the tip. Occlusion of the tip allows rapid aspiration of the lens material and potentially the posterior capsule by the phaco tip.

Chopping

Complications may occur from incorrect positioning of the phaco tip inside the heminucleus. The tip must be placed into the central part of the nucleus, using ultrasound to achieve good occlusion and maintain stable aspiration. If the tip is too superficial and asymmetric from the center of the heminucleus, it is more difficult for the surgeon to complete chopping the lens fragments, which tend to rotate, using the phaco tip as the fulcrum.

Another complication is a tear in the anterior capsule due to contact with the chopper. If the volume of the nucleus is small, the tear will be localized and not extend peripherally, allowing the surgeon to continue phacoemulsification using the stop and chop technique. If the tear of the capsule extends toward the equator, the surgeon should use the chopping technique to divide the lens into smaller fragments, or prolapse the nucleus into the AC to avoid additional stress on the capsule and zonules (see Figures E1 to E6).

Chop and Flip Technique

The chop and flip technique involves direct separation of the quadrants through a combined action using the chopper and phaco tip. The steps include only the nucleus leaving the epinucleus behind to protect the posterior capsule. The epinucleus will be later removed. The phaco tip is placed in a bevel-down position for the first crack of the cataract into 2 sections. It is then rotated into a bevel-up position to further split the heminucleus. Good hydrodelineation of the nucleus from the epinucleus is essential in this technique. The advantage is a greater degree of safety and less ultrasound is needed.[10]

Chopping

With chopping, the chopper is positioned at the "golden ring"; it is then moved centrally as though trying to touch the phaco tip. A vertical vector force is applied to engage and elevate the nucleus, allowing the chopper to reach the posterior fibers of dense nuclei. If the phaco tip has not occluded the nucleus, this step will not be successful. The complication here may result from excessive stress to the zonules. Thus, the surgeon should engage and elevate the lens and present it for chopping.

Removal of the Epinucleus

An epinucleus that is not freely mobile may lead to complications. The surgeon will need to perform repeated manipulations on this softer lens material while protecting the capsule. The surgeon should separate the epinucleus from the cortex using a dispersive viscoelastic. A dense epinucleus is easily removed with irrigation/aspiration (I/A); the surgeon may instead opt to use the phaco tip in an I/A mode to achieve greater linear aspiration with better control, using no ultrasound.

Flip and Tilt Technique

The flip and tilt technique involves mobilization, then prolapse of the entire nucleus out of the capsular bag. The surgeon must achieve complete cortical cleaving hydrodissection.[11] Prior to manipulation of the nucleus, the surgeon must ensure that the lens rotates freely inside the bag (Figure 5-6).

A larger capsulorrhexis of at least 5.5 mm should be made in order to allow prolapse of the nucleus into the AC.

Mobilization of the lens requires peripheral positioning of the spatula that is then rotated and pushed downward. This force changes the position of the lens, positioning it at an angle of 45 degrees to the iris plane. At this point, using an angled tip, the lens is engaged and emulsified from the periphery inward. These steps are performed at the level of the anterior capsule.

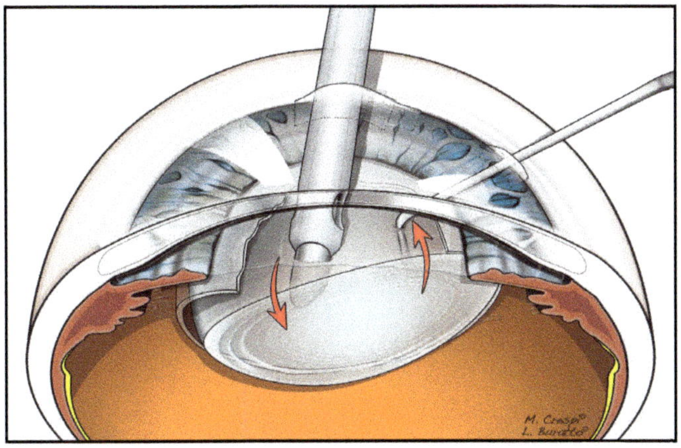

Figure 5-6. Bimanual mobilization of the nucleus. Prior to initiating the phaco flip technique, the surgeon should begin with bimanual mobilization of the nucleus. Hydrodissection is required with complete separation of the epinucleus from the cortex. The surgeon attempts to rotate the nucleus by pushing peripherally on the nucleus.

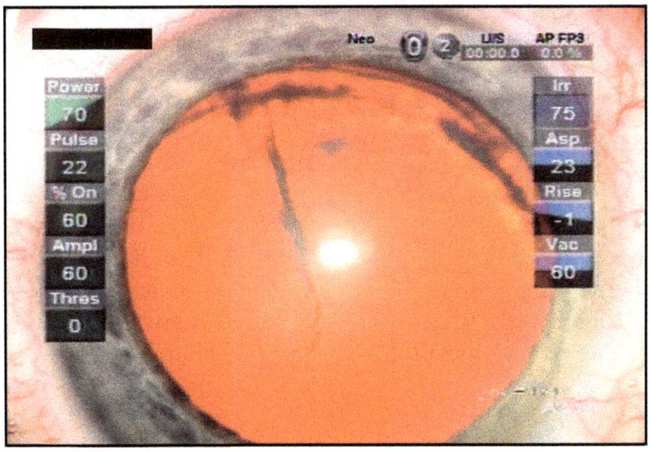

Figure E1. Dislocation of the lens before beginning surgery.

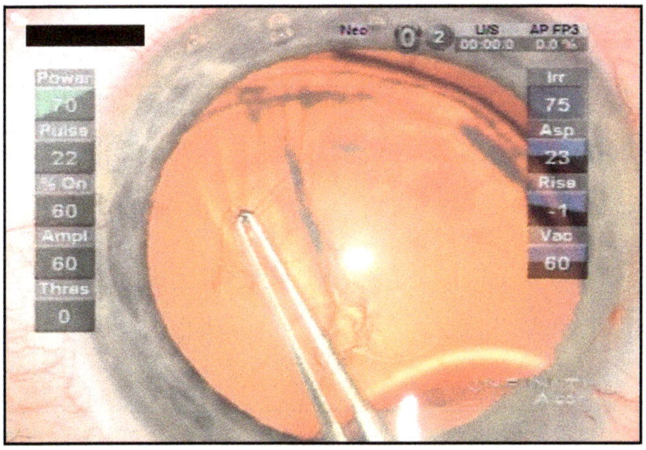

Figure E2. Capsulorrhexis is performed and then followed by hydrodissection without any particular difficulty.

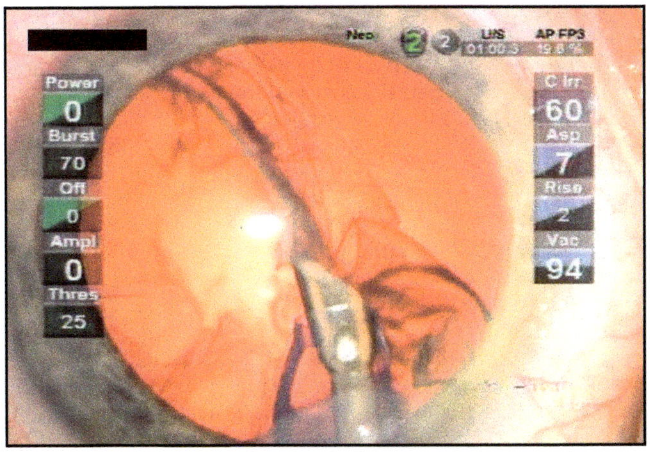

Figure E3. At the completion of phacoemulsification, the capsular bag is aspirated with U/S.

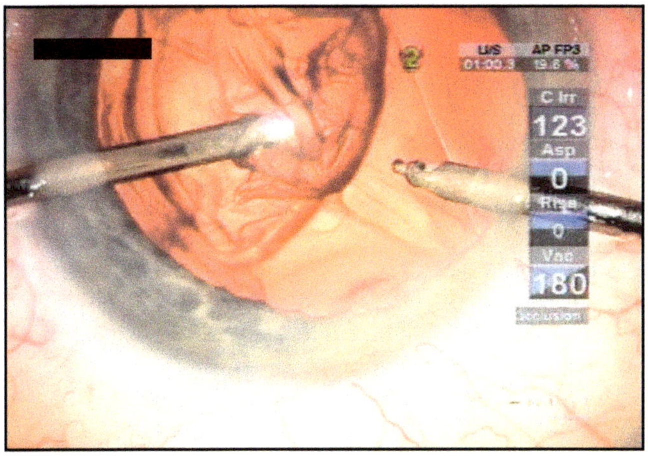

Figure E4. I/A completes the dislocation of the capsular bag, which is then removed.

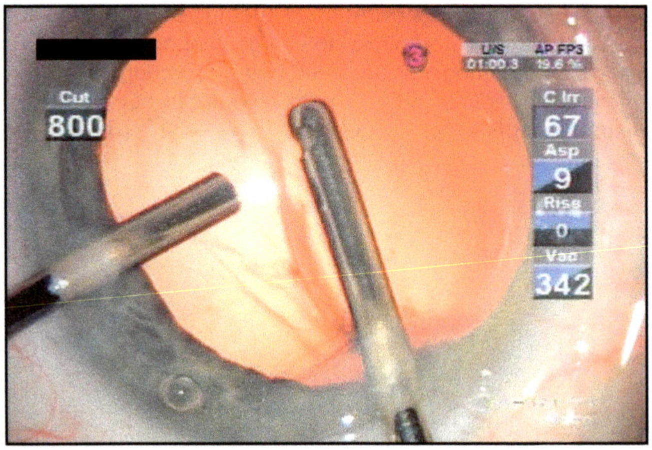

Figure E5. Anterior vitrectomy is then performed.

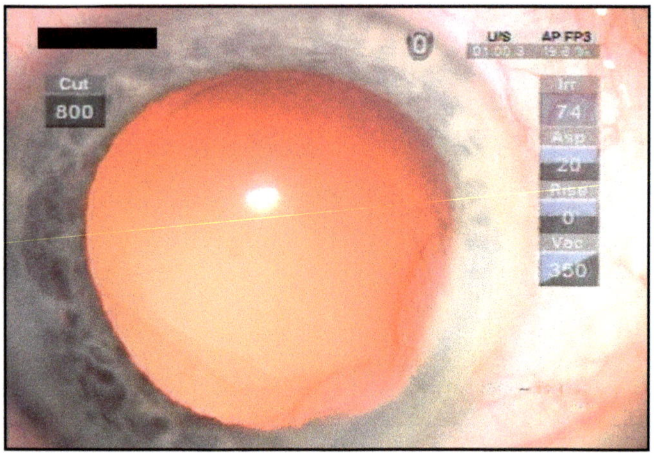

Figure E6. The operation ends without IOL implantation, which will be done several weeks later.

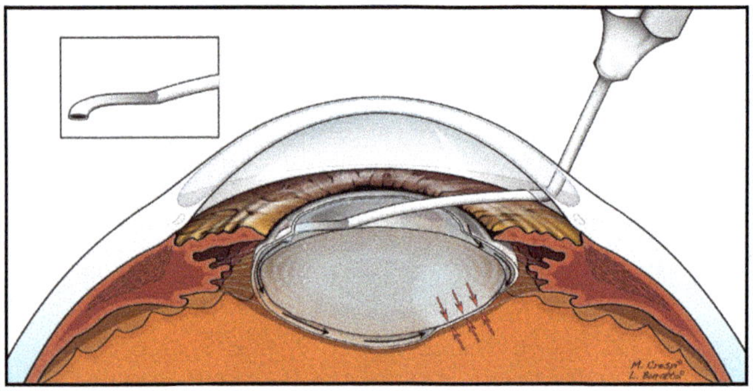

Figure 5-7. Posterior adhesions. Posterior adhesions between the lens and the posterior capsule resulting from inadequate hydrodissection will force the surgeon to use unnecessary rotation maneuvers with potential damage to the zonules and the capsule due to mechanical stress.

Flipping Step

Flipping maneuvers are performed using a blunt spatula, though this may occasionally tear the posterior capsule. It may also damage the endothelium because of contact between the lens and corneal endothelium; it may damage the zonules through mechanical stress by improper maneuvers used to mobilize the nucleus, in the presence of posterior adhesions that require detachment with greater force (Figure 5-7). With loose zonules, the surgeon should perform the flipping motion in the stronger area of the zonules to avoid stressing the weaker zonules.

Phacoemulsification

With this technique the nucleus is emulsified from the periphery toward the center. The surgeon should maintain aspiration until he or she is certain that the nucleus has been engaged and emulsification can begin. The surgeon should avoid this technique in eyes with shallow chambers or an axial length of less than 20 mm because of potential damage from ultrasound to the endothelium in such small spaces.

References

1. Li W, Zhao Y, Zheng Q, et al. Phacoemulsification complication. *Ophthalmology.* 2010;117(6):1275 e1271-1273.
2. Woodfield AS, Gower EW, Cassard SD, Ramanthan S. Intraoperative phacoemulsification complication rates of second- and third-year ophthalmology residents a 5-year comparison. *Ophthalmology.* 2011;118(5):954-958.
3. Elnaby EA, El Zawahry OM, Abdelrahman AM, Ibrahim HE. Phaco prechop versus divide and conquer phacoemulsification: a prospective comparative interventional study, Middle East. *Afr J Ophthalmol.* 2008;15(3):123-127.
4. Tsorbatzoglou A, Modis L, Kertesz K, Nemeth G, Berta A. Comparison of divide and conquer and phaco-chop techniques during fluid-based phaco-emulsification. *Eur J Ophthalmol.* 2007;17(3):315-319.
5. Wong T, Hingorani M, Lee V. Phacoemulsification time and power requirements in phaco chop and divide and conquer nucleofractis techniques. *J Cataract Refract Surg.* 2000;26(9): 1374-1378.
6. Ram J, Wesendahl TA, Auffarth GU, Apple DJ. Evaluation of in situ fracture versus phaco chop techniques. *J Cataract Refract Surg.* 1998;24(11):1464-1468.
7. DeBry P, Olson RJ, Crandall AS. Comparison of energy required for phaco-chop and divide and conquer phacoemulsification. *J Cataract Refract Surg.* 1998;24(5):689-692.
8. Park JH, Lee SM, Kwon JW, et al. Ultrasound energy in phacoemulsification: a comparative analysis of phaco-chop and stop-and-chop techniques according to the degree of nuclear density. *Ophthalmic Surg Lasers Imaging.* 2010;41(2):236-241.

9. Sachdev N, Brar GS, Sukhija J, Gupta V, Ram J. Phacoemulsification in vitrectomized eyes: results using a 'phaco chop' technique. *Acta Ophthalmol.* 2009;87(4):382-385.
10. Fine IH, Packer M, Hoffman RS. Use of power modulations in phacoemulsification. Choo-choo chop and flip phacoemulsification. *J Cataract Refract Surg.* 2001;27(2):188-197.
11. Tam DY, Ahmed II. The phaco hemi-flip: a method of lens removal in nuclei of soft to moderate density. *Ophthalmic Surg Lasers Imaging.* 2011;42(2):170-174.

6

Complications With Intraocular Lens Implantation

Lucio Buratto, MD; Stephen F. Brint, MD, FACS; and Mario R. Romano, MD, PhD

Intraocular lens (IOL) implantation has the primary objective of restoring new optics to the eye. Currently, IOLs are injected through increasingly smaller corneal incisions with minimal induced astigmatism. They attempt to eliminate lower order aberrations, reduce or prevent the increase in spherical aberration, and reduce posterior capsule opacity (PCO). It should be remembered that the complications from an IOL may cause damage to the zonules and capsule that can destabilize the implant. We will now examine potential damage to intraocular structures during IOL implantation (see Figures A1 to A2 and B1 to B6).

Damage to Intraocular Lens

Intraoperative Complications

Forceps Damage

IOLs are folded and delicately inserted using forceps or a cartridge and injected through ever smaller corneal incisions.

Folding the IOL with forceps depresses the anterior surface of the IOL in contact with the forceps. This crease may still be visible 72 hours after implantation and will be more obvious if the IOL has been stored at 36°C prior to implantation. This can be prevented by placing ophthalmic viscoelastic device (OVD) onto the IOL before it is folded.[1] Rarely, forceps can deform and crack the haptics or the optic of the IOL.

Cartridge Damage

Currently, the majority of presbyopia correcting intraocular implants (PC IOLs) are injected using cartridges corresponding to the incision size. The most significant damage to an IOL occurs when it is loaded into and then injected from the cartridge. The haptic is damaged with greatest frequency. Each manufacturer recommends precise positioning of the IOL in the cartridge prior to pushing the IOL into the tip to avoid friction at the junction between the haptic and the optic. Prior to injecting the lens into the eye, the surgeon should ensure that the IOL has been folded correctly inside the cartridge and that the plunger has engaged the optic. The haptic of the IOL is often damaged during injection, but the surgeon only recognizes this when the lens is inside the anterior chamber (AC). The IOL must be removed, the primary incision must be enlarged to 3.5 mm, and the optic is cut into halves or thirds to facilitate the rotary extraction. A new lens is then implanted (Figure 6-1). Additional friction occurs with excessive resistance of the lens inside the cartridge due to inadequate OVD in the cartridge. The lens should be injected slowly with continuous pressure; the surgeon should monitor the progression of the IOL as it moves along the cartridge and passes into the AC (see Figures C1 and C2).

Buratto L, Brint SF, Romano MR.
Cataract Surgery Complications (pp 47-56).
© 2013 Taylor & Francis Group.

Figure 6-1. IOL removal. The haptic of the IOL may be damaged and the surgeon is aware only once the IOL has been injected into the AC. In these cases, it is necessary to enlarge the main incision to 3.50 mm, cutting the optic at least two-thirds of its diameter. A rotary extraction is then performed by grasping half of the optic, and the remainder rotates and follows.

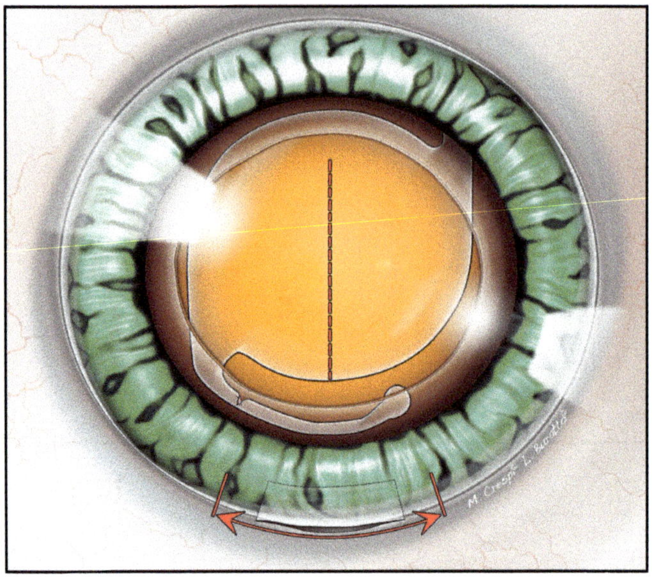

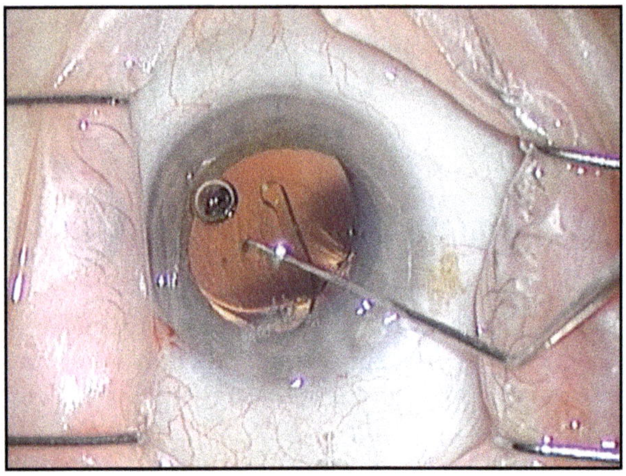

Figure A1. After insertion of the IOL in the bag, the loop can still adhere to the optic plate.

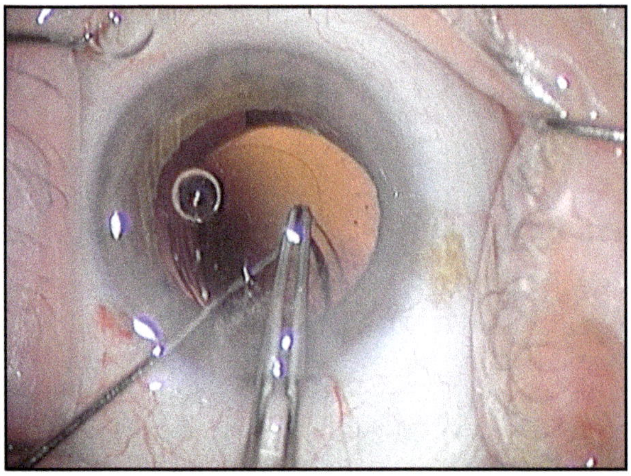

Figure A2. Using a McPherson forceps and spatula to stabilize the optic plate, you can easily pull the loop.

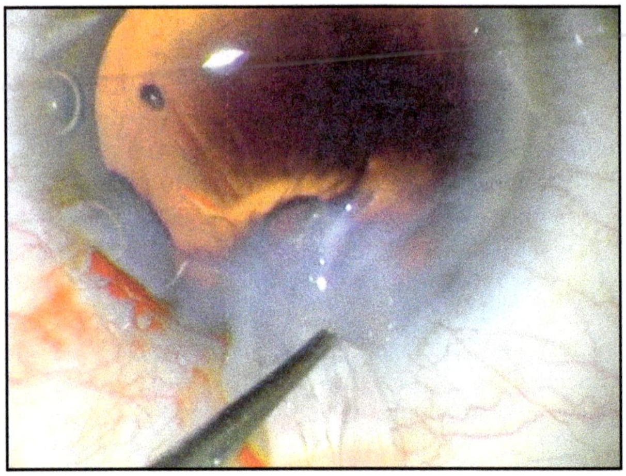

Figure B1. The incision is narrow, but the surgeon tries to inject the IOL.

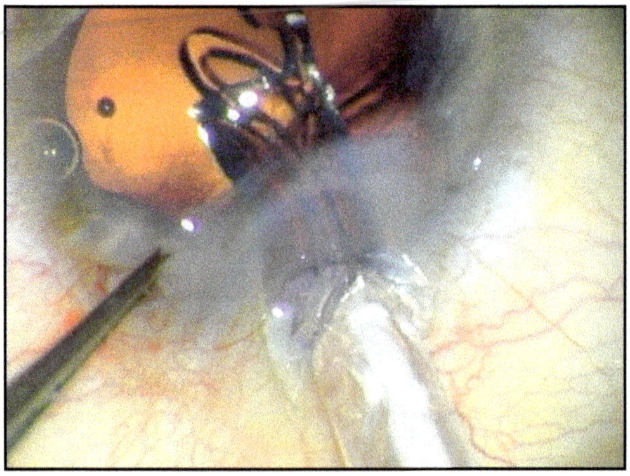

Figure B2. The IOL, however, remains trapped within the tunnel, neither inside nor outside.

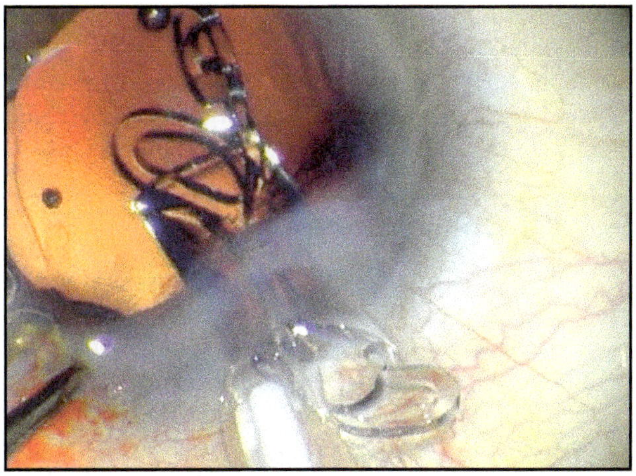

Figure B3. The surgeon tries to extend the incision.

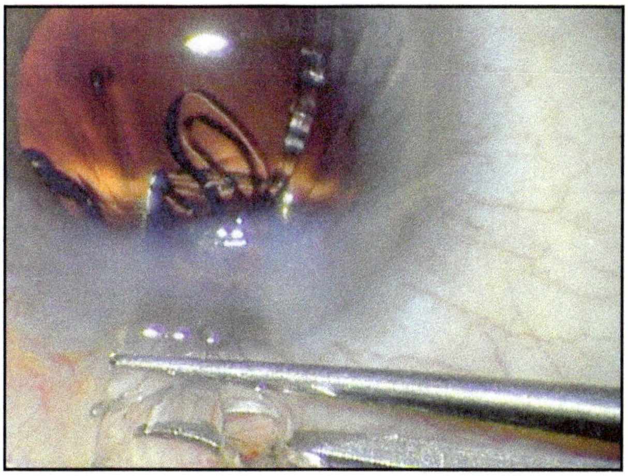

Figure B4. Using a forceps, exerting a counterforce with a spatula, the IOL can be removed from the corneal incision.

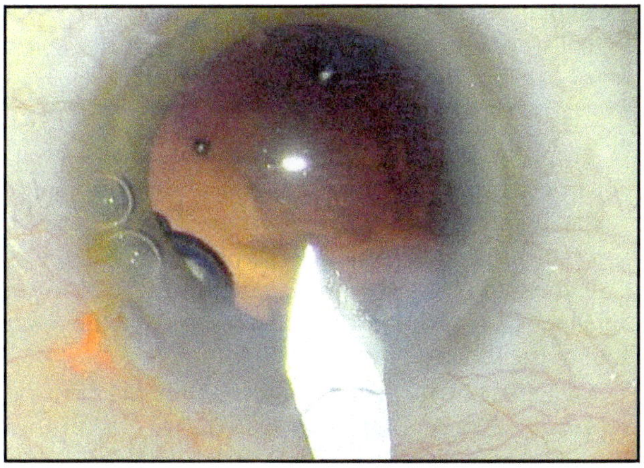

Figure B5. The incision is extended a little longer.

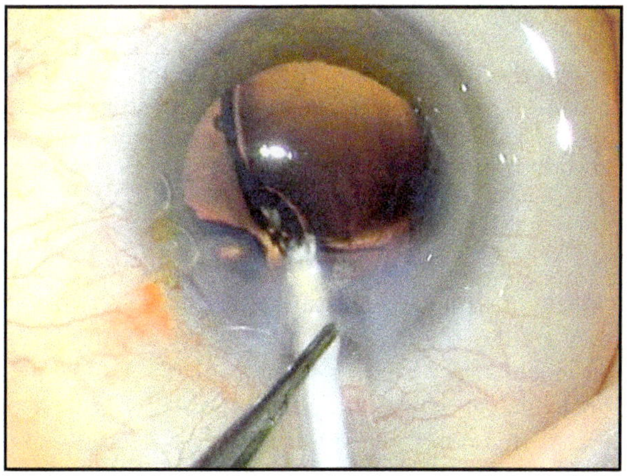

Figure B6. A new IOL is injected.

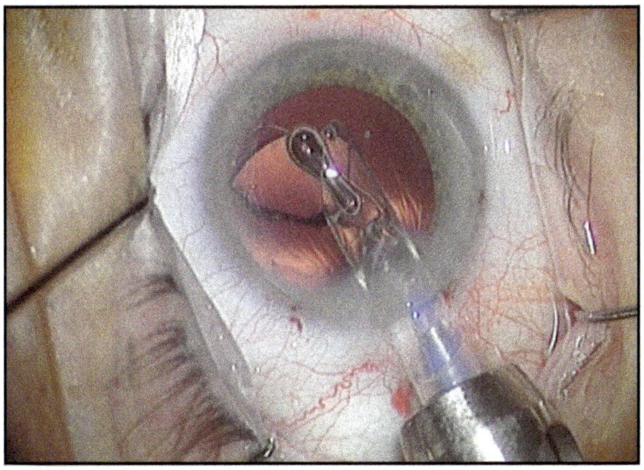

Figure C1. The IOL is broken during insertion and a piece of IOL is in the AC.

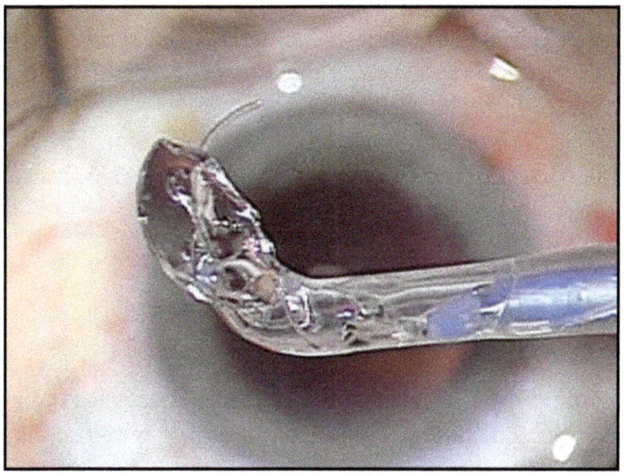

Figure C2. The other piece is still in the injector.

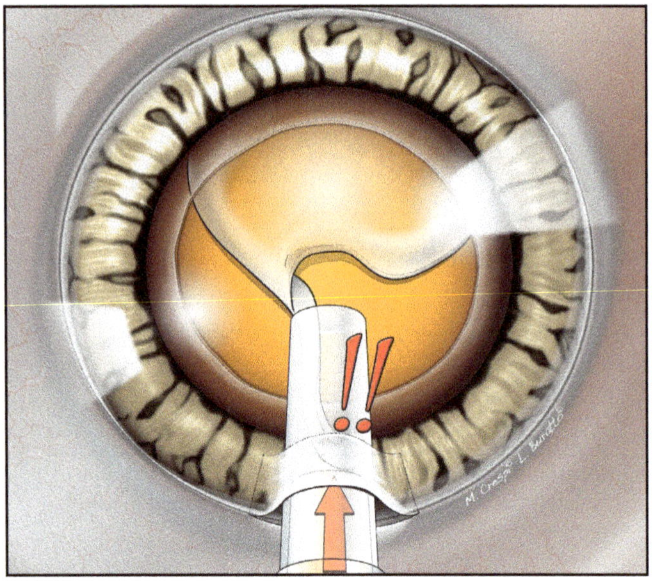

Figure 6-2. Lodging of the proximal haptic in the cartridge. The proximal haptic of the IOL may be lodged inside the cartridge. The surgeon should leave the cartridge in position, withdrawing the plunger with a reverse rotation. A second instrument through the side port incision may sometimes be required to free the haptic from the cartridge.

Another critical moment is the injection of the trailing haptic of the IOL; it can remain stuck inside the cartridge (Figure 6-2) after the optic has entered the AC. Here, the surgeon must be very careful, maintaining the cartridge in position while retracting the plunger slowly with reverse rotation. At this point, the surgeon tries to inject the IOL again, engaging the haptic. Occasionally, a second instrument may be helpful, introduced through a side port; this may facilitate the release of the trapped haptic from the cartridge.

Finally, damage to the IOL can occur from the IOL having been loaded into the cartridge too early. A silicone IOL will stick to the walls of the cartridge, creating strong resistance to movement of the lens inside the injector. The IOL should be loaded in the cartridge during cortical aspiration and not at the beginning of surgery.

Postoperative Complications

Opacification of the Intraocular Lens

Polymethylmethacrylate (PMMA) has always been considered the gold standard of biocompatibility material, having been used since the very first implantation of IOLs. In the early 1990s, deposits were seen on the surface of the IOL and were confirmed with the electron microscope. These appeared 8 to 15 years after the lens implantation. Initially, they did not affect visual acuity. In advanced stages, these deposits created a "snowflake" formation with a reduction in contrast sensitivity.[2,3] The damage appears to have been caused by ultraviolet exposure that led to the release of nitrogen (N_2) from the polymer with successive cavitation inside the IOL.[3] Currently, PMMA is considered stable and biocompatible. However, it has largely been abandoned because of the use of foldable IOLs (see Figures D1 to D4).

IOL Opacification

Foldable hydrophilic acrylic lenses are produced from acrylic copolymers with a water content varying from 18% to 28%. These lenses are biocompatible, foldable, and injectable through incisions smaller than 2.0 mm. The long-term complication associated with these lenses is precipitation of calcium granules along parallel lines on the lens surface.[4] This was frequently seen with the Memory Lens (Ciba Vision, Duluth, Georgia) implanted between 1999 and 2000. One possible explanation is that under certain conditions, these IOLs absorb proteins with subsequent deposition of calcium on the surface of the protein.[4]

Progressive opacification has also been observed with silicone lenses, sometimes immediately after implantation, probably due to impurities of gas or detergents used during the sterilization and storage procedures of the IOLs.[5] Calcium and phosphate precipitates have also been seen on silicone IOLs, seeming to be responsible for the opacification of the IOLs.

Opacification of the implant requires the removal and replacement of the IOL. Surgical "dusting" with the YAG laser has proved to be ineffective.[7]

Silicone oil, used as an intraocular tamponade in patients undergoing vitreo-retinal surgery, may adhere to the IOL, modifying the optics of the lens. It was recently shown that in some cases a semifluorinate alkane (F4H5) is good when used to remove residue of silicone oil from the surface of the IOL.[8]

Damage to the Zonules and the Bag

Intraoperative Complications

The most common mistake is that both haptics are not placed inside the capsular bag. At the end of IOL insertion and removal of the OVD, the surgeon may notice a certain amount of tilt and decentration of the IOL. This is not always obvious; thus, the surgeon should rotate the IOL in the bag at the end of the implantation to ensure correct positioning. If the haptics are not positioned correctly, the lens will not rotate. Inadequate filling of the bag or

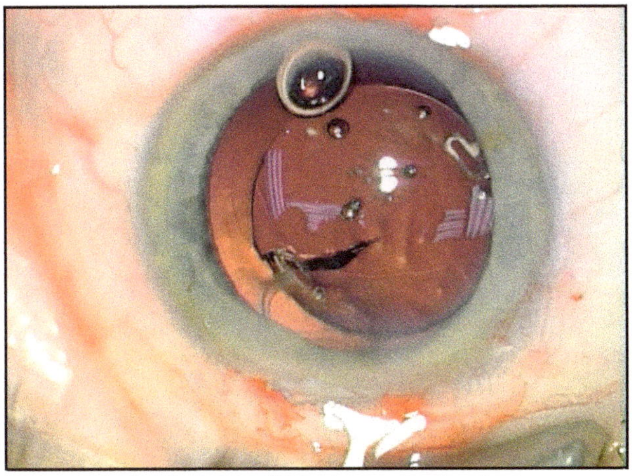

Figure D1. Break down of IOL during the implant.

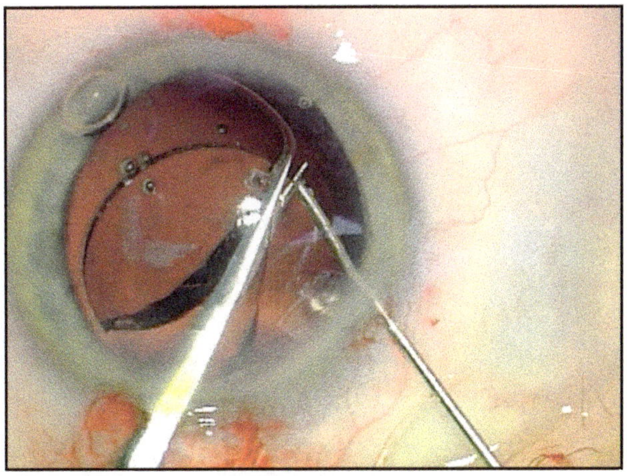

Figure D2. The IOL should be cut into 2 pieces.

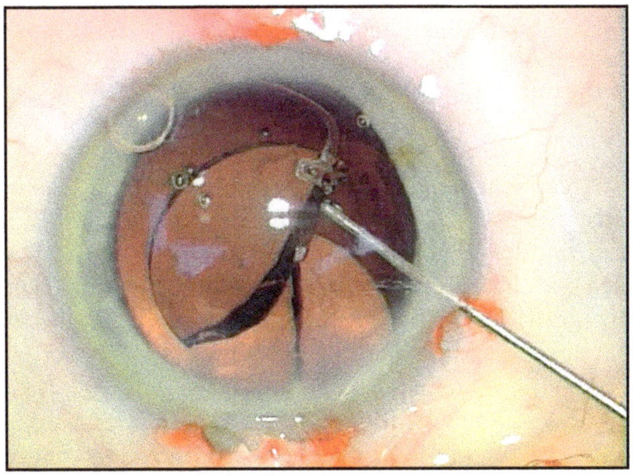

Figure D3. Remove the first piece.

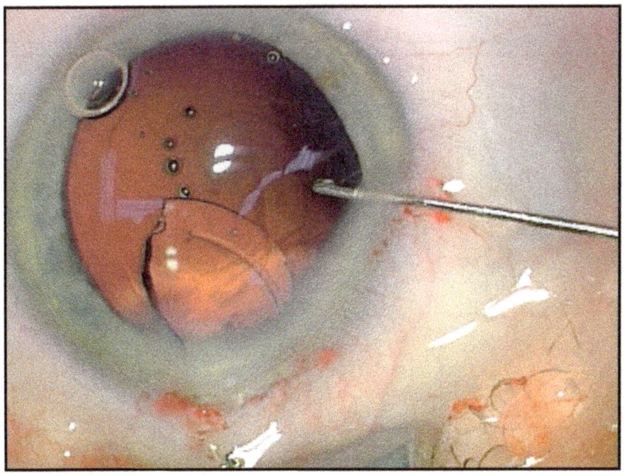

Figure D4. Remove the second piece.

aggressive manipulation to rotate and position the haptics of the IOL in the bag will stress the zonules and the capsular bag with potential loss of support of the IOL.

If there is zonular dialysis present at implantation, the lenses may dislocate from the posterior chamber to the vitreous chamber or anteriorly into the sulcus, creating vitreous or angle damage.

In these cases, a capsular tension ring (CTR) should be inserted prior to IOL implantation.[9]

Postoperative Complications

Dislocation, decentration, and tilt of the IOL are complications that may appear postoperatively (sunrise syndrome: upward dislocation of the IOL [Figure 6-3A]; sunset syndrome: downward dislocation of the IOL [Figure 6-3B]), normally due to capsulorrhexis asymmetry, lack of centration of the lens during insertion, contraction of a capsulorrhexis smaller than 4 mm diameter, iatrogenic stress to the zonules, or structural damage to the haptics (see Figure 6-3).

Decentration

Usually even with correct implantation of the IOL, tilt of 2 to 3 degrees and 0.2 to 0.3 mm occur. This is not clinically significant and does not create problems. In approximately 10% of pseudophakic patients, tilt of 10 degrees and decentration of 1 mm is seen. Higher-order astigmatic and chromatic aberrations may occur, and that can cause deterioration of visual quality.[10-12] These errors are increased with spherical, toric, and multifocal lenses.

If the zonules are damaged, the surgeon should insert a CTR prior to IOL insertion. This will reduce decentration and tilt of the IOL.[13]

The results of a recent comparative study of 111 eyes using the femtosecond laser in cataract surgery created significant reduction in decentration induced by asymmetry and irregularity of the anterior capsulorrhexis, independent of the eye type, keratometry values, diameter of the

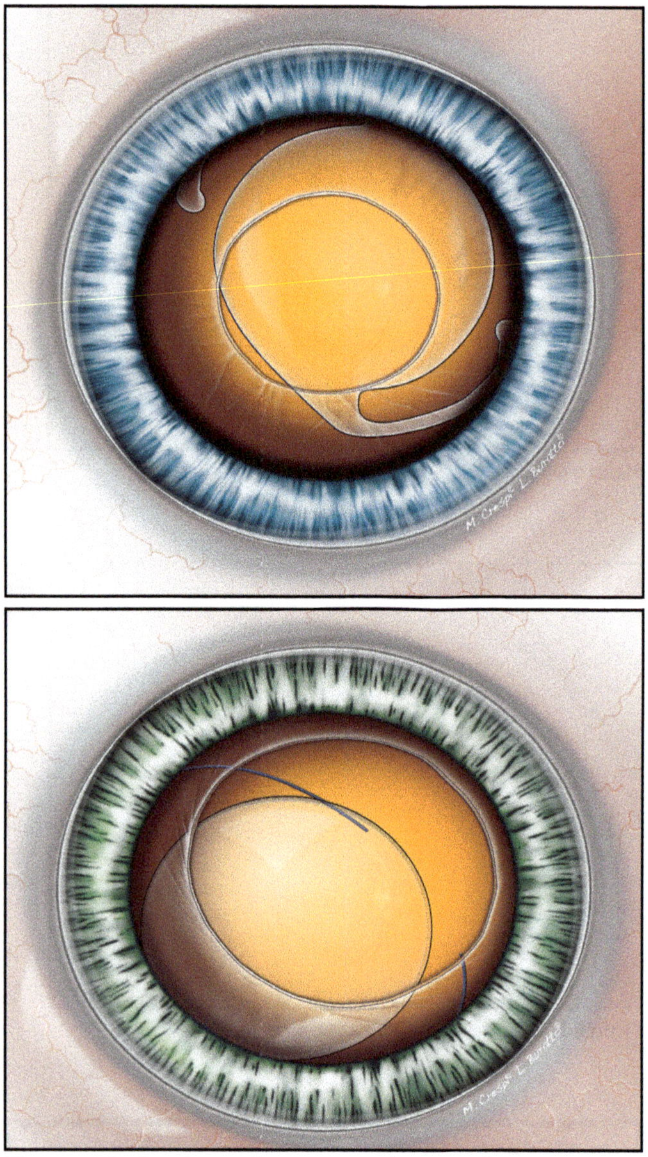

Figure 6-3. Sunrise and sunset syndromes. The sunrise syndrome, or upward dislocation of the IOL (A), and sunset syndrome, or downward displacement of the IOL (B) may be caused by asymmetry of the capsulorrhexis, poor centration during IOL implantation, contraction of a too small anterior capsulorrhexis, iatrogenic stress on the zonules, or damage to the haptics. In approximately 10% of pseudophakic patients, tilt of 10 degrees and decentration of 1 mm is seen. High order astigmatic and chromatic aberrations occur with this amount of tilt or decentration, causing a marked deterioration in visual quality.

anterior capsulorrhexis, and variables that determine the symmetry of manual capsulorrhexis.[14]

Early and late dislocation of the IOL into the vitreous is one of the most serious complications; this can cause rhegmatogenous retinal damage and pupillary block syndrome.[15] This may be caused by ocular trauma, anterior capsulorrhexis with a diameter larger than 6.5 mm, implantation on excessively small capsular remnants, iridotomy, loose zonules, and intravitreous injection.[16,17]

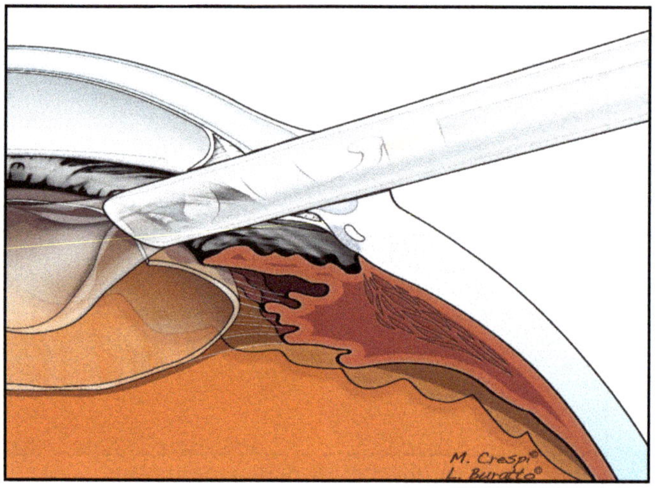

Figure 6-4. Detachment of Descemet's membrane during cartridge insertion. This occurs as the cartridge or IOL pass through the corneal tunnel. If the cartridge or IOL is forced through a tunnel that is too small, or if the incision is not cut cleanly through Descemet's or intersects Schwalbe's line, the injection of the IOL or the cartridge may lead to a Descemet's detachment.

Treatment ranges from repositioning of the implant to exchange of the IOL. Repositioning is done with intact IOLs and zonules. The surgeon should enter the eye cautiously, free both haptics from adhesions with the iris and capsule, and position both haptics into the same plane (in the sulcus or bag), depending on residual support.

Removal is recommended if damage to the lens or zonules may lead to incorrect positioning of the lens. Removal of the lens is advised if there is active infection or inflammation that will improve if the IOL is removed.[18]

Endothelial Damage

Implanting an IOL can cause endothelial damage through tears and potential detachment of Descemet's membrane. This complication occurs as the IOL passes through the corneal incision, particularly with forceps. If the IOL is forced through a small tunnel or if the corneal incision is not smooth across Descemet's or crosses Schwalbe's line, the passage of the IOL or cartridge may create a Descemet's detachment (Figure 6-4). The damage is usually localized but can rarely extend as far as the visual axis, causing significant functional damage. If there is extension of the detachment, the surgeon should suture the corneal incision and create another one. At the end of the procedure, the surgeon should inject air or gas (C3F8 12%) in the AC to facilitate reattachment of Descemet's to the cornea.[19]

Sometimes endothelial damage can also be caused by rotation of the haptics in the AC, or chamber shallowing due to loss of OVD as the lens is being implanted with endothelial contact with the IOL (see Figures E1 to E6, F1 to F6, and G1 to G3).

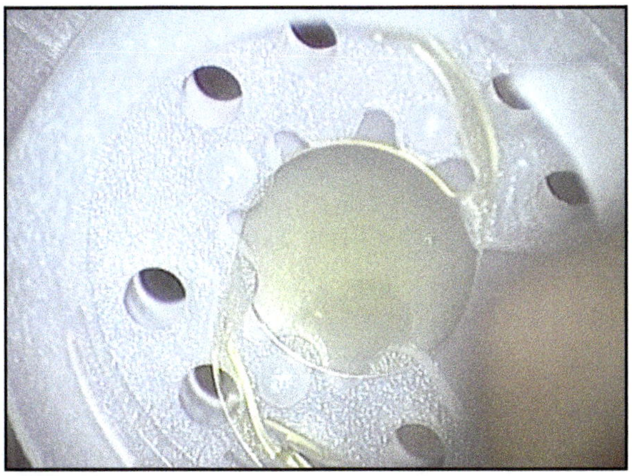

Figure E1. The IOL is in its container.

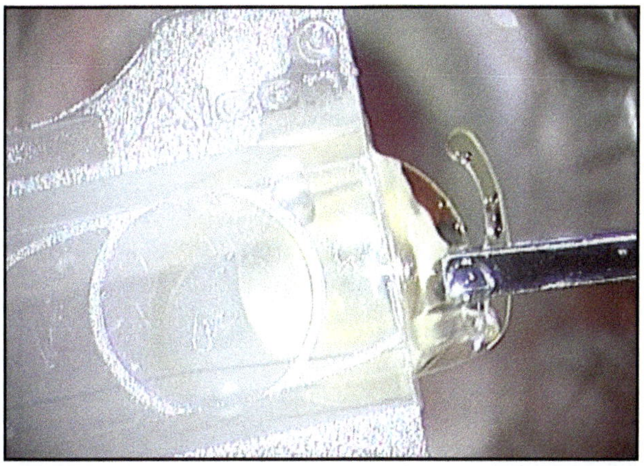

Figure E2. The IOL is withdrawn and apparently correctly loaded.

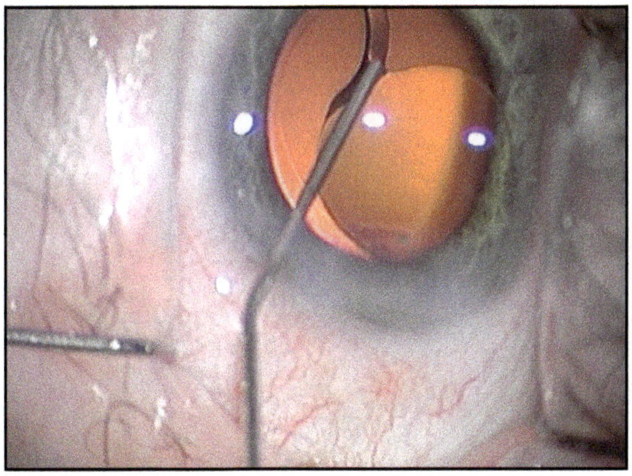

Figure E3. After the injection, the IOL appears with a loop bent backwards.

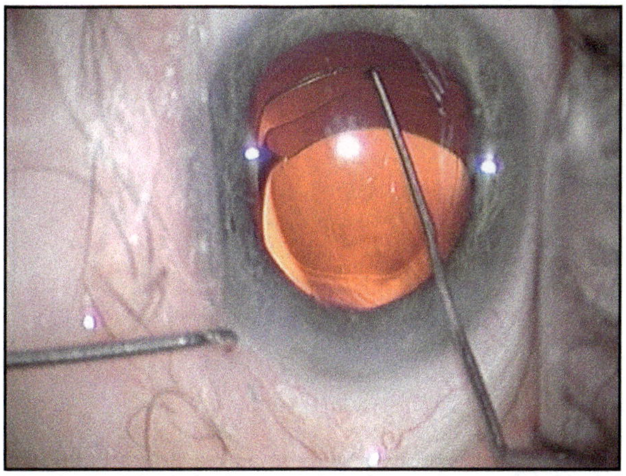

Figure E4. The loop is rotated and straightened in the AC but now the lens is reversed.

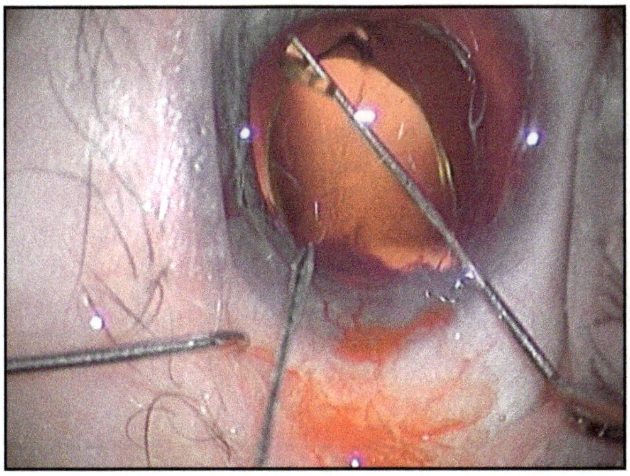

Figure E5. OVD is injected in order to outdistance the endothelium and the posterior capsule from the IOL. The IOL is then inverted.

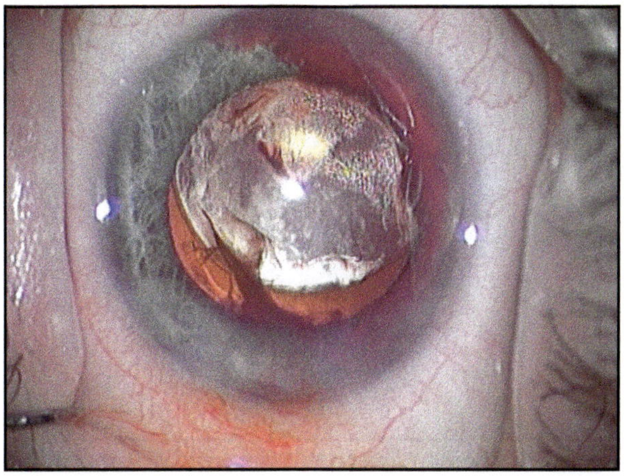

Figure E6. During this step, a loop damages the peripheral iris and blood appears in the AC. Once the blood and OVD are aspirated, the lens appears to be properly placed in the bag.

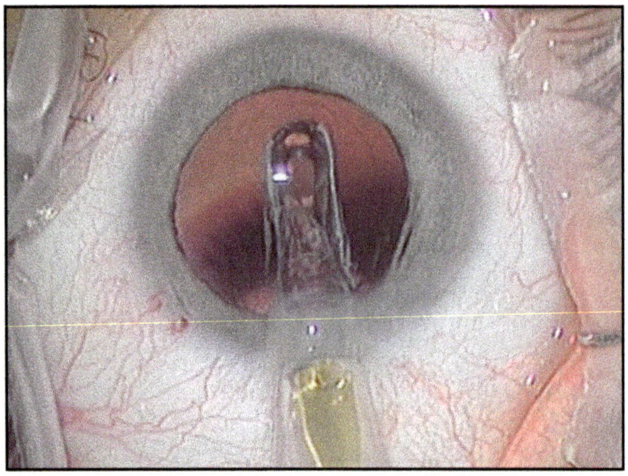

Figure F1. Implant of single-piece acrylic IOL.

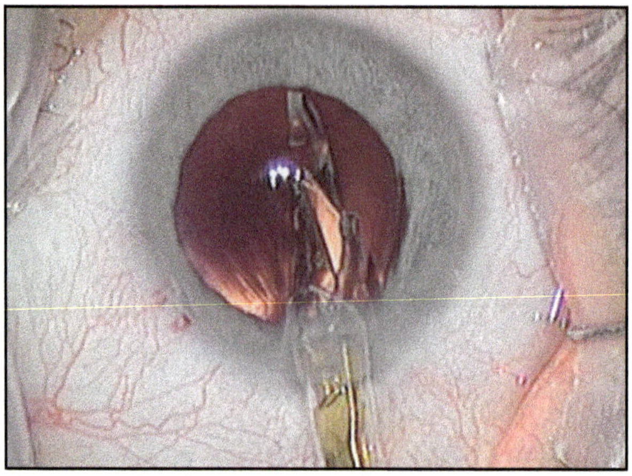

Figure F2. The IOL opens vertically into the AC.

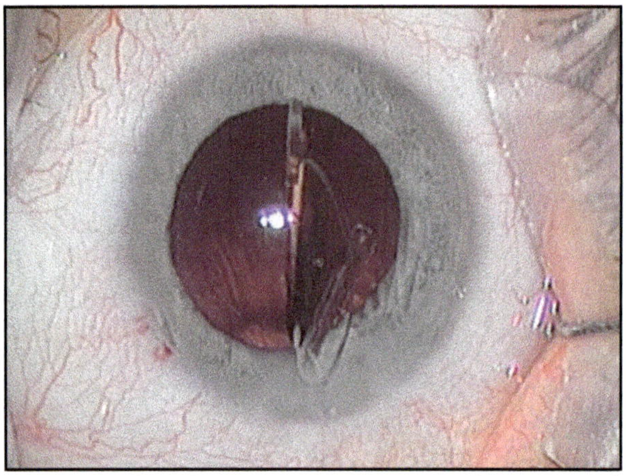

Figure F3. It is first necessary inject an OVD to avoid contact with the endothelium.

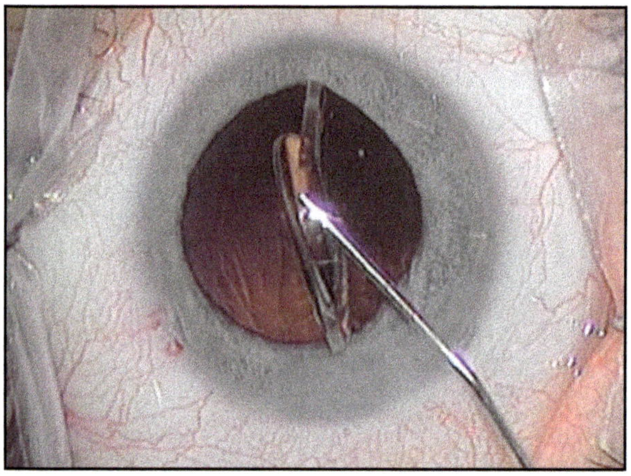

Figure F4. Then the IOL is slowly rotated horizontally.

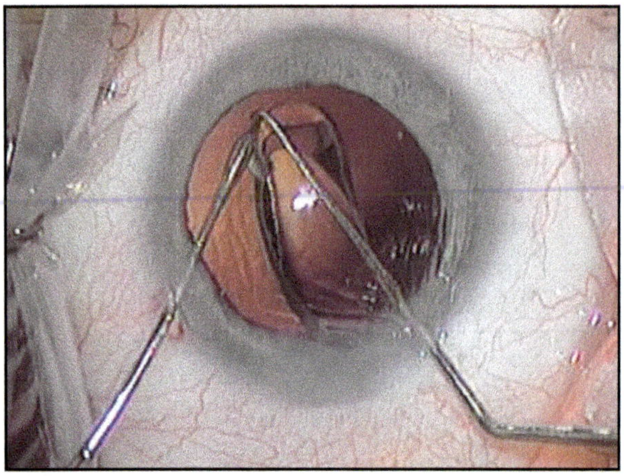

Figure F5. Then the first loop is placed in the bag.

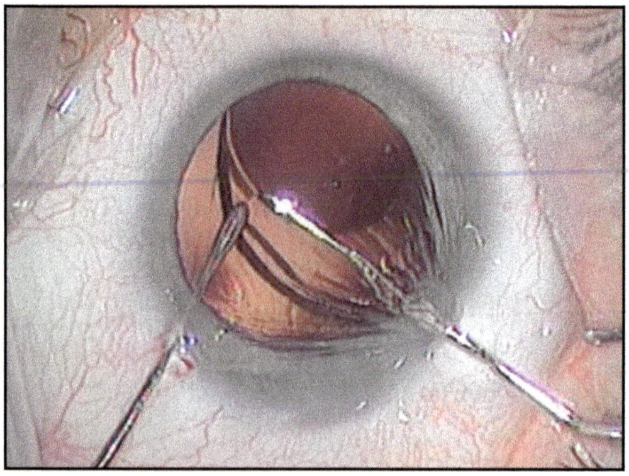

Figure F6. Finally the second loop of IOL is placed.

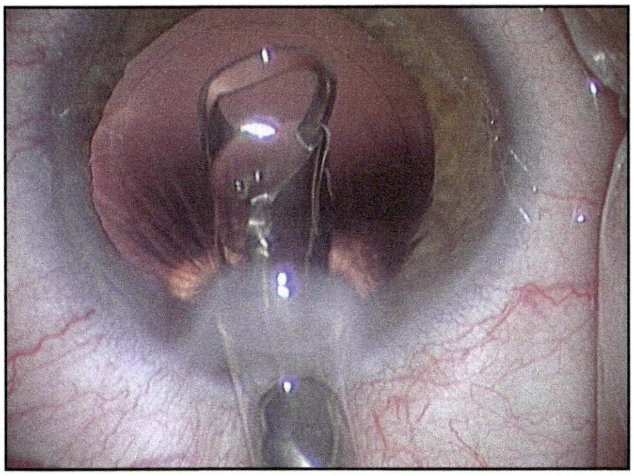

Figure G1. The IOL is injected into the AC.

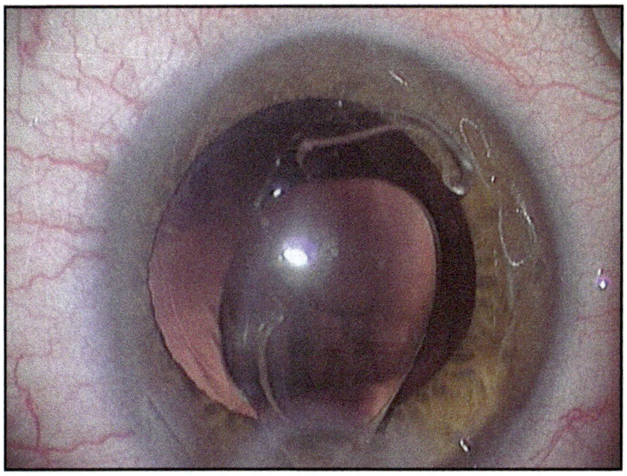

Figure G2. It opens upside down.

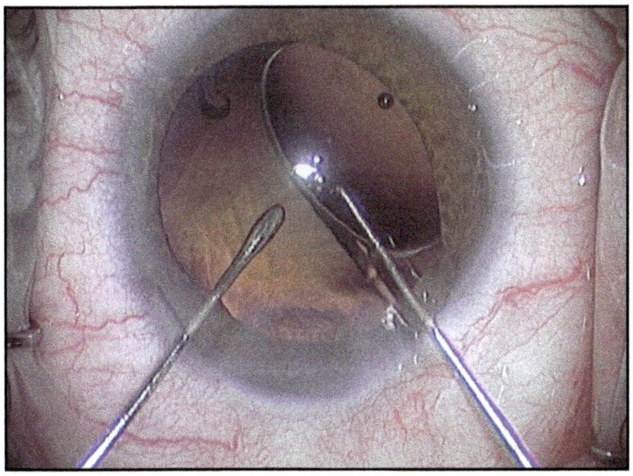

Figure G3. The IOL is straightened using 2 spatulas after OVD injection.

Iris Damage

Iris prolapse is common and may occur as the IOL is being implanted. It may sometimes lead to irreversible iris damage. The etiology may be a short corneal tunnel or an excessively scleral incision. Eyes with an axial length of less than 20 mm, shallow ACs, previous filtering surgery, or iris atrophy may be predisposing factors.[20] Over-filling of the AC with OVD will increase AC pressure with further prolapse of the iris. Moreover, an incision too small for IOL insertion creates excessive stress, with a greater incidence of iris prolapse.[20]

Sometimes the iris may prolapse into the tip of the cartridge that has just been placed in the incision. The cartridge opens the tunnel and with positive intraocular pressure allows prolapse of the iris into the tip (Figure 6-5A). Thus, the cartridge should be introduced into the incision in a bevel-up position. The tip is then rotated downward once it has entered the AC. The surgeon may also use a spatula through the side port incisions to disengage the iris from the tip of the cartridge (Figure 6-5B). If iris prolapse

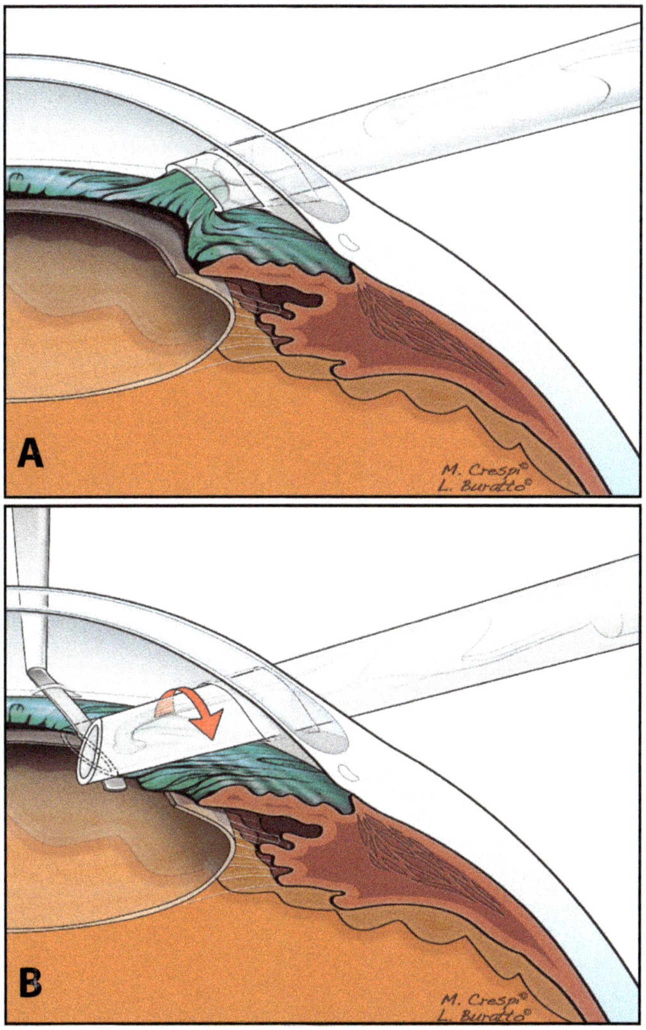

Figure 6-5. Iris engaged by the cartridge. (A) The cartridge opens the corneal tunnel, and with positive intraocular pressure, the iris may prolapse into the cartridge tip. To avoid this problem, the cartridge should be introduced bevel-up, rotating the tip downward as soon as it has entered the AC. (B) The surgeon may also use a spatula to assist, introduced through the side port incision to disengage the iris from the cartridge tip.

persists, there will be progressive pigment dispersion with loss in sphincter tone and iris atrophy. The surgeon should reposit the iris with a spatula through the side incision, and if the prolapse persists, the initial incision should be sutured and the lens implanted through a new incision. Excessive force on the iris during lens implantation may cause iridodialysis[21] and more rarely hyphema with vascularization of the corneal incision, rupture of iris vessels, and dislocation of the IOL.[22,23]

References

1. Erie JC, Newman B, Mahr MA, Khan AR, McIntosh M. Acrylic intraocular lens damage after folding using a forceps insertion technique. *J Cataract Refract Surg.* 2010;36(3):483-487.
2. Schmidbauer JM, Apple DJ, Peng Q, Arthur SN, Vargas LG. Cloudiness of a PMMA intraocular lens. "Snowflake" degeneration. *Ophthalmologe.* 2002;99(4):306-307.
3. Peng Q, Apple DJ, Arthur SN, Merritt JH, Escobar-Gomez M, Hoddinott DS. Snowflake opacification of poly(methyl methacrylate) intraocular lens optic biomaterial: a newly described syndrome. *Int Ophthalmol Clin.* 2001;41(3):91-107.
4. Werner L, Apple DJ, Escobar-Gomez M, et al. Postoperative deposition of calcium on the surfaces of a hydrogel intraocular lens. *Ophthalmology.* 2000;107(12):2179-2185.
5. Chew JJ, Werner L, Mackman G, Mamalis N. Late opacification of a silicone intraocular lens caused by ophthalmic ointment. *J Cataract Refract Surg.* 2006;32(2):341-346.
6. Wackernagel W, Ettinger K, Weitgasser U, et al. Opacification of a silicone intraocular lens caused by calcium deposits on the optic. *J Cataract Refract Surg.* 2004;30(2):517-520.
7. Parkin B, Pitts-Crick M. Opacification of silicone intraocular implant requiring lens exchange. *Eye (Lond).* 2000;14(pt 5):794-795.
8. Stappler T, Williams R, Wong D. F4H5: a novel substance for the removal of silicone oil from intraocular lenses. *Br J Ophthalmol.* 2010;94(3):364-367.
9. Menapace R, Findl O, Georgopoulos M, Rainer G, Vass C, Schmetterer K. The capsular tension ring: designs, applications, and techniques. *J Cataract Refract Surg.* 2000;26(6):898-912.
10. Khan JM, Romano MR, Groenewald C. Recurrent hypopyon due to methicillin-resistant staphylococcus aureus after cataract surgery. *Eye (Lond).* 2009;23(5):1235.
11. Mannan R, Pruthi A, Om Parkash R, Jhanji V. Descemet membrane detachment during foldable intraocular lens implantation. *Eye Contact Lens.* 2011;37(2):106-108.
12. Taguri AH, Sanders R. Iris prolapse in small incision cataract surgery. *Ophthalmic Surg Lasers.* 2002;33(1):66-70.
13. Walker NJ, Foster A, Apel AJ. Traumatic expulsive iridodialysis after small-incision sutureless cataract surgery. *J Cataract Refract Surg.* 2004;30(10):2223-2224.
14. Pavlin CJ, Harasiewicz K, Foster FS. Ultrasound biomicroscopic analysis of haptic position in late-onset, recurrent hyphema after posterior chamber lens implantation. *J Cataract Refract Surg.* 1994;20(2):182-185.
15. Odufuwa TO, Bolger J. Late hyphema after small incision cataract surgery. *J Cataract Refract Surg.* 1994;20(3):342-343.

7

Complications Arising From Equipment and Tubing

Lucio Buratto, MD; Stephen F. Brint, MD, FACS; and Mario R. Romano, MD, PhD

Modern phacoemulsification techniques are increasingly dependent on the correct functioning of the machine. The results are usually excellent; however, unexpected complications may occur.

The best results depend on efficient, quick techniques performed with minimal use of ultrasound and decreased fluid flow in the anterior chamber (AC). Modern equipment attempts to create dynamic equilibrium between the fluid entering the eye (modulated by infusion pressure) and fluid leaving the eye (modulated by aspiration) to ensure stability of the AC and provide smooth removal of the lens fragments.[1]

The system must be able to balance stroke and cavitation effects that the ultrasound induces; this repels as opposed to aspirating lens fragments. Longitudinal movements and rotation of the tip are optimized by variable duty cycles potentially creating localized heating and repulsion of lens fragments. During phacoemulsification, energy is created and dispersed in the AC.

Surgical maneuvers are performed in an open system. Constant flow from the sleeve avoids overheating the corneal incision from ultrasonic energy.

Modern systems also significantly reduce surge using hardware and software improvements.

Hardware improvements include reduction in the elasticity and internal diameter of the aspiration tubing (less compliant). Some systems also have an Aspiration Bypass System (ABS) located on one side of the phaco tip, ensuring aspiration flow even when the tip is occluded. This ensures minimal constant flow to cool the tip and allows reduced vacuum levels.

Modern software in some phaco devices also changes the pump speed and ultrasound using requested dynamic rise (amount of pump speed desired according to different situations, nuclear density, etc).

Once the preset threshold of vacuum has been reached (occlusion), a burst of longitudinal ultrasound waves releases material from the tip. The vacuum is reduced, pulling lens material to the tip with no shallowing of the AC.

Complications Associated With Inadequate Fluid Balance

The fluid aspirated is measured in cc/min and depends on the speed of rotation of the peristaltic pump, allowing independent control of aspiration and vacuum. Venturi pumps are independent of vacuum created in the tubing, and this is the only variable parameter. Flow leaving the

Buratto L, Brint SF, Romano MR.
Cataract Surgery Complications (pp 57-62).
© 2013 Taylor & Francis Group.

eye is also dependent on other factors not directly under control of the equipment, such as the corneal incision, the relationship between the sleeve diameter and incision size, and the size of the corneal incision.

Safety in Anterior Chamber Management

- Reduce vacuum levels.
- Set preocclusion limits with micropulse to avoid complete occlusion.
- With marked anterior chamber (AC) instability, use an AC maintainer allowing constant infusion from a different location.
- Use pressurized infusion if available, as this can minimize pressure variations in the AC. In a recent comparative study, it was concluded that pressurized infusion induced significantly less endothelial loss and shorter irrigation/aspiration times.

In the various steps of lens fragmentation and aspiration, occlusion of the tip by lens material leads to blockage of fluid aspiration with increased vacuum levels in the tubing and tubing contraction. This is followed by release (surge) with high levels of vacuum created by previous occlusion, augmented with expansion of previously collapsed tubing (Figure 7-1A). This leads to uncontrolled surge from the AC unbalanced by adequate inflow, resulting in dangerous shallowing of the AC with forward movement of the posterior capsule with irreversible damage[1] (Figure 7-1B).

Less compliant (stiffer) tubing is used with more resistance to high vacuum levels. Modern phacoemulsification devices can shut off aspiration when occluded (avoiding further increases) and can instantaneously reverse the pump.

Instability of the posterior chamber may come from poor positioning or a tear in the infusion sleeve with resulting difficulty in lens removal.[2] The surgeon should always check the integrity, position, and size of the sleeve, matching it to the size of the corneal incision.

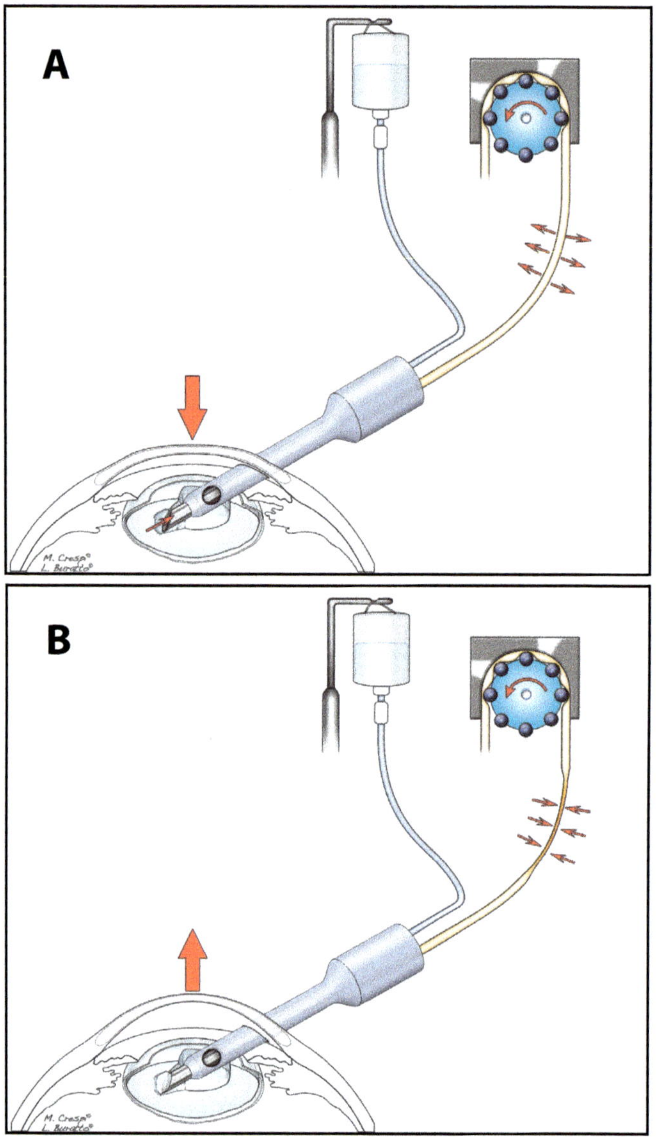

Figure 7-1. Surge. (A) Occlusion of the phaco tip by lens material stops fluid flow through the phaco hand piece and slight collapse of the tubing. (B) When the occlusion is broken, high levels of vacuum build up, and expansion of the previously collapsed tubing may collapse the AC and cause potential damage.

Ultrasound Complications

Ultrasound emulsifies the lens through the direct effect of the stroke on the nucleus and through induced cavitation. Ultrasound power is the result of frequency of the tip (35,000 to 45,000 cycles/sec) and length of elongation (2 to 4 mm).[1]

This energy may sometimes release microfragments of titanium from the phaco tip into the aqueous. These are well tolerated and do not create clinically significant damage.[4]

Increased Temperature of the Phaco Tip

Increased temperature of the phaco tip is caused by high ultrasound power required to emulsify dense cataracts. Under these conditions, ultrasound can cause endothelial damage, damage to the corneal tunnel, and damage to the blood-aqueous barrier of the iris. In order to minimize damage, the power of the ultrasound should be reduced and optimized.

Newer strategies: New phaco devices include pulsed ultrasonic bursts with short intervals of aspiration alone.

In the "pulse" or "burst" modes, the ultrasound has a duration of 50 to 150 milliseconds interrupted with short aspirations allowing tip cooling and more efficient aspiration of lens fragments with less repulsion. An additional advantage is greater security provided with occlusion. The tip with microinterruptions creates less trauma to the adjacent structures. The latest generation of machines also have software that optimizes duty cycles through micropulse (ie, time lapse cycling, on/off of the ultrasound). These settings ensure that the temperature does not exceed 55°C even with an extremely dense nucleus (cold phaco).[1]

Longitudinal movements, now accompanied by torsion (Ozil) of the tip, emulsify the lens, reducing heat effects and repulsion by the longitudinal component. The surgeon should use intraoperative OVD to reduce oxidative damage induced by ultrasound.[5]

Damage Induced by Cavitation

Elongation of the tip induces ultrasonic vibrations, generating areas of high and low pressure. When the tip returns to the starting position, the low pressure generates micro bubbles that tend to implode with successive changes of high pressure waves. This cavitation occurs in 6 to 25 milliseconds. Increase in pressure creates an implosion of approximately 75% of the microbubbles with a cavitation wave of 75,000 PSI. The remaining 25% of the bubbles are too large for implosion and are pushed back by the tip.[1] The energy from ultrasound bursts in excess of 25 milliseconds generates a sustained cavitation wave that cannot emulsify. Thus, new phaco devices use micropulses to maximize transitory cavitation without dissipating energy.

The direction of cavitation changes depending on the angle of the tip used (45 degrees, 30 degrees, and 15 degrees). Zero-degree tips create frontal cavitation with a focal point 0.5 mm from the tip (Figure 7-2A). Taking the angle of cavitation into account, the surgeon must orient the cavitation wave toward the nucleus[1] (Figures 7-2B and 7-2C). Different orientations may lead to damage to the iris and the endothelium (Figure 7-3).

With low endothelial cell density, it is necessary to consider the damage induced by cavitation. Thus, the tip should be oriented to produce complete occlusion with minimal damage to adjoining structures. With a 0-degree tip, complete occlusion occurs by positioning the tip perpendicular to the heminucleus (Figure 7-4A). To achieve complete occlusion with a 30- or 45-degree tip, the inclination must be changed (Figure 7-4B).

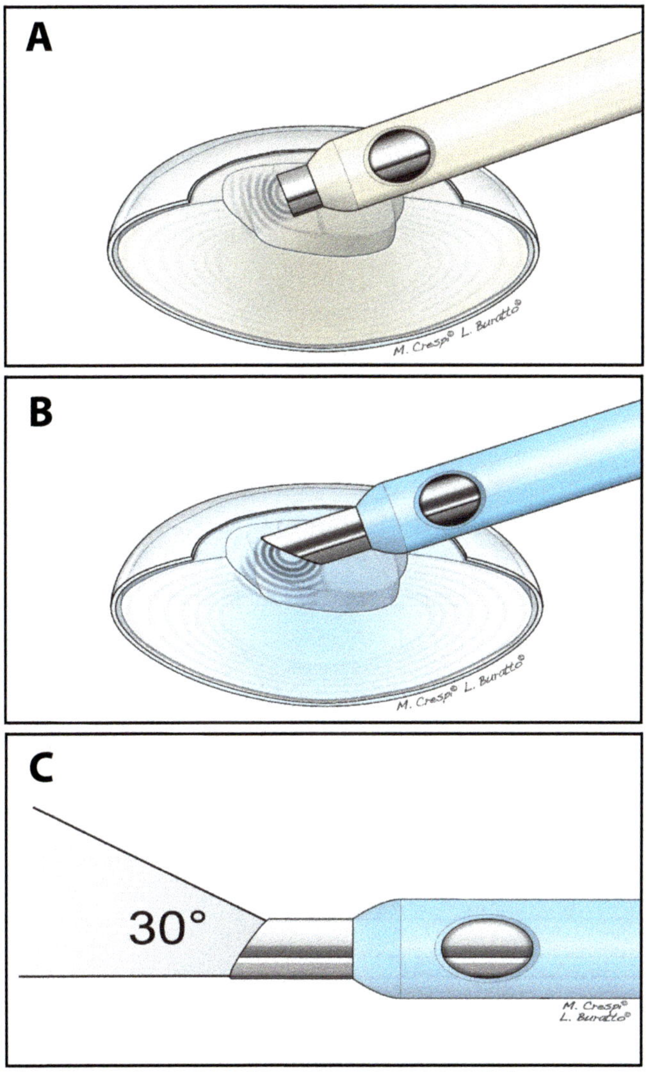

Figure 7-2. Cavitation. The ultrasonic stroke of the phaco tip creates areas of high and low pressure. This cavitation occurs in 6 to 25 milliseconds and amount depends on the angle of the phaco tip. (A) Zero-degree tips create frontal cavitation with a focal point 0.5 mm from the tip. (B) Considering the angle of cavitation, the surgeon should orient the cavitation toward the nucleus. (C) Cavitation angle. Cavitation using a 30-degree phaco tip.

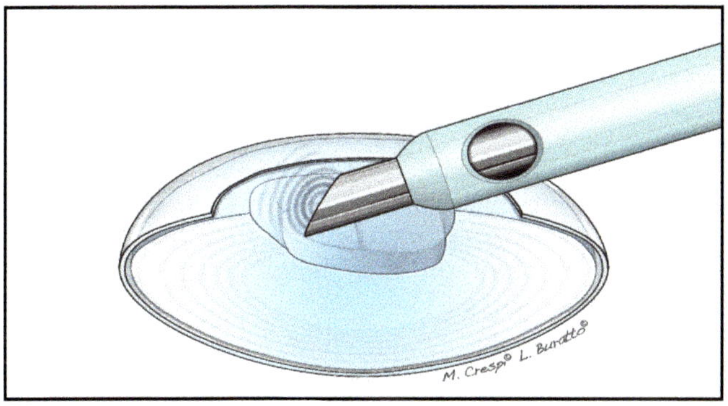

Figure 7-3. Different orientations of the phaco tip may damage the iris or endothelium.

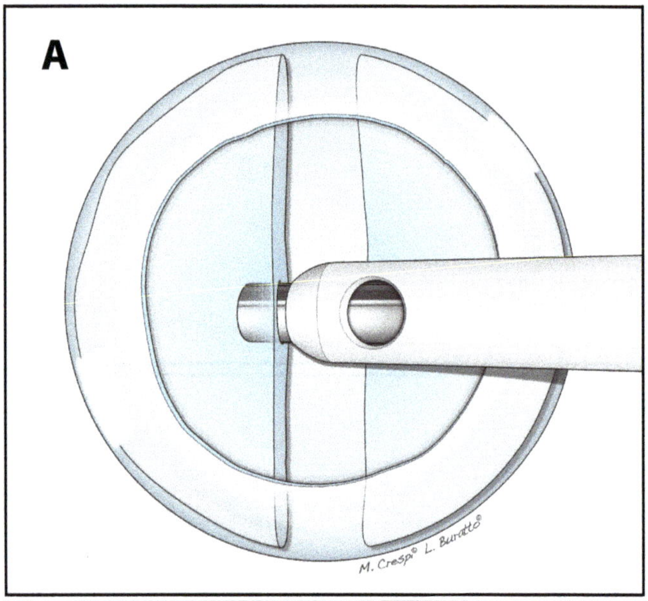

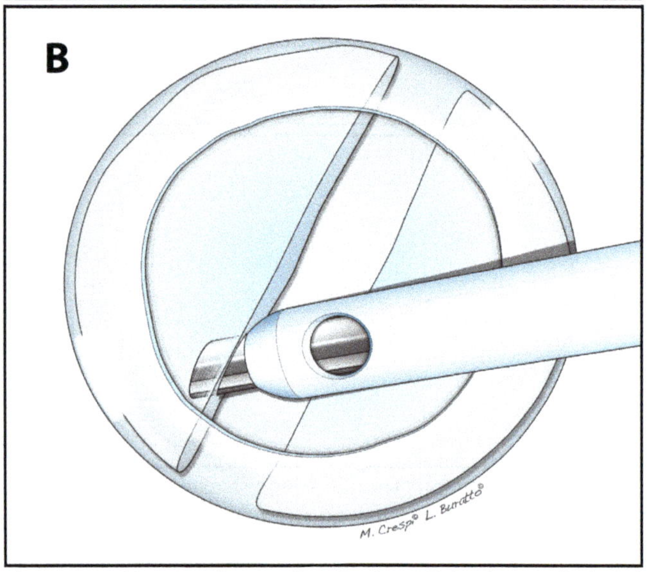

Figure 7-4. Heminucleus and cavitation. With a low endothelial cell count, the surgeon must plan for cavitation. The phaco tip should be oriented for complete occlusion with minimal collateral damage. (A) With a 0-degree tip, complete occlusion is easily achieved by positioning the tip perpendicular to the heminucleus. (B) With a 30- or 45-degree tip, to achieve complete occlusion, the tip needs to be inclined. Cavitation affects the edges of the lens, offering less resistance to phacoemulsification.

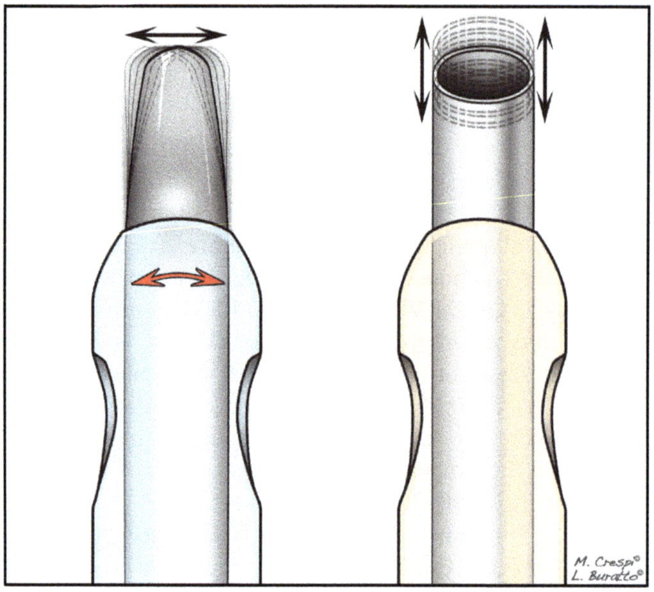

Figure 7-5. Longitudinal versus Ozil. Longitudinal phaco has been joined by Ozil torsional movement. This emulsifies the lens, reducing thermal effects and repulsion associated with longitudinal phaco.

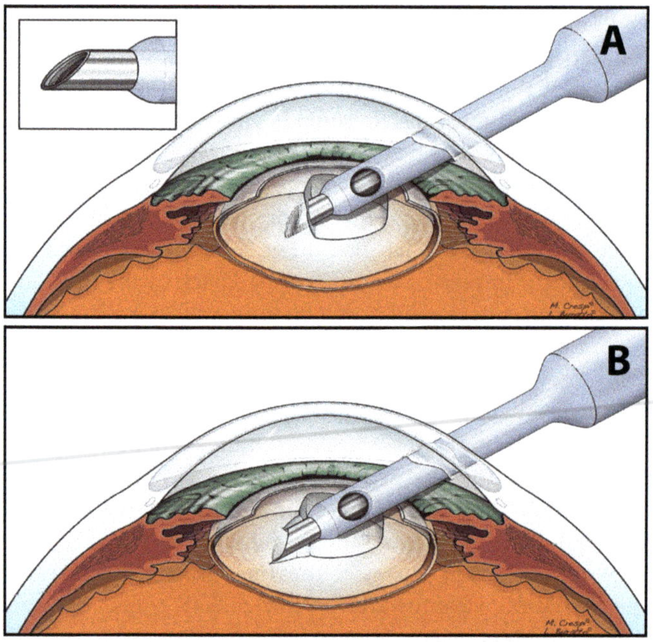

Figure 7-6. Ridged tips with grooves. High-speed digital imaging shows that ridged tips (A) create greater cavitation than standard tips. (B) Once the nucleus has been grasped, the lens material is more stable at the tip, with better followability and shorter phaco times.

The ultrasound produced by torsional movements (Ozil) allows better orientation and location of cavitation waves, with a Kelman 45-degree angled tip. Torsional phaco also has less lens repulsion than longitudinal movements[6] (Figure 7-5).

Recently, ridged tips, which have grooves inside the tip, have developed. High-speed digital photography has shown that ridged tips create greater cavitation than standard phaco tips (Figure 7-6A). Moreover, the nucleus is much more engaged (Figure 7-6B) and tends to follow the ridging of the tip with greater efficiency, reducing operating times.[7]

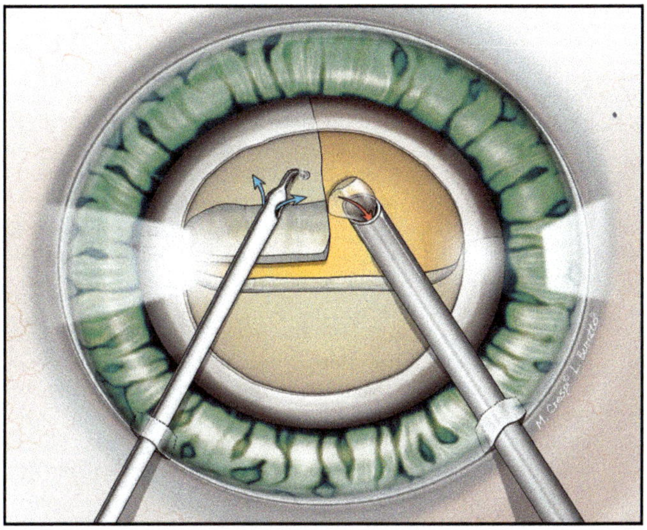

Figure 7-7. Bimanual microincision technique. The bimanual technique requires an irrigating chopper, allowing separate infusion from that of the phaco tip, maintaining the infusion separate from aspiration, and creating less turbulence.

Complications of Microincisional Technique

The bimanual approach uses an irrigating chopper, which provides continuous infusion and is separate from the phaco tip (Figure 7-7). The advantage to this approach is that the infusion and aspiration lines are separated to minimize energy from the phaco tip. With the coaxial technique, both irrigation/aspiration (I/A) use the same incision. The irrigating chopper creates greater AC stability with constant independent irrigation.

The "cold phaco" technique (C-MICS) and the bimanual microincision technique (B-MICS) are both safe and effective techniques and have comparable results.[8]

Fluid loss from the AC was analyzed comparing the use of an irrigating chopper as a second instrument.[9]

The loss of liquid through a side port incision is 127 mL ± 60 (SD), correlated with surgical time. Fluid loss through the side port incision is approximately 67% (SD 11).[9] The loss of fluid through the primary incision is 75% when the in situ chopper is used during the entire phacoemulsification, and 59% when the chopper is removed immediately after nuclear chopping.[9]

With the coaxial mini-invasive technique, the surgeon should remove the chopper once chopping is completed; this will reduce fluid loss and maintain AC stability.

A study of endothelial cell loss using microincision cataract surgery (MICS) versus standard phacoemulsification demonstrated no statistical difference. Endothelial cell loss was significant in both groups but there was no significant difference between the 2 groups: 9.5% (MICS) versus 7.6% (standard phaco).[8]

A randomized prospective study recently demonstrated that the parameters of vacuum (200 mm Hg versus 400 mm Hg) and flow (20 cc/min versus 40 cc/min) do not significantly affect mean endothelial cell loss; the cell loss was correlated to the total energy used.[10]

With the bimanual MICS technique, it is difficult to emulsify hard nuclei. Here, the surgeon should use pulse mode rather than burst mode and less ultrasound energy; wound burn and endothelial cell loss are minimized.[11]

Complications With the Femtosecond Laser Used in Refractive Cataract Surgery

The infrared 800-nm femtosecond laser offers precise incisions in designated targets, including the lens, without collateral damage[12] (Figure 7-8). Despite early promising results and popularity in refractive cataract surgery, safety studies have not yet been published. There have been reports of sporadic complications like posterior capsule rupture with lens dislocation,[13] macular edema not statistically significant from the control group,[14] and capsular block.[13]

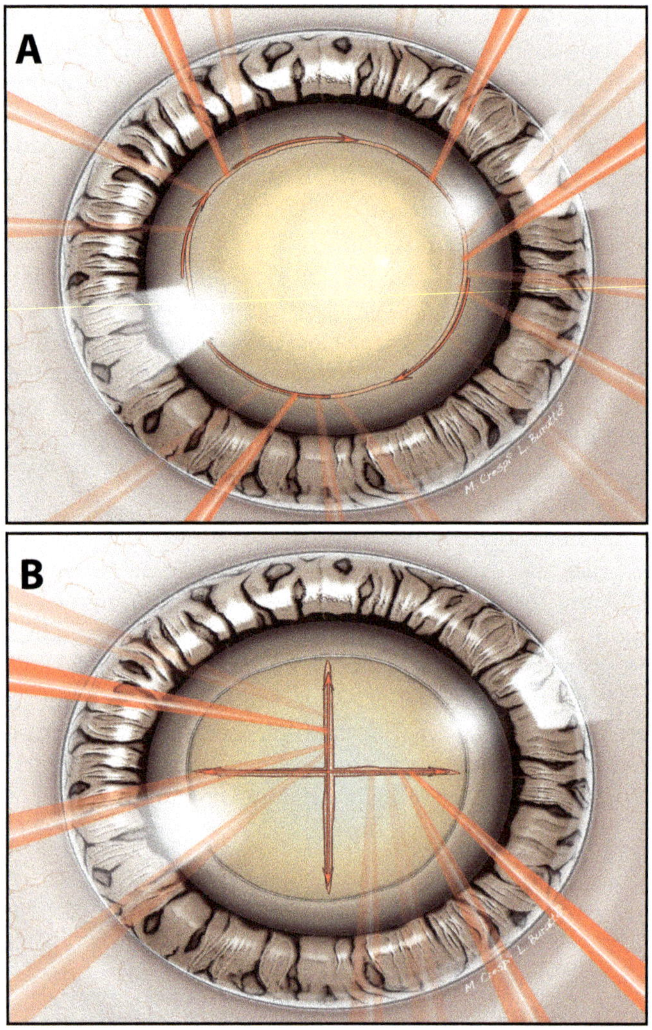

Figure 7-8. Femtosecond laser-assisted cataract surgery. The IR 800-nm femtosecond laser allows the creation of precise incisions (A), including the lens (B), without collateral damage. A handful of cases with complications, including posterior capsule rupture with lens dislocation, have been reported. This is felt to be a learning curve issue, avoiding excessive hydrodissection with this perfect capsulorrhexis.

References

1. Packer M, Fishkind WJ, Fine IH, Seibel BS, Hoffman RS. The physics of phaco: a review. *J Cataract Refract Surg.* 2005;31(2):424-431.
2. Shum JW, Chan KS, Wong D, Li KK. Intraoperative fracture of phacoemulsification sleeve. *BMC Ophthalmol.* 2010;10:29.
3. Chaudhry P, Prakash G, Jacob S, Narasimhan S, Agarwal S, Agarwal A. Safety and efficacy of gas-forced infusion (air pump) in coaxial phacoemulsification. *J Cataract Refract Surg.* 2010;36(12):2139-2145.
4. Kose S, Mentes J, Uretmen O, Topcuoglu N, Kokturk U, Yilmaz H. The nature and origin of intraocular metallic foreign bodies appearing after phacoemulsification. *Ophthalmologica.* 2003;217(3):212-214.
5. Augustin AJ, Dick HB. Oxidative tissue damage after phacoemulsification: influence of ophthalmic viscosurgical devices. *J Cataract Refract Surg.* 2004;30(2):424-427.
6. Krey HF. Ultrasonic turbulences at the phacoemulsification tip. *J Cataract Refract Surg.* 1989;15(3):343-344.
7. Watanabe A. New phacoemulsification tip with a grooved, thread-ed-tip construction. *J Cataract Refract Surg.* 2011;37(7):1329-1332.
8. Kahraman G, Amon M, Franz C, Prinz A, Abela-Formanek C. Intraindividual comparison of surgical trauma after bimanual microincision and conventional small-incision coaxial phacoemulsification. *J Cataract Refract Surg.* 2007;33(4):618-622.
9. Liyanage SE, Angunawela RI, Wong SC, Little BC. Anterior chamber instability caused by incisional leakage in coaxial phacoemulsification. *J Cataract Refract Surg.* 2009;35(6):1003-1005.
10. Baradaran-Rafii A, Rahmati-Kamel M, Eslani M, Kiavash V, Karimian F. Effect of hydrodynamic parameters on corneal endothelial cell loss after phacoemulsification. *J Cataract Refract Surg.* 2009;35(4):732-737.
11. Liu Y, Jiang Y, Wu M, Zhang T. Bimanual microincision phacoemulsification in treating hard cataracts using different power modes. *Clin Experiment Ophthalmol.* 2008;36(5):426-430.
12. He L, Sheehy K, Culbertson W. Femtosecond laser-assisted cataract surgery. *Curr Opin Ophthalmol.* 2011;22(1):43-52.
13. Roberts TV, Sutton G, Lawless MA, Jindal-Bali S, Hodge C. Capsular block syndrome associated with femtosecond laser-assisted cataract surgery. *J Cataract Refract Surg.* 2011;37(11):2068-2070.
14. Ecsedy M, Mihaltz K, Kovacs I, Takacs A, Filkorn T, Nagy ZZ. Effect of femtosecond laser cataract surgery on the macula. *J Refract Surg.* 2011;27(10):717-722.

8

Posterior Capsule Rupture

Lucio Buratto, MD; Stephen F. Brint, MD, FACS; and Mario R. Romano, MD, PhD

Posterior capsule rupture (PCR) is one of the most troublesome intraoperative complications because of loss of capsular support for bag implantation of the implant, loss of separation between the posterior capsule and the vitreous, possible dislocation of lens material into the vitreous, retinal tears, inflammation, etc. Risk factors associated with PCR are age, sex (male), glaucoma, diabetic retinopathy, brunescent cataracts, phacodonesis, pseudoexfoliation, axial length (>26 mm), use of alpha-blockers, and poorly visualized ocular fundus because of dense vitreous opacities.[1,2]

Ideally, PCR is not complicated by rupture of the anterior hyaloid face; the vitreous remains compartmentalized without inducing further traction to the vitreous base. There is a low incidence of dislocation of lens fragments into the vitreous varying from 0.06% to 0.20% even in the hands of expert surgeons. The incidence of PCR itself is higher, in some cases as much as 4% (see Figures A1 to A4).[3,4]

Rupture of the Posterior Capsule During Hydroseparation

The most common cause of PCR at this step is strong adhesion between the cortex and posterior capsule, reported in up to 40% of cases of posterior polar cataracts.[5] To prevent PCR with a posterior polar cataract, hydrodelineation is done to preserve the posterior adhesion and, at the same time, begin the surgery using protection by the epinucleus.

Hydrodissection just up to the equator of the lens is advised, avoiding fluid flow reaching the posterior pole of the lens. The surgeon should then viscodissect the posterior adhesions, which is not entirely risk free.

If the posterior polar adhesion persists after cortical aspiration, once IOL implantation is done, the surgeon may perform an intraoperative posterior capsulotomy using a 25- or 27-gauge vitrectomy with infusion into the anterior chamber (AC) or a subsequent YAG capsulotomy.

The risk of PCRs increases when the capsulorrhexis is smaller than 4.5 mm due to increased resistance in hydroseparation and increased pressure on the posterior capsule (see Chapter 4). It is extremely important that the surgeon

Buratto L, Brint SF, Romano MR.
Cataract Surgery Complications (pp 63-74).
© 2013 Taylor & Francis Group.

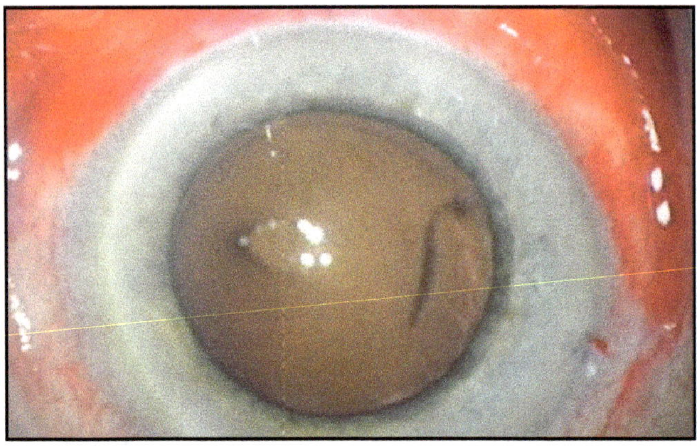

Figure A1. At the end of phacoemulsification, the anterior capsulorrhexis is intact, but irrigation from the U/S tip stops and the chamber is flattened.

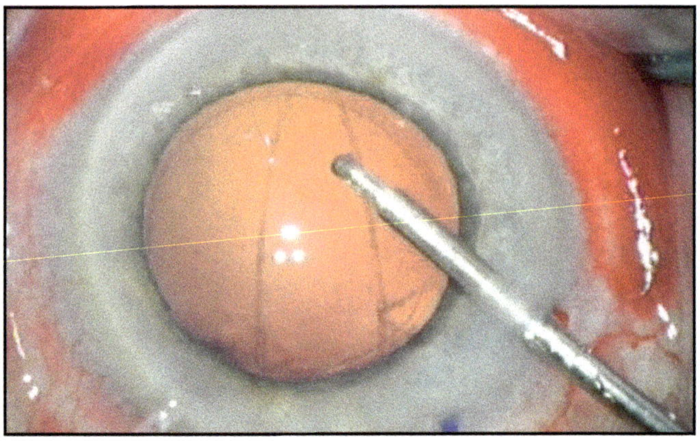

Figure A2. Before removing the irrigation cannula from the AC, OVD is injected to keep the vitreous back.

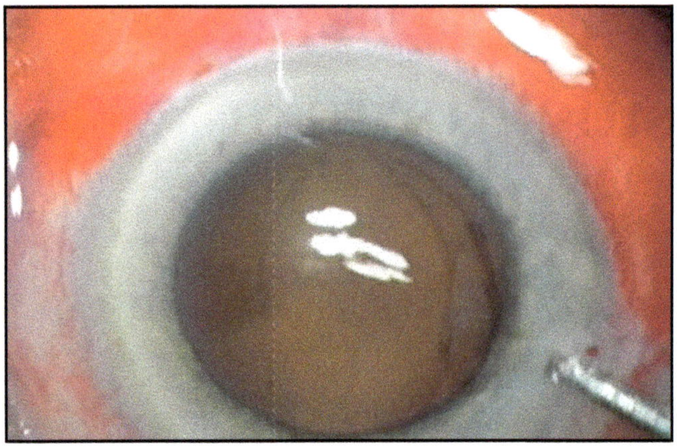

Figure A3. The posterior capsule spontaneously breaks.

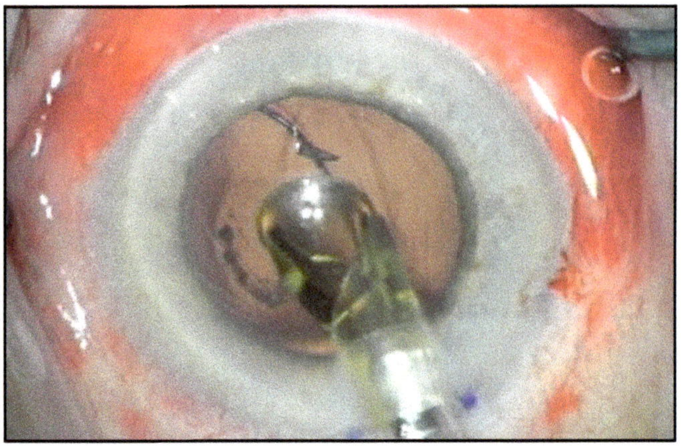

Figure A4. The IOL is then injected and placed in the sulcus.

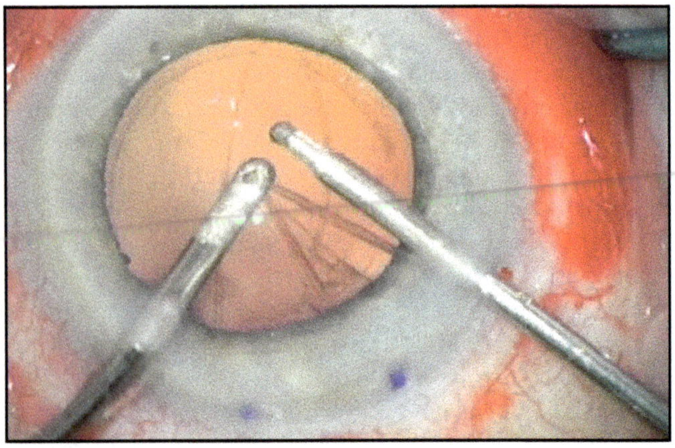

Figure A5. Irrigation/aspiration (I/A) is performed with a bimanual technique and the anterior hyaloid remains intact.

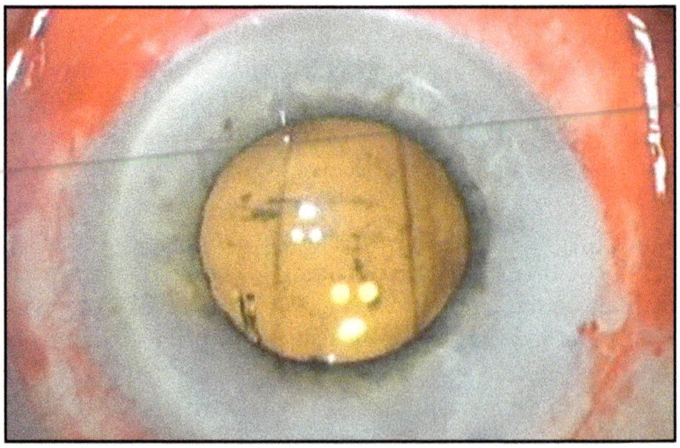

Figure A6. IOL properly placed in the bag.

recognizes the signs of PCR early to avoid a dropped lens from the pressure of hydrodissection or insertion of the phaco tip into the AC.

> **Signs of Posterior Capsule Rupture During Hydroseparation**
>
> The signs of PCR during hydroseparation include the following:
>
> - Excessive lateral displacement of the nucleus
> - Increase in AC depth and space between the posterior iris and the anterior lens surface
> - Sudden and prominent red reflex

Early recognition provides a variety of options: visco-expression of the nucleus after enlargement of the corneal incision to at least 5 mm, followed by bimanual anterior vitrectomy with IOL implantation in the sulcus. The surgeon should perform pars plana posterior vitrectomy with a dropped lens or refer to a vitroretinal surgeon promptly.

Posterior Capsule Rupture During Phacoemulsification

Increased lens density leads to an increase in nuclear thickness and reduction in epinuclear thickness.

All steps performed near the posterior capsule create a greater risk of PCR, particularly sculpting and cracking (see Figures B1 to B6).

> **Signs of Posterior Capsule Rupture During Phacoemulsification**
>
> Signs of PCR during phacoemulsification include the following:
>
> - Sudden increase in AC depth
> - Change in fluidics with poor mobility of the lens
> - Asymmetrical iris due to vitreous prolapse
> - Posterior or lateral dislocation of lens fragments

Rapid recognition of a torn PC improves the prognosis and simplifies management. With a PCR, the surgeon should stop phacoemulsification while avoiding chasing lens fragments. If the surgeon does not recognize the rupture, aspiration generated by phaco will pull vitreous into the AC to the phaco tip (Figure 8-1A). Vitreous prolapse and pressure from the infusion allow sudden loss of residual lens fragments into the vitreous (Figure 8-1B). Increased traction on the vitreous base may lead to tears of the peripheral retina (Figure 8-2).

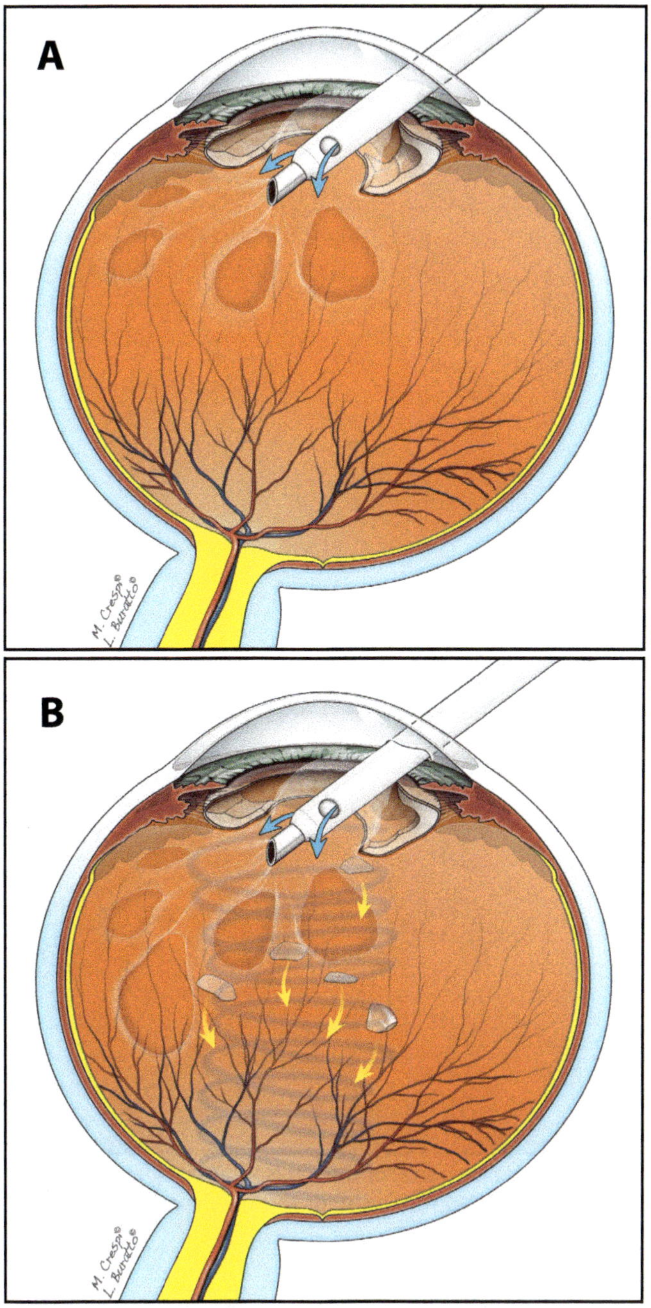

Figure 8-1. Phaco with PCR. With PCR, the surgeon must stop phaco, avoiding "chasing" lens fragments. If the surgeon persists with phacoemulsification, aspiration pulls vitreous into the AC toward the phaco tip (A), allowing sudden rapid loss of lens fragments into the vitreous (B).

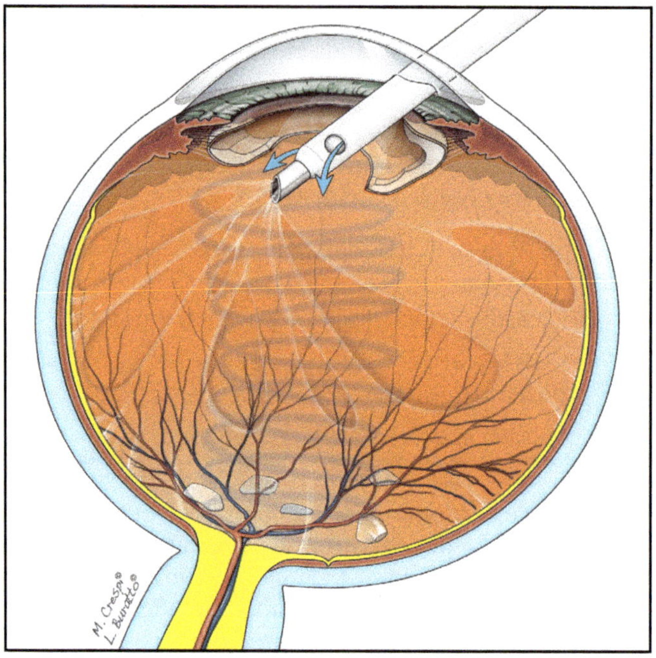

Figure 8-2. Iatrogenic vitreous traction. Phaco when vitreous is present increases traction on the vitreous base, potentially damaging the peripheral retina.

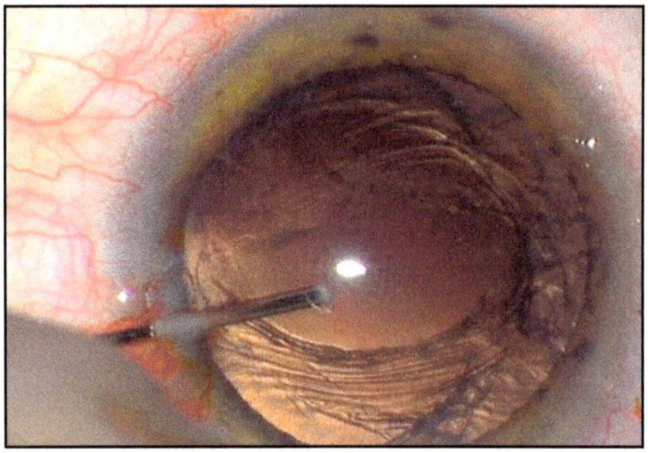

Figure B1. With removal of the ultrasound tip from the AC, the AC is flattened and the posterior capsule is opened spontaneously.

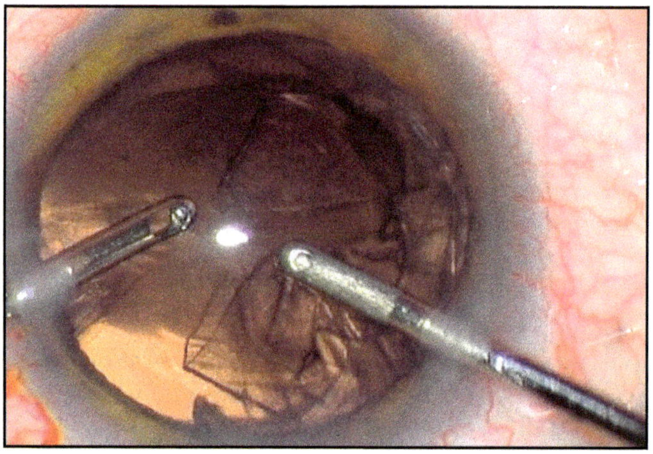

Figure B2. Bimanual cortex removal is performed and the vitreous face remains intact.

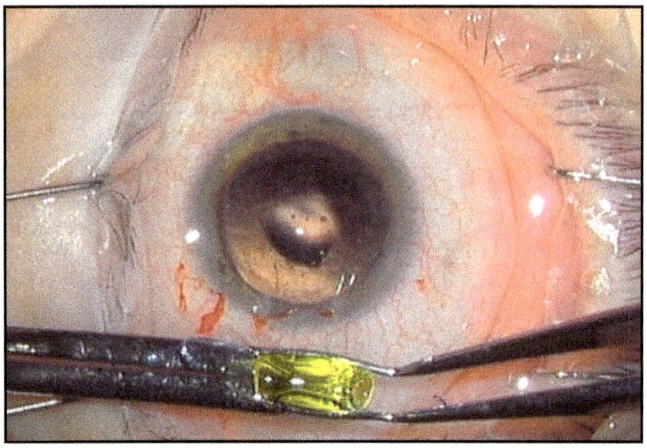

Figure B3. The IOL is folded and inserted with forceps with a manual technique. Better control of IOL opening is possible, avoiding breaking the anterior hyaloid.

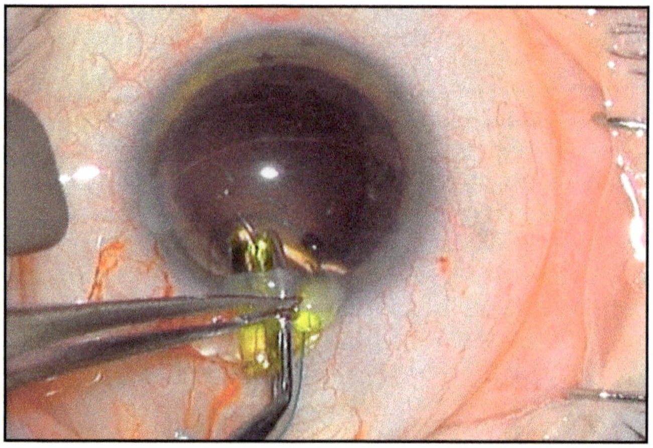

Figure B4. The IOL is inserted.

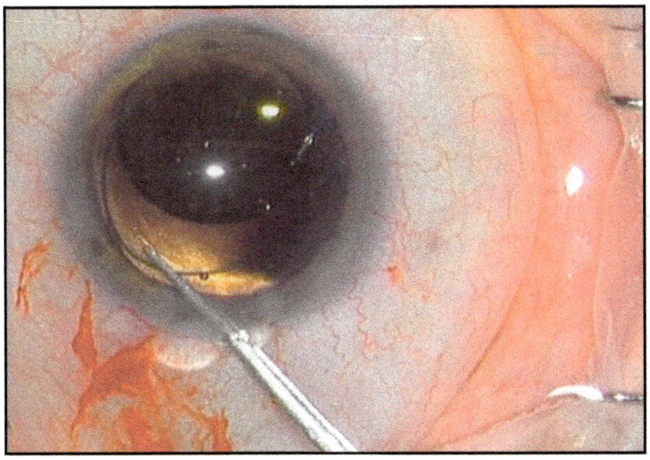

Figure B5. The IOL is positioned in the bag (3 pieces IOL).

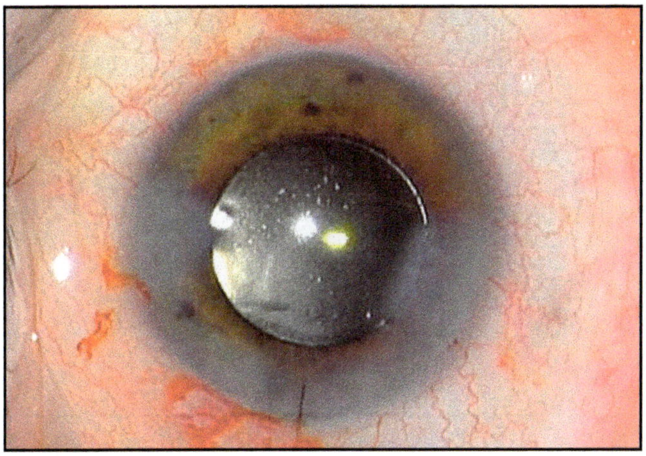

Figure B6. The IOL is properly centered and positioned in the bag.

> **Posterior Capsule Rupture During Phacoemulsification**
>
> With PCR during phacoemulsification, the surgeon should do the following:
>
> - Maintain adequate pressure in the AC to minimize vitreous loss.
> - Avoid aspiration or emulsification.
> - Stop infusion through the tip.
> - Keep the primary corneal incision closed using the tip, removing only once positive pressure has been created in the AC, and using OVD injected below the nucleus through the side port incision.

Posterior Capsule Rupture With an Intact Anterior Hyaloid

PCR with an intact anterior hyaloid usually develops after idiopathic zonular disinsertion, or because of an extension in the creation of the rhexis extending out past the equator. It is important to preserve the integrity of the anterior hyaloid face, even with PCR, to prevent vitreous prolapse and subsequent vitreo-retinal traction. The surgeon should proceed cautiously with additional OVD to equalize pressure between the AC and the vitreous face.

With a soft nucleus: Inject a dispersive viscoelastic (eg, Viscoat [Alcon Laboratories Inc, Fort Worth, TX]) under the nucleus to create a barrier between the nucleus and the hyaloid. The OVD buffers irrigation flow and relative turbulence. The OVD should be injected slowly; a rapid or excessive injection may extend the tear or rupture the hyaloid face. The surgeon may proceed with phacoemulsification using low values (low bottle height and low flow rate).

With dense residual nuclear material: The surgeon utilizes viscoexpression of the lens material. After injecting additional dispersive OVD to protect the vitreous face, the nucleus is expressed using an OVD. This can be performed dry, with coaxial irrigation, or by using a separate corneal incision.

The "dry" technique uses low molecular weight OVD, usually about 6 mL, to maintain AC depth, and to elevate the lens fragments into the AC. Aspiration or infusion are not used.[6] During the OVD injection, the surgeon should gently depress the posterior lip of the corneal incision to facilitate expression of the lens material.

A loop may assist expression of the nucleus through an incision (approximately 5 mm in length, varying on the lens density). The surgeon removes the residual cortex using manual Simcoe cannula aspiration.

Posterior Capsule Rupture With Disruption of the Vitreous Face

Disruption of the vitreous face almost always leads to vitreous in the AC.

Various surgical techniques are used to remove lens fragments from the vitreous without creating traction on the base and avoiding loss of fragments into the vitreous. The approach depends on the experience of the surgeon and the size and density of the fragments.

For large nuclei of medium density, viscoexpression of the lens fragments is recommended. This has been described above, protecting the endothelium with OVD, and a minimal (preferably dry) vitrectomy may be required.

The surgeon may need to enlarge the incision to accommodate the size of the lens fragment.

A loop may facilitate the removal of larger lens fragments. With smaller lens fragments, good surgeons may proceed

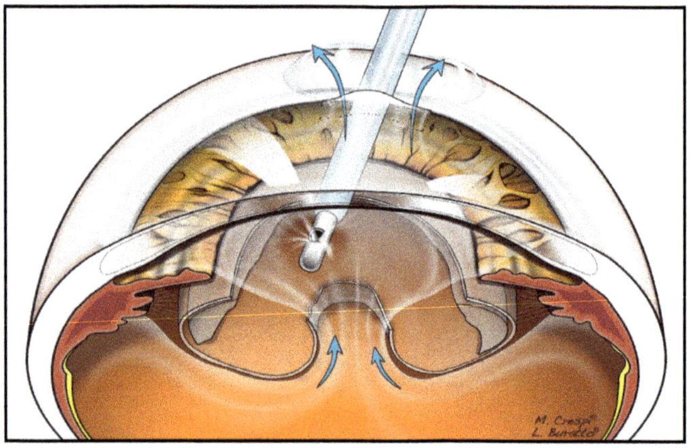

Figure 8-3. Coaxial vitrectomy. Coaxial vitrectomy has the advantage of being a one-handed procedure. The major disadvantage is the repulsion of the vitreous fibers from the mouth of the cutter and greater vitreous hydration. Hydration of the vitreous tends to extend the PCR, increasing vitreous prolapse. Another disadvantage is vitreous to the wound.

with phacoemulsification of the residual material in the AC. The surgeon then injects OVD and performs a dry anterior vitrectomy to allow free access for phaco in the AC. The flow rate should be reduced to 18 cc/min with a bottle height of approximately 50 cm and vacuum reduced to 100 mm Hg. Phacoemulsification should be done using dispersive OVD around the nucleus. Infusion should be off to avoid losing lens material before approaching it. Once there is nuclear occlusion with the tip, low flow aspiration (low flow irrigation has now been activated) can begin. Once occlusion occurs, emulsification in the AC with low ultrasound (30%) is used. This can be assisted using a Sheets glide (2.5 mm tapered to 1.75 mm x 20 mm) positioned below the fragments to avoid losing them posteriorly.

Following the removal of the nucleus, the surgeon should perform a bimanual anterior vitrectomy with separate infusion through a paracentesis using a high cut rate (at least 800 cuts/min).

Infusion into the AC may be coaxial with the vitrector or preferably through a separate incision. Coaxial vitrectomy (Figure 8-3) has the advantage of being one-handed and is familiar to the anterior segment surgeon. Its main limitation is repulsion of the vitreous, poorer vitrectomy, excess tugging on the vitreous with possible vitreous traction, retinal tears, etc (see Chapter 9). The opening of the vitrector should be oriented centrally, possibly using the side port incision (Figure 8-4A). Using the vitrector in the primary incision tends to bring more vitreous to the incision (Figure 8-4B).

The bimanual technique uses 2 paracentesis incisions—one for the infusion cannula and the other for the vitrectomy probe (small gauge is better).

With vitreous loss through the primary incision, the incision should be sutured following good vitrectomy (Figure 8-5). The technique of anterior vitrectomy will be discussed in a dedicated chapter.

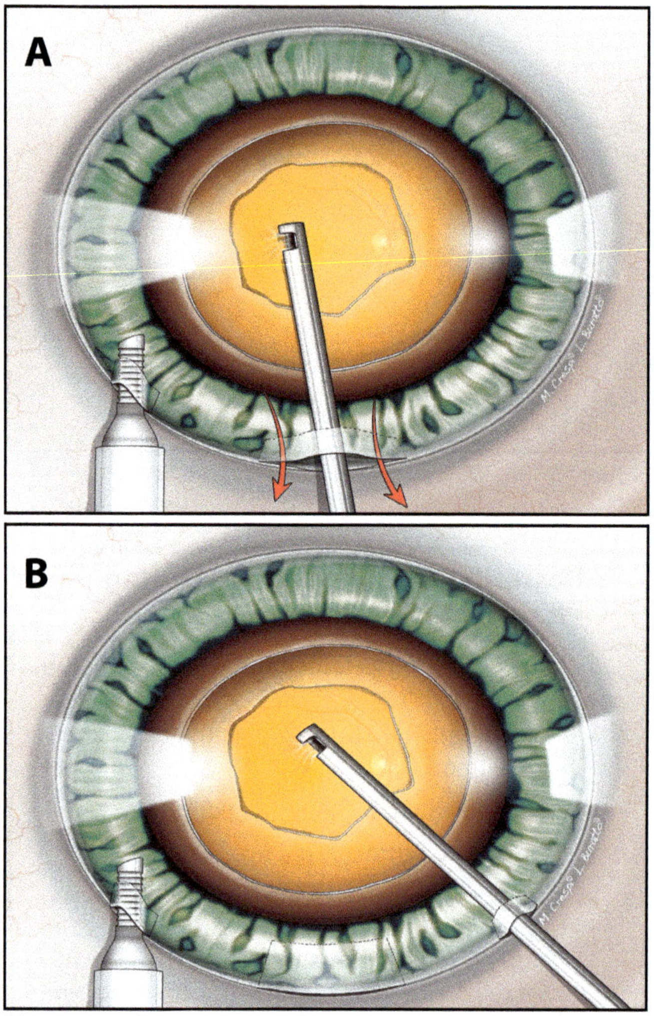

Figure 8-4. Orientation of the vitrectomy probe and corneal access. The opening of the vitrectomy probe should be oriented toward the center of the vitreous chamber, possibly through a paracentesis (A). The orientation of the vitrector directed toward the AC using the main incision will draw vitreous forward, encouraging vitreous prolapse through the primary incision (B).

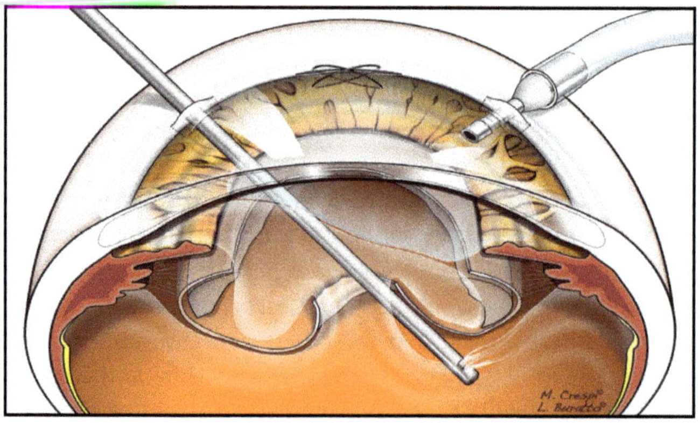

Figure 8-5. Bimanual vitrectomy. The bimanual technique involves using 2 side port incisions, an infusion cannula on one side, and the vitrector (preferably small gauge) on the other. With vitreous prolapse through the main incision, the surgeon should use a suture. The vitrector is placed posteriorly and peripherally with the opening toward the vitreous base.

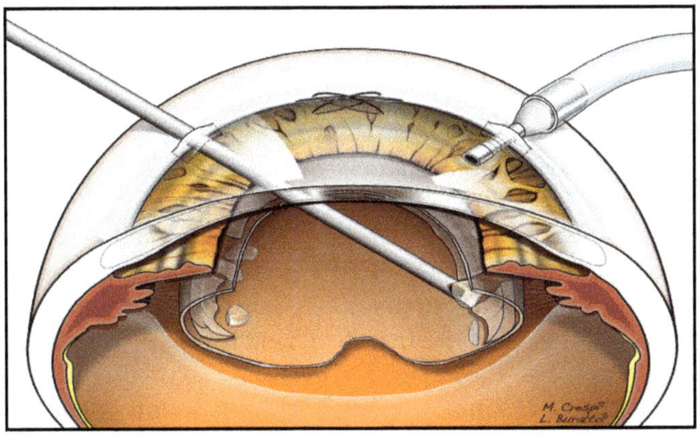

Figure 8-6. Cortical removal with the vitrectomy probe. Once vitrectomy is complete, the cutting action can be stopped and the probe can be used to remove cortex.

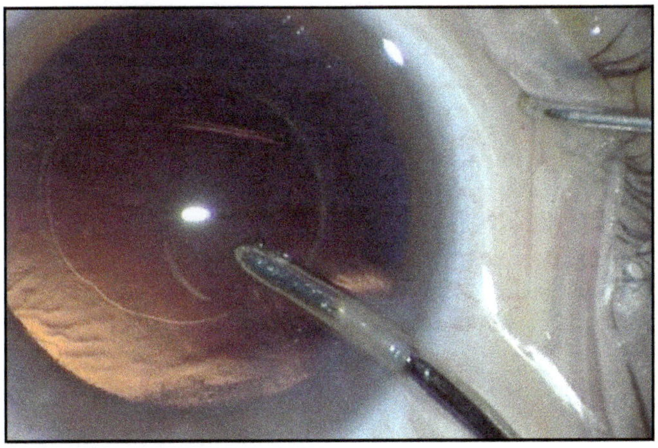

Figure C1. During the cleaning of the posterior capsule with I/A, the posterior capsule opens.

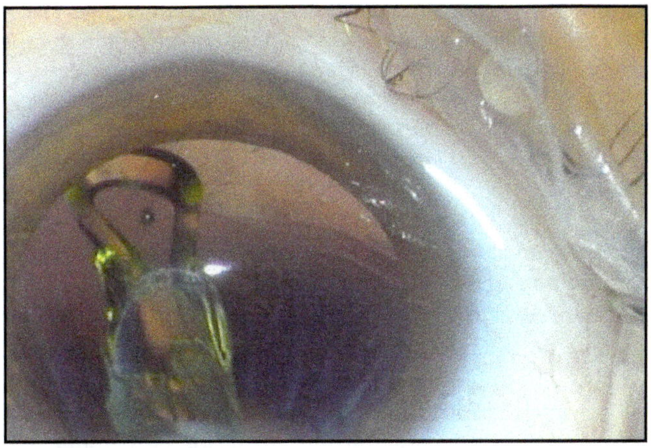

Figure C2. One-piece IOL is implanted in the capsular bag.

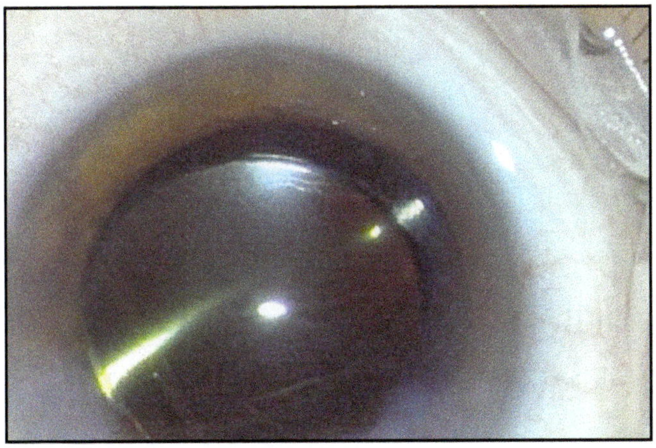

Figure C3. The IOL is properly positioned.

Once the vitrectomy is complete, cortical removal can proceed with low flow (infusion 20 to 30 mm Hg; vacuum 150 mm Hg with a 20-gauge vitrectomy [Figure 8-6]). If there is adequate capsular support, the surgeon can implant an IOL in the ciliary sulcus (a 3-piece is preferable with a minimum length of 12.5 mm; see Figures C1 to C3).[7]

Posterior Capsule Rupture With Loss of Lens Fragments Into the Vitreous

This may occur in the initial steps of surgery (during hydrodissection or rotation of the nucleus, usually loosing the entire nucleus and not just fragments) or during final emulsification of the quadrants. If the procedure is under topical anesthesia, the surgeon may elect to convert to local sub-Tenon's anesthesia.

The primary objective is to engage the nucleus in the AC without excessive vitreous traction. The preferred maneuver under these circumstances is anterior vitrectomy assisted with a loop under the nucleus.

The surgeon then makes 2 paracentesis incisions, extending the primary incision to 5 mm.

An AC maintainer is placed in one of the side incisions. A loop, introduced through the main incision, is placed under the nuclear material to be expressed.

The vitrector is introduced through a second side port incision facilitating vitrectomy while maintaining the nucleus in the AC with the loop avoiding vitreous traction (Figure 8-7).

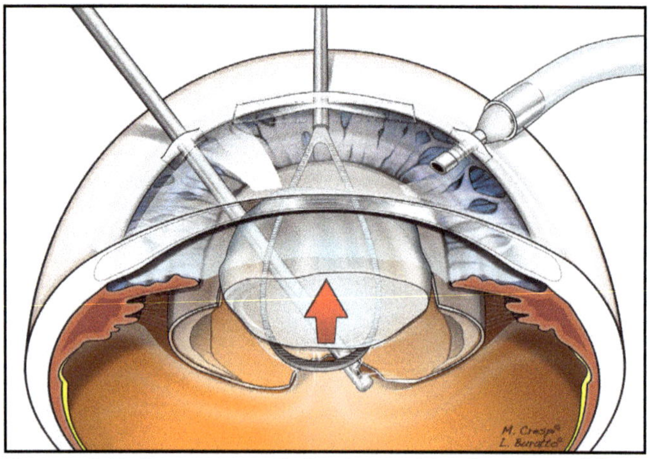

Figure 8-7. Expression of the lens with vitrectomy. Visco-expression can be assisted by a loop for larger fragments. The vitrectomy probe is placed through a second paracentesis so that it can facilitate movements of the loop, helping to avoid vitreous traction on the retina.

If the nucleus is completely dropped into the vitreous, the surgeon should use a pars plana approach with an AC maintainer, removing both the dropped nuclear material as well as the vitreous. The lens material is removed using emulsification directly in the posterior chamber or, rarely, with an extremely dense nucleus, through bringing of the nucleus into the AC, expression, followed by injection of liquid perfluorocarbon. Posterior vitrectomy will be discussed in depth in a specific chapter. These cases are typically referred to a vitreo-retinal surgeon, as the anterior segment surgeon rarely has these skills.

Vitrectomy Assisted With Triamcinolone

Use of triamcinolone may be useful to assist visualization of the vitreous. Triamcinolone acetonide (TA, 4 mg/0.1 mL) is a steroid characterized by insoluble crystals integrated in the collagen matrix, useful for visualization of the vitreous collagen fibers.[8] TA also has a proven anti-inflammatory effect further justifying its use. Recent studies have shown that a good vitrectomy, assisted with TA, greatly reduces complications.[8] Its preparation is simple, passing the TA contained in a 40-mg/mL vial through a 5-μ filter, to separate the particles of TA from its carrier.

Prognosis

Proper management of PCRs allows good functional recovery over the first 3 months with visual acuities better than 20/40 in 70% of cases.

The most common postoperative complication is cystoid macular edema, with an incidence of 9% to 35% and increased intraocular pressure on day 1 in excess of 30 mm Hg in 20% of cases.[10]

The incidence of retinal detachment was 4% after 3 years; axial length greater than 26 mm and dislocation of residual lens fragments into the vitreous increase the risk (see Figures D1 to D6, E1 to E6, and F1 to F6).[11]

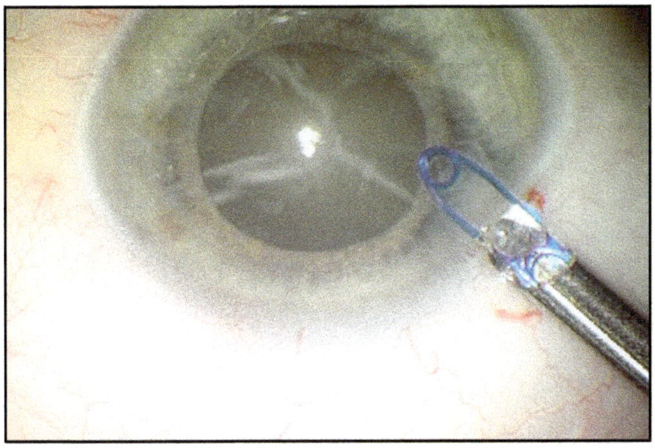

Figure D1. In a hard cataract with moderately dilated pupil, the surgeon injects a pupil dilator.

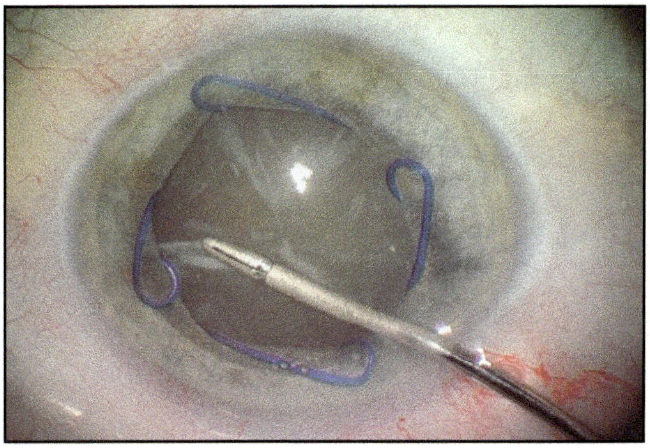

Figure D2. The pupillary dilator is in place and the capsulorrhexis is initiated with coaxial rhexis forceps.

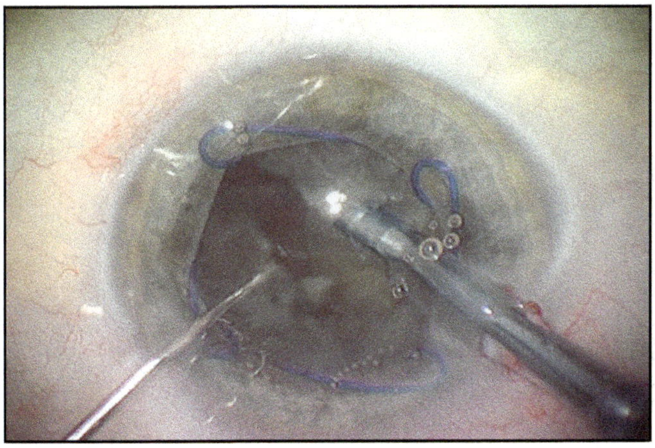

Figure D3. Phaco chop is then performed.

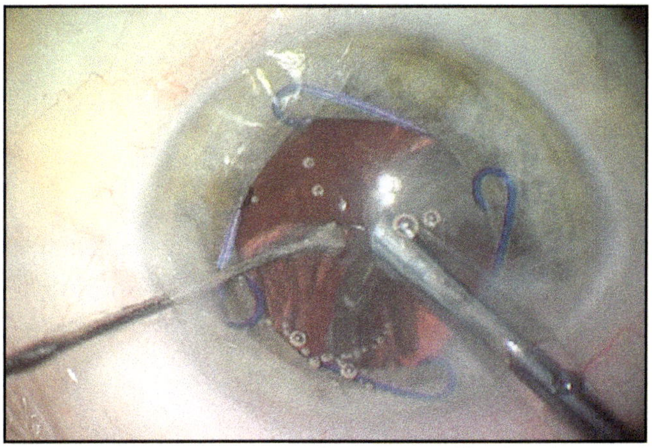

Figure D4. The posterior capsule is aspirated by the ultrasound tip and broken.

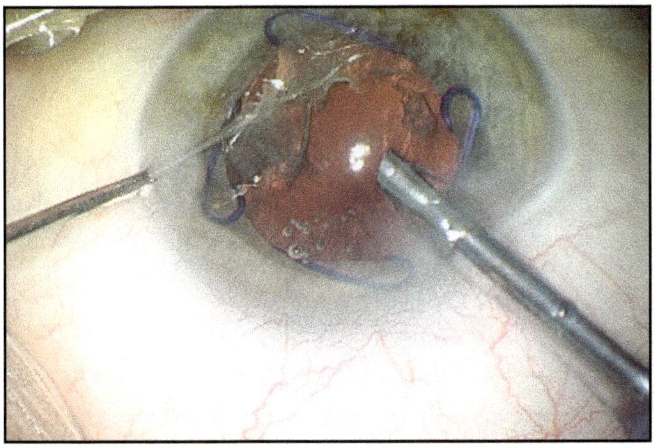

Figure D5. The nucleus is, however, largely removed. In the AC there are still some fragments.

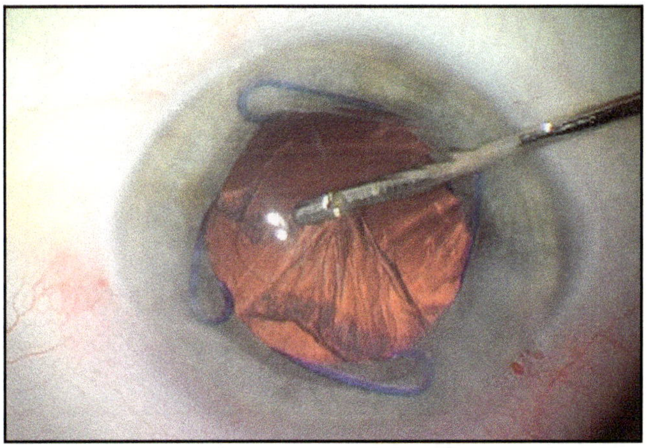

Figure D6. The fragments and the cortex are removed with I/A.

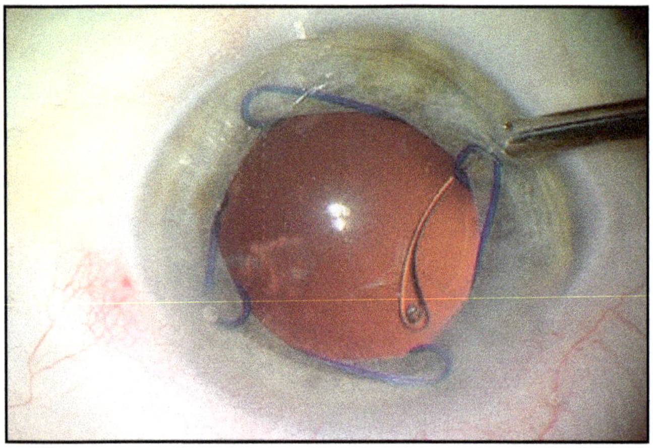

Figure E1. The surgeon decides to place a capsular tension ring even though the posterior capsule is open.

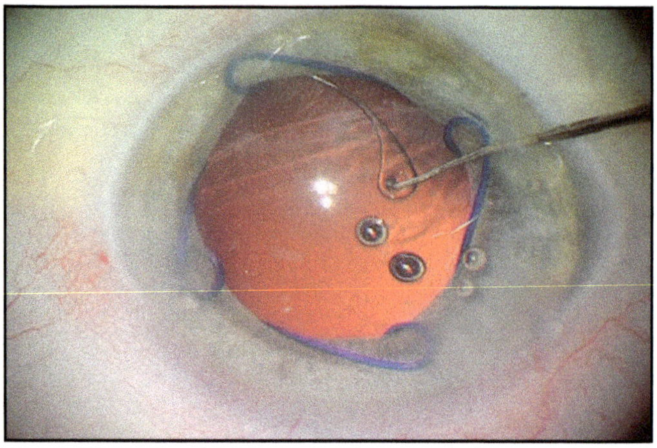

Figure E2. During this maneuver, the capsular bag is dislocated.

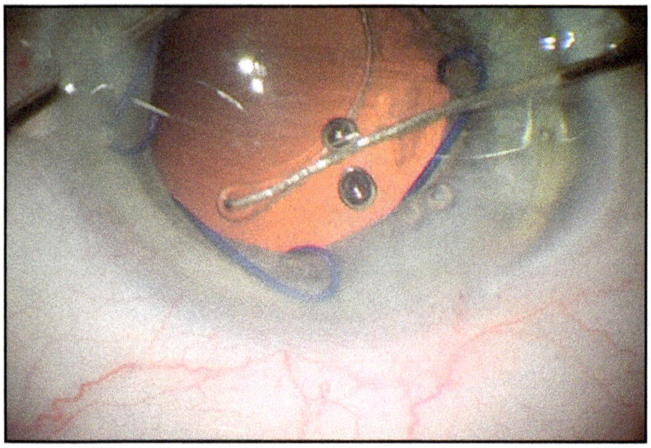

Figure E3. The surgeon, however, attempts to place the ring.

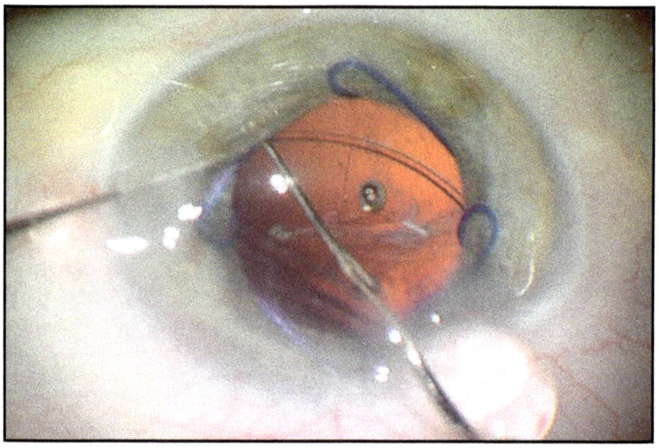

Figure E4. The capsular bag is dislocated even more.

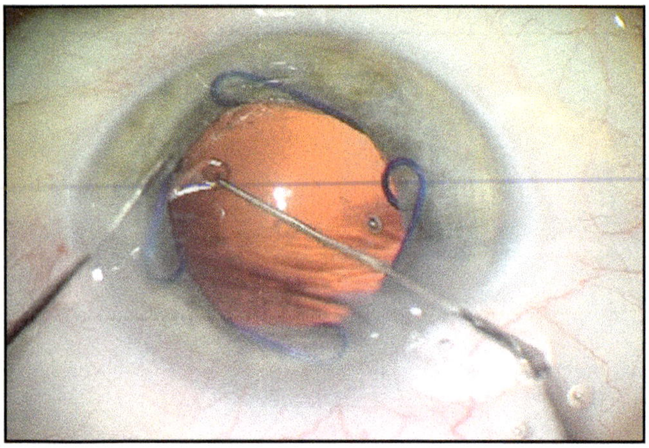

Figure E5. The surgeon decides to remove the ring.

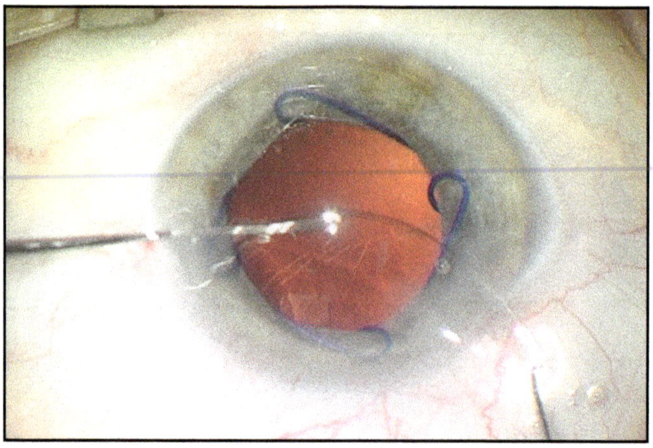

Figure E6. The ring is removed.

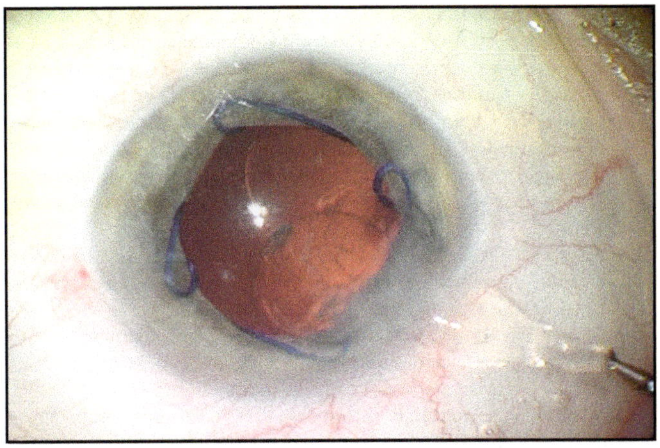

Figure F1. The surgeon decides to remove the capsular bag. He performs an intracapsular extraction through a 2.75-mm incision.

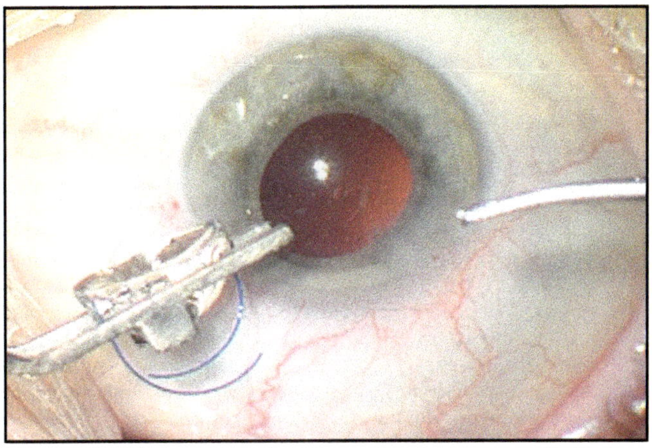

Figure F2. The surgeon decides to implant an acrylic 3-piece IOL in the posterior chamber despite the absence of the capsular bag.

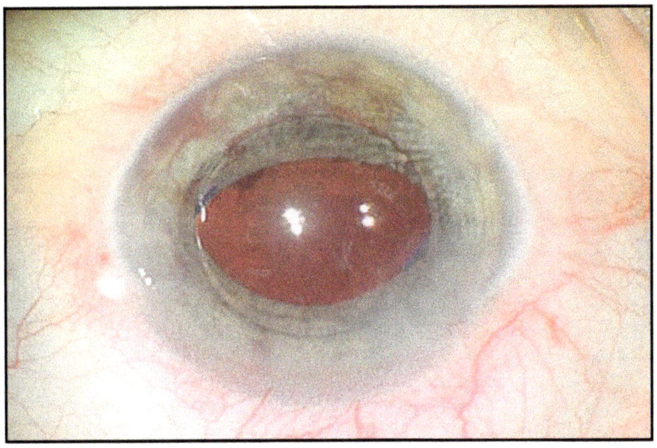

Figure F3. The surgeon places the loop behind the iris and the optic plate in front.

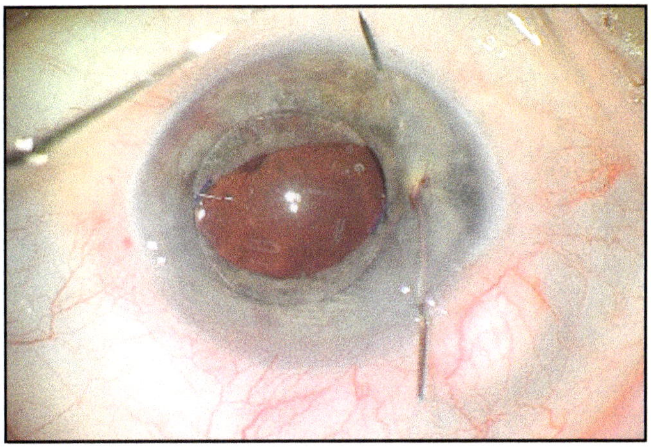

Figure F4. The surgeon performs a suture through cornea and iris, passing under the loop (probably also engaging vitreous in the suture).

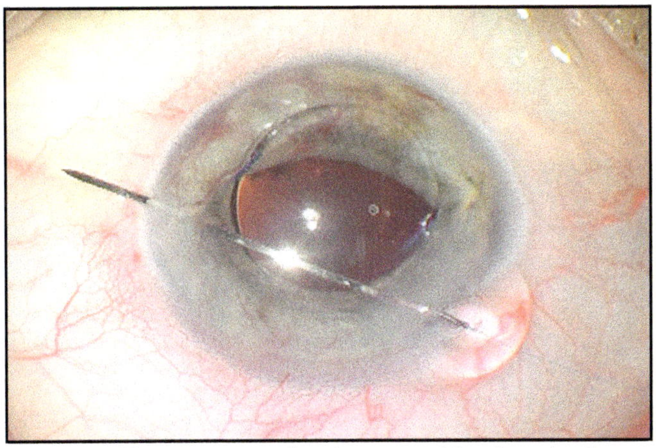

Figure F5. The same procedure is repeated for the other loop.

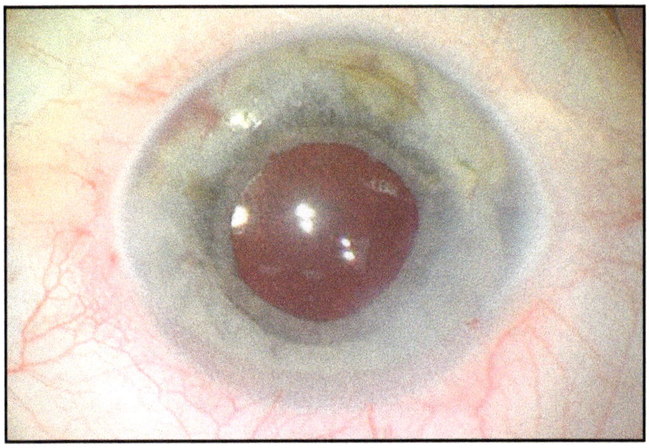

Figure F6. At the end of surgery, the IOL is placed in the posterior chamber with the 2 loops attached to the iris. Vitrectomy was not performed.

References

1. Narendran N, Jaycock P, Johnston RL, et al. The Cataract National Dataset electronic multicentre audit of 55,567 operations: risk stratification for posterior capsule rupture and vitreous loss. *Eye (Lond).* 2009;23(1):31-37.
2. Osborne SA, Adams WE, Bunce CV, Fraser SG. Validation of two scoring systems for the prediction of posterior capsule rupture during phacoemulsification surgery. *Br J Ophthalmol.* 2006;90(3):333-336.
3. Ang GS, Whyte IF. Effect and outcomes of posterior capsule rupture in a district general hospital setting. *J Cataract Refract Surg.* 2006;32(4):623-627.
4. Ionides A, Minassian D, Tuft S. Visual outcome following posterior capsule rupture during cataract surgery. *Br J Ophthalmol.* 2001;85(2):222-224.
5. Siatiri H, Moghimi S. Posterior polar cataract: minimizing risk of posterior capsule rupture. *Eye (Lond).* 2006;20(7):814-816.
6. Akura J, Hatta S, Kaneda S, et al. Management of posterior capsule rupture during phacoemulsification using the dry technique. *J Cataract Refract Surg.* 2001;27(7):982-989.
7. Brazitikos PD, Balidis MO, Tranos P, et al. Sulcus implantation of a 3-piece, 6.0 mm optic, hydrophobic foldable acrylic intraocular lens in phacoemulsification complicated by posterior capsule rupture. *J Cataract Refract Surg.* 2002;28(9):1618-1622.
8. Chang CJ, Chiang SY, Chen CL, Wang TY. Clinical outcomes of combined sutureless vitrectomy with triamcinolone stain to manage vitreous loss resulting from posterior capsule rupture during phacoemulsification. *J Cataract Refract Surg.* 2006;32(12): 2054-2059.
9. Nikica G, Ljerka HP, Jelena P, et al. Cystoid macular edema in anterior chamber lens implantation following posterior capsule rupture. *Doc Ophthalmol.* 1992;81(3):309-315.
10. Chan FM, Mathur R, Ku JJ, et al. Short-term outcomes in eyes with posterior capsule rupture during cataract surgery. *J Cataract Refract Surg.* 2003;29(3):537-541.
11. Jakobsson G, Montan P, Zetterberg M, et al. Capsule complication during cataract surgery: retinal detachment after cataract surgery with capsule complication: Swedish Capsule Rupture Study Group report 4. *J Cataract Refract Surg.* 2009;35(10):1699-1705.

9

Anterior Vitrectomy

Lucio Buratto, MD; Stephen F. Brint, MD, FACS; and Mario R. Romano, MD, PhD

Rupture of the capsular bag and vitreous prolapse into the anterior chamber (AC) requires basic knowledge of anterior vitrectomy that may be needed during surgery, having an incidence of 0.45% to 3.6%.[1-3] The surgeon's primary concern with capsular rupture is to prevent nuclear dislocation into the vitreous. Not understanding vitreous anatomy, surgeons may induce iatrogenic damage.

Chains of glycosaminoglycans and hyaluronic acid give the vitreous a gelatinous consistency that may trap lens and cortical remnants. The surgeon must remove the lens fragments without inducing vitreous traction on the retina.

Regardless of the presence or absence of residual lens material, the objective of anterior vitrectomy is to remove vitreous prolapse and sever adhesions between the vitreous and AC structures.

Complete removal of the vitreous from the AC also avoids engaging strands in the corneal incisions (responsible for traction on the vitreous base) and possibly leaving a wick from the incision to the vitreous, leading to endophthalmitis.

Vitreous prolapse can also cause corneal edema and secondary glaucoma with direct contact between the vitreous with the related structures. Finally, anterior inflammation from residual vitreous traction can lead to vitritis and cystoid macular edema. The incidence of these complications decrease with meticulous vitrectomy.[4]

Setting the Parameters

Vitrectomy requires aspiration to bring vitreous to the mouth of the vitrector, allowing the guillotine cutter to cut the vitreous. The vitreous is removed in single bites; the quantity of vitreous removed with each cut cycle is directly proportional to aspiration and inversely proportional to the cutting rate. The surgeon can control the following parameters: intraocular infusion, cut rate, aspiration, and duty cycle. Appropriate settings will minimize traction and potential damage induced by vitrectomy (Tables 9-1 and 9-2).

The anterior vitrectomy cutter is 20 gauge and has a cut rate of approximately 800 cuts/min, whereas posterior cutters are smaller (27 gauge) and can reach speeds up to 7500 cuts/minute, significantly reducing vitreous traction during vitrectomy.

With systems designed for both the anterior and posterior segments, an anterior vitrectomy may be performed with a cutter having the same cut and aspiration rate as used in posterior vitrectomy.

If available, the surgeon should perform a 25- or 27-gauge pars plana vitrectomy. By reducing the diameter of the cutter, the traction from the vitrectomy will be reduced. Another advantage of "small-gauge vitrectomy" is intraocular access through a smaller corneal paracentesis

Buratto L, Brint SF, Romano MR.
Cataract Surgery Complications (pp 75-80).
© 2013 Taylor & Francis Group.

Table 9-1

Settings for Anterior Vitrectomy

Vitrectomy	Infusion (mm Hg)	Cuts/min	Vacuum (mm Hg)
20 gauge	20 to 25	800	100 to 200

Table 9-2

Settings for Posterior Vitrectomy

Vitrectomy	Infusion (mm Hg)	Cuts/min	Vacuum (mm Hg)
20 gauge	20 to 25	3000 to 5000	100 to 200
23 gauge	25 to 30	3000 to 5000	250 to 450
25 gauge	30 to 35	3000 to 5000	400 to 600
27 gauge	35 to 40	2500 to 5000	550 to 750

incision. Using traditional 20-gauge pneumatic vitrectomy, vitreous traction increases by 4.96 dynes (7.90 dynes with electrical cutters) with each vacuum increase of 100 mm Hg. For 25-gauge pneumatic vitrectomy, vitreo-retinal traction increases by 3.40 dynes with each vacuum increase of 100 mm Hg.[5,6]

The flow leaving the cutter, in the 2 steps—liquid and viscous (vitreous)—is inversely proportional to the fourth power of the opening size and cut rate (that may reach 7500 cuts/minute). In other words, by reducing the diameter of the 25-gauge cutter and increasing the cut rate to 5000, vitrectomy will be safer with less traction, but longer surgical times.

The recent introduction of variable duty cycles allow control of cut rate, on/off time, and optimization of flow maintaining a nontractional constant flow of vitreous gel.

Adjustment of the duty cycle permits quick removal of the vitreous. For a 20-gauge vitrectomy, the surgeon sets a 75/25 on/off duty cycle with 5000 cuts for central vitrectomy; this can be reduced to 25/75 on/off duty cycle with 5000 cuts/min for a peripheral vitrectomy when close to the iris and other anterior structures.

There is not a big difference in flow in terms of the duty cycle for a 25-gauge vitrectomy with a cut rate of 5000 cuts/min. The new 25-gauge systems provide excellent performance through openings of 0.45 mm with rapid vitrectomy (flow rate of 7.8 mL/min without traction; the settings are 5000 cuts/min, 50/50 duty cycle, and vacuum of 650 mm Hg).[5,6]

Vitreous traction also depends on the quality of the vitrectomy cut. The cutter may be pneumatic (compressed air used for opening and closing with a duty cycle independent of the cut speed)[7] or electric, which currently does not allow independent regulation of the parameters. Pneumatic cutters produce a cut quality superior to that of electric cutters.

With anterior lens material, a 20-gauge approach may assist with removal of the lens fragments, adjusting aspiration flow (0 to 20 cc/min) independent of the vacuum level (useful with occlusion). If the surgeon elects to remove the lens material with the cutter, the surgeon should reduce the cut rate (1000 to 3000 cuts/min) to more easily engage lens material in the mouth of the cutter and reduce repulsion induced by a high cut rate. Finally, inflow can be compressed if the system permits (irrespective of the size of the vitrectomy instrument). Compression maintains desired intraocular pressure (IOP), reducing AC fluctuation and risk of further vitreous prolapse. If the infusion flow falls by gravity, the IOP should be kept above 20 mm Hg.

Operating in a Closed System

Vitrectomy requires a closed system in which the surgeon has direct control of settings and is able to avoid collapse of the globe and further prolapse of the vitreous.

Once a capsule rupture has been recognized, the surgeon should immediately create a closed system by doing the following:

- Stop aspiration, trying to recover lens material (aspiration only increases vitreous prolapse enlarging the capsular rupture, and increasing traction on the vitreous base [see Chapter 8 on posterior capsule rupture]).
- Maintain the phaco tip in the AC in the 0 position, remove vitreous from the primary corneal incision using a blunt spatula introduced through a paracentesis incision (rapid removal of the phaco tip induces further vitreous prolapse due to negative AC pressure).
- Remove the phaco tip slowly after having injected ophthalmic viscoelastic device (OVD) into the AC to avoid further loss of vitreous induced by negative pressure created with tip removal.
- Suture the primary corneal incision with 10-0 nylon once the tip is removed and the incision has been cleaned using a blunt spatula sweep of the incision.
- Insert an AC maintainer. The AC maintainer is positioned in the corneal side incision or in a new incision created as far as possible from the main incision and positioned so that its flow is directed toward the angle to avoid damage to the endothelium or creating turbulence further displacing lens material.

Localized Posterior Capsule Rupture

An example of localized posterior capsular rupture with moderate prolapse of vitreous in the AC, and absence of nuclear material and residual cortex involves the following:

- Introduce an AC maintainer or an infusion cannula (30 mm Hg) into the side port incision; a 25-gauge cutter with a cut rate of 5000, vacuum of 400 to 600 mm Hg.
- The main incision should be closed with 10.0 nylon. The cutter should be placed beneath the capsule rupture to avoid increasing its size induced by pulling the vitreous forward (Figure 9-1).
- After having reduced the vitreous prolapse, the surgeon examines the anterior segment; using the cutter and spatula to identify residual strands of vitreous in the AC, trapped in corneal incisions, and on the anterior iris face (Figures 9-2 and 9-3).
- The movement of the spatula must be radial to the anterior surface of the iris and the surgeon should identify individual vitreous traction forces that may distort the pupil.
- He or she should proceed with the cutter in the vitreous using external scleral indentation approximately 5 to 8 mm from the limbus. The vitreous base is cleaned (and any retinal tears treated with laser or cryotherapy). The cutter can enter through a paracentesis incision (Figure 9-4A) or for those who have greater experience with vitrectomy, through a pars plana approach using small-gauge trocars (Figure 9-4B).
- If a 25-gauge posterior vitrectomy is not available, the surgeon performs the same maneuvers, introducing the cutter through the primary incision with a greater risk of encouraging vitreous prolapse and inducing traction.

- Initially maintain a low level of positive infusion pressure (15 to 20 mm Hg) to avoid turbulence leading to dislocation of residual lens material into the vitreous.[1,8]
- Begin vitrectomy using bimanual or coaxial infusion through the corneal side port incision or through the primary incision (depending on the gauge of vitrectomy).

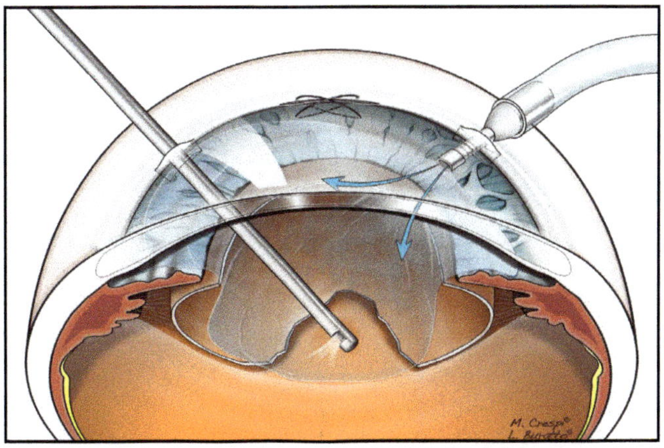

Figure 9-1. Vitreous prolapse into the AC. With PC rupture and a dropped nucleus, the surgeon should suture the primary incision with 10-0 nylon. The cutter should be positioned below the capsule tear to avoid enlarging the tear.

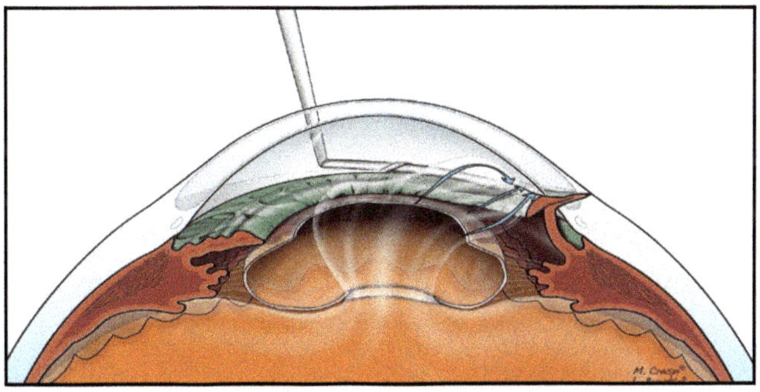

Figure 9-2. Reduction of iris distortion from trapped vitreous strands. The surgeon uses a spatula to sweep the AC from the incision to the pupil using the side port incision.

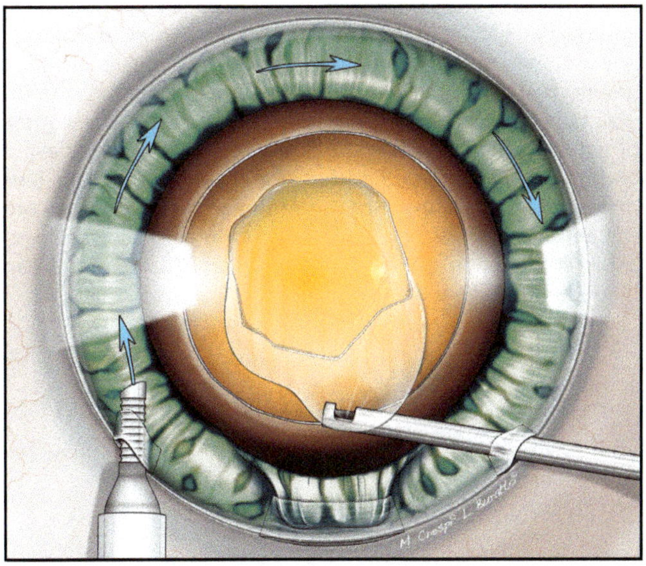

Figure 9-3. Prolapse of vitreous and iris through the primary incision. With vitreous through the primary incision, the surgeon should first remove vitreous prolapse using the vitrectomy probe through a corneal side port incision. The cutter must engage the vitreous strands with movement from the edge of the iris toward the pupil, cutting prolapsed vitreous. Then the surgeon reduces iris prolapse using a blunt spatula.

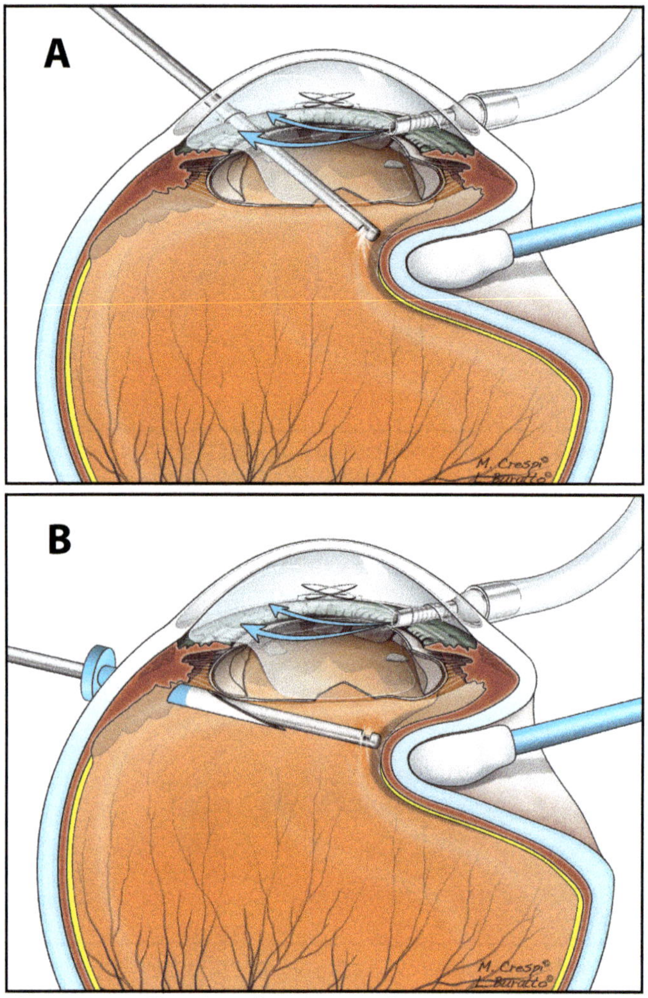

Figure 9-4. Cleaning the vitreous base. The cutter enters through a (A) corneal paracentesis or (B) pars plana using a small-gauge trocar. The procedure continues with the cutter in the vitreous with simultaneous external scleral indentation approximately 5 to 8 mm from the limbus. An AC maintainer is positioned in a paracentesis allowing adequate infusion, freeing both hands to perform a bimanual technique. The AC maintainer should be placed in an existing incision in the cornea or a new incision directing the flow toward the angle to avoid endothelial damage and turbulence that can dislocate lens material. The opening of the cutter should be oriented toward the peripheral retina. Cleaning the vitreous base allows release of vitreous traction and allows detection of retinal tears that can be treated with laser or cryotherapy.

Anterior Vitrectomy Strategy

Bimanual Approach

A bimanual technique is recommended, including an anterior infusion line, an AC maintainer, and 2 corneal paracentesis incisions, one for the cutter and another for a second instrument[9] (see Figure 9-4). Alternately, the surgeon can hold the infusion cannula in one hand and the cutter in the other (see Figure 9-3).

The advantages of this technique include the following:

- Greater freedom of movement for the 2 instruments inside the AC.
- Separate infusion allows the surgeon to maintain constant IOP without obstructing vitreous removal by the cutter. Infusion pressure varies from 20 to 30 mm Hg depending on the gauge of the cutter used (see previous).
- The vitrectomy probe without coaxial irrigation (particularly if it is small-gauge) will have a diameter smaller than the phaco tip and may also be inserted through a side port incision; this has the advantage of reducing traction and vitreous involvement (see Chapter 8 on posterior capsule rupture).
- Separate the aspiration/cutter from the infusion.
- Keep the infusion line anteriorly to keep the flow forward to avoid hydrating the vitreous, which will encourage more prolapse.
- Clean the vitreous base by using external scleral indentation, orienting the opening of the cutter toward the extreme peripheral retina. Three-hundred and sixty degrees of the retinal base should always be cleaned. The surgeon should move the AC maintainer into the second corneal incision then insert the cutter through the first incision (see Figure 9-4).

Disadvantages of the bimanual technique include the following:

- Additional side port incisions are required.
- More experience with the instrumentation is needed with a bimanual approach.

One-Handed Technique

The vitrectomy uses coaxial infusion with an anterior vitrectomy and is normally used by the cataract surgeon. This approach, however, is no longer recommended.

Advantages associated with this approach include the following:

- Infusion and vitreous removal with a single instrument.
- The anterior segment surgeon is more comfortable with a single instrument through the main corneal incision.

Disadvantages of the one-handed technique include the following:

- Coaxial infusion pushes the vitreous away from the mouth of the cutter.
- The infusion movements parallel those of the cutter (even when the cutter is behind the pupil) with hydration of the vitreous extending the capsular rupture and increasing vitreous prolapse.

- Placing the cutter in the primary incision allows escape of the vitreous, enhanced by positive intraocular pressure.

In cases where it is not possible to perform a vitrectomy, the surgeon must treat vitreous prolapse by wecking the vitreous to the outside of the incision with Merocel wecks, cutting the vitreous strands with scissors. This maneuver should be done only when there is no alternative, as it will exert significant traction on the vitreous.

Intraoperative Adjuvants

The use of substances that enhance visibility of a semitransparent structure like the vitreous allows better management of the anterior vitrectomy. The most popular is triamcinolone (TA), a steroid well known for its anti-inflammatory properties.[11] In 2003, Burk was the first to describe the use of TA in the management of complications in cataract surgery.[10] The water insoluble crystals of TA bind to the collagen matrix and enhance vitreous fibrils.

Preparation requires passage through a 5-micron filter to separate the TA particles from the carrier. The surgeon should initially inject approximately 0.5 mL of TA to visualize the vitreous fibers.

Injection of TA can be repeated during vitrectomy; this allows the surgeon to ensure that all vitreous traction has been removed. If a large amount of TA is injected at the first sign of vitreous, the surgeon loses anatomical references and actually has poorer visualization.

Advantages associated with the use of TA include the following:

- Improvement of anterior vitrectomy in terms of efficiency and time required.
- Avoidance of steps that increase vitreous traction.
- Inhibition of biosynthetic pathways of arachidonic acid reducing inflammation and stabilizing the internal blood retinal barrier.[11]

Completing the Operation

Once the anterior segment and pupil are free of vitreous, and the vitreous is below the pupil, the surgeon proceeds with cortical removal. Aspiration of the cortex can be performed with irrigation/aspiration (I/A) or by using the cutter with cutting turned off (300 to 500 mm Hg). Infusion is from the AC maintainer or the infusion cannula (Figure 9-5). If the vitrectomy is performed correctly, OVD is not required. Prior to lens implantation, the space between the anterior capsule (hopefully with the rhexis intact) and the posterior iris is opened with OVD immediately under the iris. Implantation of a 1-piece IOL is not recommended; a large 3-piece lens is preferable and should be implanted in the sulcus.

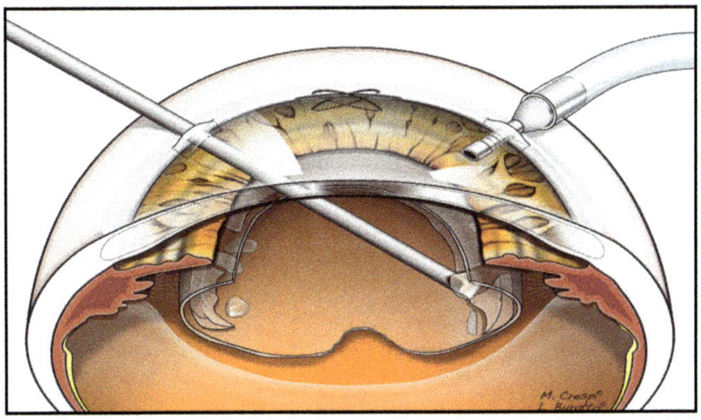

Figure 9-5. Removal of lens/cortex remnants. Aspiration of the cortex can be performed using I/A or with the cutter (cutting inactive; 300 to 500 mm Hg) with continuous infusion by the AC maintainer or the infusion cannula.

Finally, the surgeon should use an intraoperative miotic to highlight residual strands of vitreous that may distort the pupil margin. An air bubble injected in the AC may prove useful. The surface tension generated by the air liquid interface (approximately 70 mN/m) creates an air bubble, enhancing residual anterior vitreous traction.[19]

If vitreous traction is detected after implantation, the surgeon should free it using a spatula moving from the edge of the iris toward the pupil. If deformation of the iris persists, the surgeon should perform the vitrectomy again anterior and posterior to the IOL. If vitreous involvement still persists, the surgeon should proceed with a pars plana approach.

References

1. Gimbel HV, Sun R, Ferensowicz M, Anderson Penno E, Kamal A. Intraoperative management of posterior capsule tears in phacoemulsification and intraocular lens implantation. *Ophthalmology.* 2001;108(12):2186-2189; discussion 2190-2192.
2. Ng DT, Rowe NA, Francis IC, et al. Intraoperative complications of 1,000 phacoemulsification procedures: a prospective study. *J Cataract Refract Surg.* 1998;24(10):1390-1395.
3. Lundstrom M, Barry P, Leite E, Seward H, Stenevi U. 1998 European Cataract Outcome Study: report from the European Cataract Outcome Study Group. *J Cataract Refract Surg.* 2001;27(8):1176-1184.
4. Chang CJ, Chiang SY, Chen CL, Wang TY. Clinical outcomes of combined sutureless vitrectomy with triamcinolone stain to manage vitreous loss resulting from posterior capsule rupture during phacoemulsification. *J Cataract Refract Surg.* 2006;32(12):2054-2059.
5. Hubschman JP, Bourges JL, Tsui I, Reddy S, Yu F, Schwartz SD. Effect of cutting phases on flow rate in 20-, 23-, and 25-gauge vitreous cutters. *Retina.* 2009;29(9):1289-1293.
6. Hubschman JP, Gupta A, Bourla DH, Culjat M, Yu F, Schwartz SD. 20-, 23-, and 25-gauge vitreous cutters: performance and characteristics evaluation. *Retina.* 2008;28(2):249-257.

7. Peyman GA, Livir-Rallatos C, Canakis C, Easley J. A new high-speed pneumatic vitrectomy cutter. *Am J Ophthalmol.* 2002;133(4):568-569.
8. Jacobs PM. Vitreous loss during cataract surgery: prevention and optimal management. *Eye (Lond).* 2008;22(10):1286-1289.
9. Murray RG, Tipler HA. Reduction of vitreous loss in cataract surgery. *Can J Ophthalmol.* 1966;1(1):71-76.
10. Burk SE, Da Mata AP, Snyder ME, Schneider S, Osher RH, Cionni RJ. Visualizing vitreous using Kenalog suspension. *J Cataract Refract Surg.* 2003;29(4):645-651.
11. Valamanesh F, Berdugo M, Sennlaub F, et al. Effects of triamcinolone acetonide on vessels of the posterior segment of the eye. *Mol Vis.* 2009;15:2634-2648.

10

Posterior Vitrectomy

Lucio Buratto, MD; Stephen F. Brint, MD, FACS; and Mario R. Romano, MD, PhD

Rupture of the posterior capsule can result in loss of lens fragments into the vitreous. The incidence varies from 0.3% to 1.1%.[1,2] The anterior segment surgeon must be prepared to minimize the damage with broken zonules and the entire natural lens, or the intraocular lens (IOL) may dislocate. A posterior vitrectomy, necessary because of intraoperative complications, may be performed at this time or as a secondary procedure.

Simultaneous Posterior Vitrectomy

Intraoperative conversion from phacoemulsification to a posterior vitrectomy requires skills of a vitreo-retinal surgeon, staff specialized in posterior segment surgery, and dedicated equipment. Intraoperative management is preferable but cannot be improvised if the requirements described above are missing.

The first problem occurring with an intraoperative posterior approach is the necessity of local/regional anesthesia. Sub-Tenon's anesthesia is preferred as previously described.[3] This provides good analgesia but poor akinesia. It is important to remember that incorrect attempts to recover the nucleus using phaco can further complicate the situation. Phaco aspiration will engage vitreous, preventing phaco from reaching it, and emulsifying dispersed lens fragments. This may result in vitreous traction, leading to retinal tears and possible detachment.

Posterior vitrectomy must follow closure of the primary corneal incision and adequate anterior vitrectomy freeing anterior structures, removing all vitreous anterior to the anterior capsule and any vitreous strands to the corneal incisions. If performed within 7 days of the rupture, an anterior vitrectomy will significantly reduce the risk of secondary glaucoma.[4]

Anterior vitrectomy has been previously described. The surgeon prepares 3 ports for posterior vitrectomy: one is anterior, using the anterior chamber (AC) maintainer; the other 2 are pars plana 3.5 mm posterior to the limbus. The use of the AC maintainer avoids the need for an additional posterior sclerotomy but may induce corneal distortion during the vitrectomy maneuvers if not positioned correctly (the surgeon should direct the flow of the AC maintainer toward the angle and not toward the epithelium or the vitreous).[5]

Buratto L, Brint SF, Romano MR.
Cataract Surgery Complications (pp 81-88).
© 2013 Taylor & Francis Group.

AC Maintainer

The AC maintainer should not be used in the following cases:

- In patients with a low endothelial cell count as it induces turbulence that can lead to even greater endothelial cell loss.
- When there are associated retinal tears and retinal detachment (situations requiring intra- and postoperative intraocular tamponade). Here, one should avoid using an AC maintainer and create 3 pars plana ports.

Posterior Vitrectomy Later

Posterior vitrectomy can usually be postponed if the equipment, staff, etc are not readily available or if there are problems with the patient (pain, opacity of the media, choroidal detachment). With lens remnants smaller than 2 mm, anterior segment surgeons usually prefer to avoid an immediate posterior approach and postpone surgery, monitoring the clinical situation. The surgeon should proceed with removal of pieces larger than 2 mm if there is chronic inflammation, persistent macular edema, increase of intraocular pressure, or suspicion of endophthalmitis.[6]

Performing the vitrectomy later gives the surgeon the advantage of being able to plan surgery after a careful postoperative examination. The surgeon should repeat the biometry to calculate the most suitable IOL; the calculation must be adjusted for sulcus implantation (the new effective lens position), or with iris or scleral sutures if there is a lack of anterior capsular support.

Corneal edema from the previous surgery, vitreous in contact with the endothelium, and excessively high or low intraocular pressure (IOP) may be good reasons for postponing the vitrectomy due to inadequate visualization of the posterior structures. With corneal edema, the surgeon removes the epithelium prior to performing intraocular maneuvers. With marked stromal opacities and possible endophthalmitis, requiring immediate intervention, the surgeon should wait and treat the eye with osmotic and pressure-lowering drugs.

If the clinical conditions allow, he or she should also perform gonioscopy to look for lens fragments and vitreous in the angle, sometimes stimulating formation of iridocorneal synechiae (secondary glaucoma).

A "B" scan is recommended with marked media opacity. This may provide important information on location of lens fragments, characteristics of the vitreous, and unrecognized retinal detachment. It is also important with suspicion of endophthalmitis.

Surgical Technique of Vitrectomy and Phacofragmentation

The surgical technique involves a 3-way approach for complete removal of the vitreous. The surgeon proceeds initially with complete posterior detachment of the vitreous, and continues with a large-core vitrectomy to the equator and then to the periphery of the retina (Figure 10-1).

Once the lens fragments have been released from adhesions, the surgeon removes them. Even with high vacuum and a low cut rate, the cutter is able to remove the cortex of the lens; however, it is unlikely that it will be able to fragment and aspirate the harder nuclear fragments. In these cases, a posterior phacoemulsification procedure is necessary to emulsify and remove the residual fragments, freed from vitreous adhesions (Figure 10-2A). The surgeon should also clean the vitreous base using external scleral indentation to release any fragments that are adhered to the anterior vitreous (Figure 10-2B).

Vitrectomy

Vitreous removal requires a level of aspiration able to attract the vitreous to the opening of the cutter and guillotine cutting the vitreous. The vitreous is removed in single bites and the amount of vitreous removed with each cut is inversely proportional to the cut rate (see Table 9-2).

Removal of the vitreous must be performed with settings that will create low traction but also remove the vitreous rapidly and efficiently. The cutting rate of the currently available posterior vitrectomy systems can reach a speed of 7500 cuts/minute; the surgeon can adjust the speed to suit the needs of the vitrectomy. The duty cycle of the vitrectomy is defined by the "time the tip is open" by the "total time" of the cut cycle. A shave vitrectomy uses the duty cycle to further reduce induced traction; this is already low because of the high cutting speed. In surgical practice, most of the situations are managed by an "open" duty cycle that allows excellent efficiency, despite having a cut rate of 5,000 cpm, translating into very low traction.[7,8]

Prior to removal of the lens fragments, it is necessary to create a posterior vitreous detachment. This is followed by aspiration with radial movements of the peripupillary vitreous, with a cutter with the cut mode turned off starting from the margin of the optic. Posterior vitreous detachment (PVD) is an important requisite for total removal of the vitreous (avoiding incomplete PVD with vitreodissection with vitreous cortex) and vitreous traction.

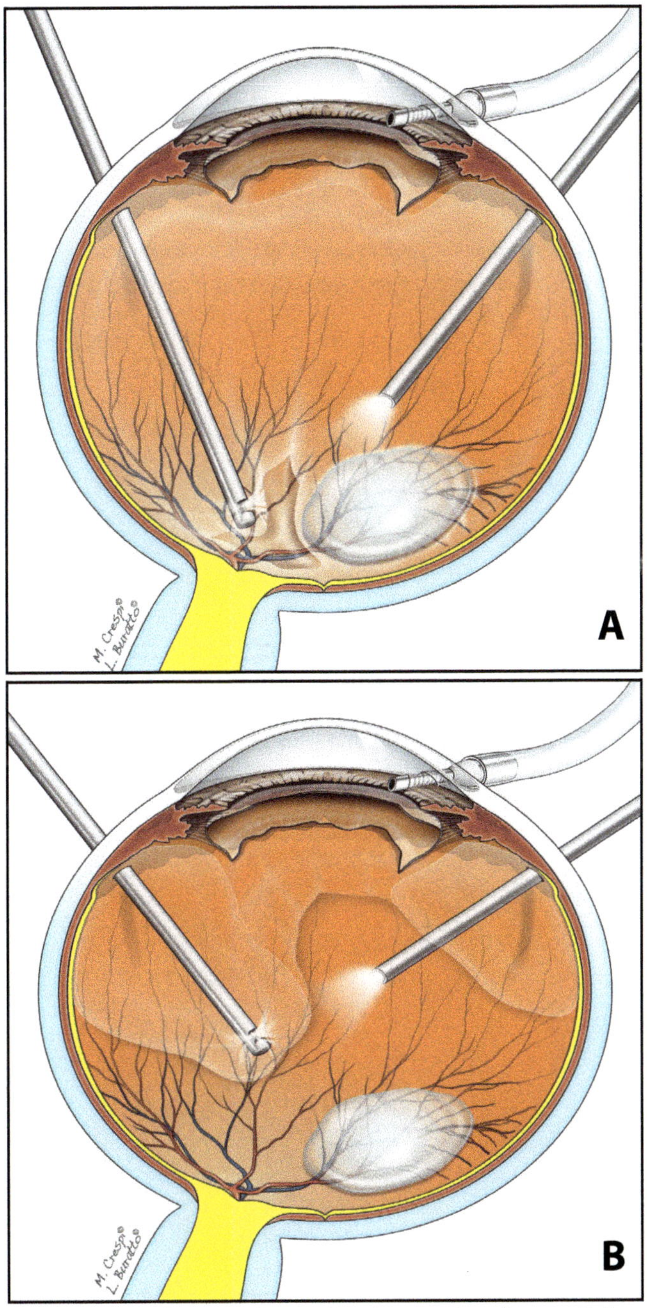

Figure 10-1. Induction of posterior vitreous detachment. Before removing lens fragments, the surgeon should induce a posterior vitreous detachment. (A) The surgeon should aspirate the peripupillary vitreous with radial movements using the cutter (cutting function turned off) starting from the edge of the optic disk to obtain total detachment from the pupil. The induction of PVD is an important step in total removal of the vitreous and vitreous tractions. The absence of PVD leads to an increased incidence of retinal tears during vitrectomy. (B) The surgeon proceeds with a central and a peripheral vitrectomy.

The removal of lens fragments with vitrectomy is possible if they are cortical or smaller than 2 mm. In order to optimize vitrectomy, the duty cycle should be set in the open mode (75% of the duty cycle with the cutter open) and a low cut rate. The cutter will then be able to aspirate more material and repel less. Additional assistance can be achieved by increasing aspiration and vacuum. These parameters create greater traction and consequently require a more accurate vitrectomy.

The Use of Perfluorocarbon Liquid

Perfluorocarbon liquid (PFCL) is a high-density semi-transparent intraoperative tamponade (1.7 to 1.9 g/dL) with a surface tension in water of 50 mN/m. The high density stabilizes the retina if it is mobile, protects the posterior pole from any touch of nuclear fragments to the macular region, and finally allows the nuclear fragments to float on the surface of the bubble. Through the Van der Waals forces at the interface, the high surface tension keeps the tamponade in a single bubble.

Aggressive aspiration and inspiration (ie, direct contact between the infusion cannula and the anterior surface of the bubble of PFCL) may split the bubble of PFCL.

The risk associated with formation of multiple tiny bubbles, or "fish eggs," is associated with the passage of the bubble into the subretinal space through any tears. The passage of PFCL beneath the retina creates direct contact between the bubble and the pigmented epithelium, inducing atrophy and irreversible damage to the retina.

Removal of PFCL must always be performed at the end of the surgery because the chemical characteristics and the low viscosity (2 to 3 cSt) stimulate postoperative inflammatory responses. The removal of PFCL should pass through an air exchange, avoiding direct PFC oil exchange particularly if a high-density oil is used (consisting of semifluorinate, alkanes, or ethers that are soluble in PFCL).

Phacofragmentation

Phacofragmentation of the lens is performed with initial aspiration parameters of approximately 150 mm Hg and ultrasound power of approximately 10%; these parameters are then changed depending on the density of the lens. The fragments can be removed from the posterior chamber or directly through the incision into the AC. Small fragments are easy to remove with linear aspiration directly from the retinal surface with the phaco tip (Figure 10-2).

If the surgeon prefers phacofragmentation in the posterior chamber, a bubble of PFCL (approximately 2 mL) should be injected to protect the posterior pole during the maneuvers of aspiration and fragmentation (Figure 10-3A). The surgical technique involves engaging the lens fragment with aspiration and with aspiration active, the surgeon can initiate fragmentation at the center of the vitreous chamber assisted by a light pipe or by a cyclodialysis spatula. This keeps the fragments close to the phaco tip and will reduce repulsion (Figure 10-3B). At the end of phacofragmentation, it is difficult to remove small lens pieces that cannot be aspirated with the Charles needle. In these cases, the surgeon should perform posterior phaco with ultrasound deactivated and low parameters of aspiration.

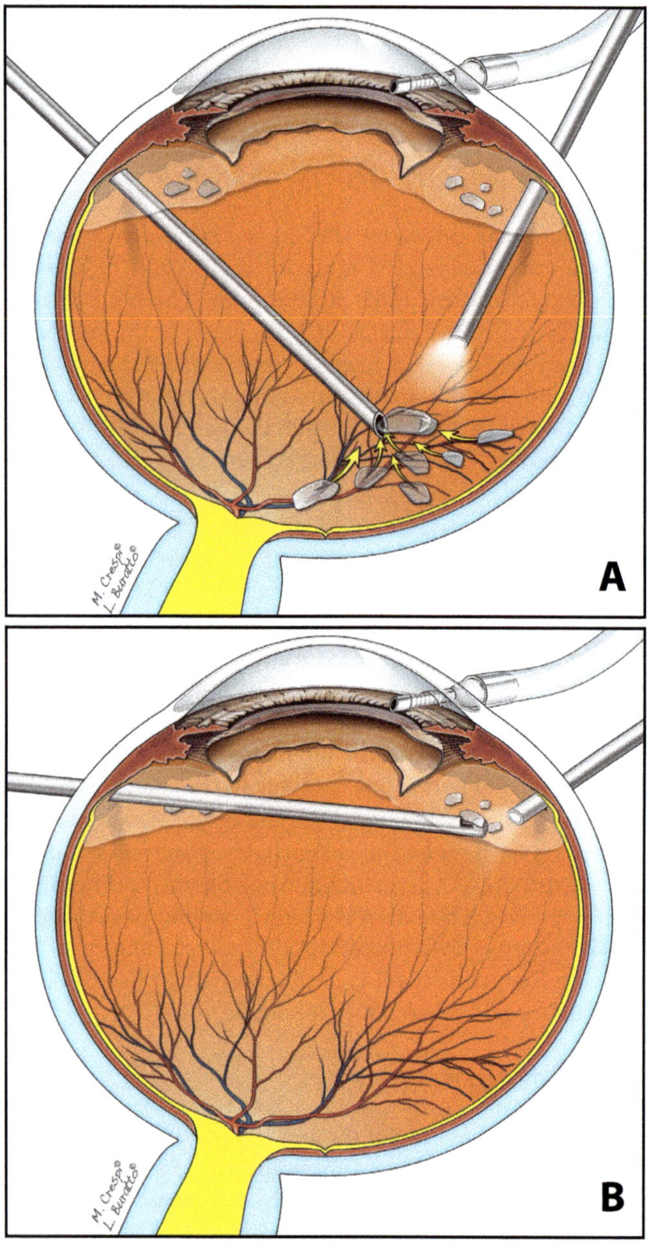

Figure 10-2. Removal of multiple lens fragments from the surface of the retina. (A) Once the vitreous has been removed, tiny residual lens fragments can be removed easily, with aspiration at approximately 150 mm Hg, directly with the phaco tip near the retina. (B) The surgeon then examines the eye very carefully, performing accurate cleaning of the periphery where the lens fragments can be trapped near the vitreous base.

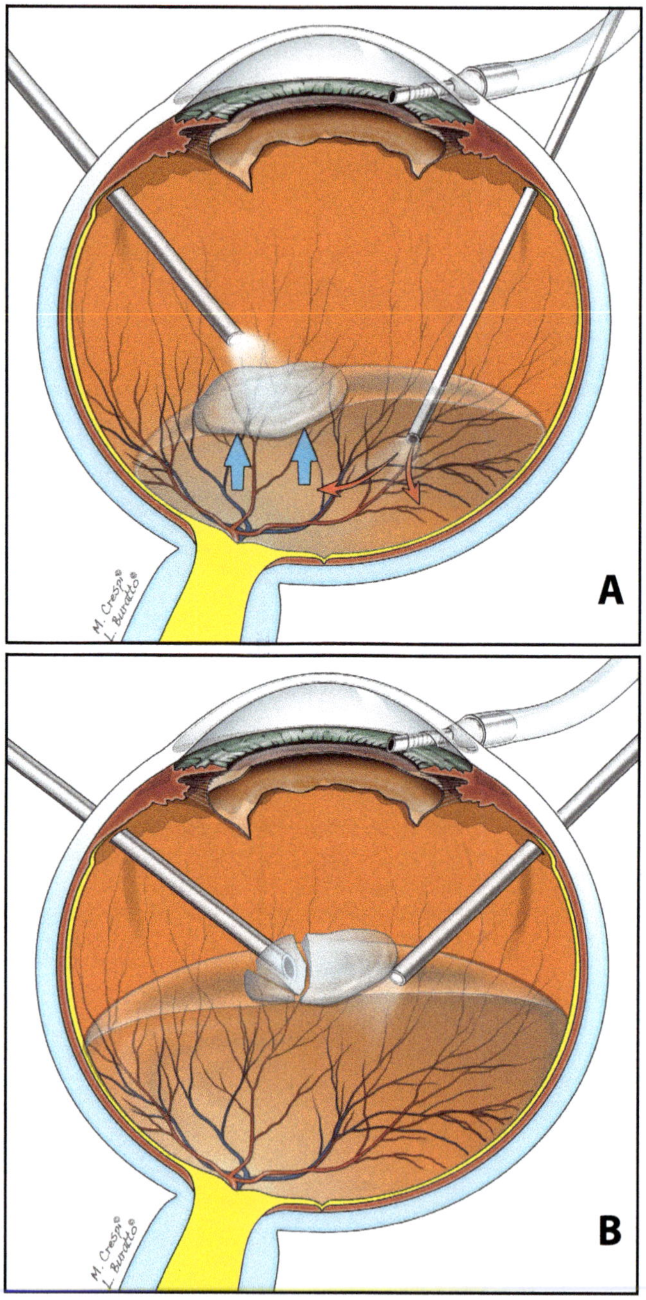

Figure 10-3. Phacofragmentation in the vitreous chamber. (A) With phacofragmentation in the posterior chamber, the surgeon should use a bubble of PFCL (approximately 2 mL) to protect the posterior pole during aspiration and fragmentation maneuvers. The surgical technique involves engaging the lens material with aspiration and, while maintaining active aspiration, beginning fragmentation at the center of the vitreous chamber. (B) This can be facilitated with a light pipe that also facilitates fragmentation and keeps the fragments close to the phaco tip, reducing repulsion.

Management of Posterior Vitrectomy

If the surgeon cannot perform posterior vitrectomy, he or she should do the following:

- Avoid chasing fragments with the phaco tip.
- Perform an anterior vitrectomy to clear the corneal incisions.
- If possible, remove lens fragments from the angle and from the AC using viscoexpression.
- Suture corneal incisions.

If the surgeon can proceed with posterior vitrectomy, he or she should do the following:

- Create a posterior detachment of the vitreous prior to manipulation or removal of lens material.
- Perform a total vitrectomy.
- Use only minimal amounts of PFCL to protect the macula.
- Remove cortical fragments with the cutter using low parameters (low cut frequency, open duty cycle, high levels of aspiration and vacuum).
- Remove nuclear fragments with posterior phaco using low ultrasound power.
- Always examine the peripheral retina at the end of the procedure.
- If there is any doubt, perform a 360-degree endolaser treatment.

Technique of Posterior-Assisted Levitation of Lens Material

Under special conditions, particularly when the nucleus is extremely dense, it is possible to fill the vitreous cavity with PFCL to elevate the lens into the AC. PFCL, injected from the sclerotomy below the fragments, has a high density that allows the lens to float on the anterior surface of the bubble (Figure 10-4A).[9,10]

During progressive filling of the vitreous chamber with PFCL, the lens fragments may disappear beneath the iris diaphragm (they are dislocated into the meniscus of the bubble) and disappear from view. In this case, the surgeon should continue filling with PFCL to the iris diaphragm and mechanically dislodge the fragments to the center of the pupil using a blunt spatula. The fragments can be emulsified and aspirated in the vitreous chamber (low parameters of vacuum and aspiration, 100 mm Hg/20 cc/min [Figure 10-4B]) or the surgeon can continue adding PFCL beyond the iris diaphragm (Figure 10-4C). When it reaches the AC, the nucleus can be expressed through an incision large enough for expression.

Retinal Detachment and Intraoperative Prophylaxis

Retinal detachment may be associated with traction induced during the cataract operation by careless vitrectomy. If the surgeon is aware of retinal detachment in the presence of the nucleus in the posterior chamber, the posterior vitrectomy will need to remove the lens fragments, avoiding the mobile retina that will require tamponade and stability.

With retinal stability, some surgeons prefer to place an indented equatorial scleral band prior to proceeding with vitrectomy. The objective is to distend the traction on the vitreous base, facilitate removal of anterior vitreous, and ensure adequate indentation of the peripheral retina. Scleral indentation is not always necessary. The use of PFCL is always recommended as it will stabilize a loose retina that may otherwise interfere with the maneuvers for removal of the lens fragments and eventually induce additional damage.

Once the lens material has been removed, the surgeon proceeds with endolaser treatment or cryo of the retinal tear under an air bubble or PFCL.

A vitreous tamponade of lower density (air, gas, light oil) or higher density (heavy oil) depending on the position and shape of the tear is performed. The surgeon should also perform an inferior or superior mechanical iridectomy, the choice depending on the tamponade used (the position of the iridectomy should be opposite from the action of the tamponade; ie, with heavy silicone oil, the surgeon should perform the iridectomy at 12 o'clock).

While the tamponade is inside the eye, the surgeon should not proceed with implantation of an IOL in the sulcus because of problems of possible dislocation.

At the end of surgery, even when there is no retinal detachment, the surgeon must examine the peripheral retina to look for any rhegmatogenous areas that can be treated intraoperatively with laser photocoagulation. It is also possible to perform a prophylactic pre-equatorial intraoperative laser treatment even when retinal tears are absent. This leads to a significant reduction in retinal detachment—namely 1.3%, compared to approximately 10% ($P = 0.024$).[11]

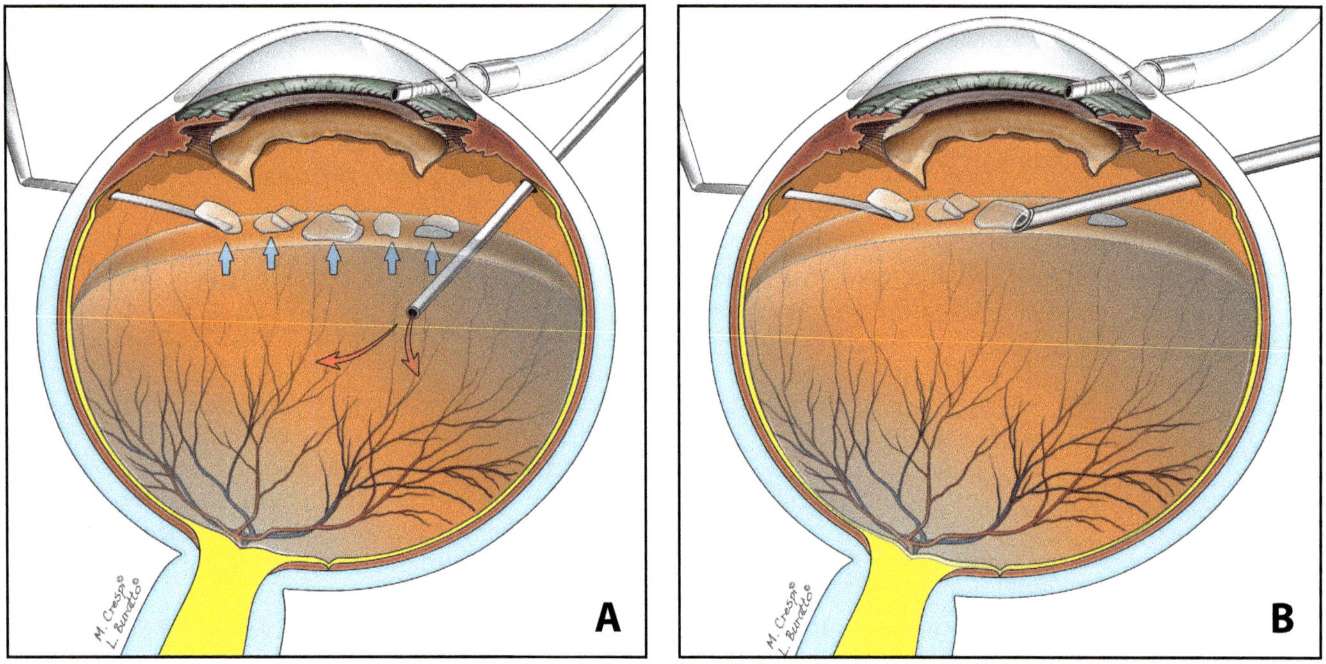

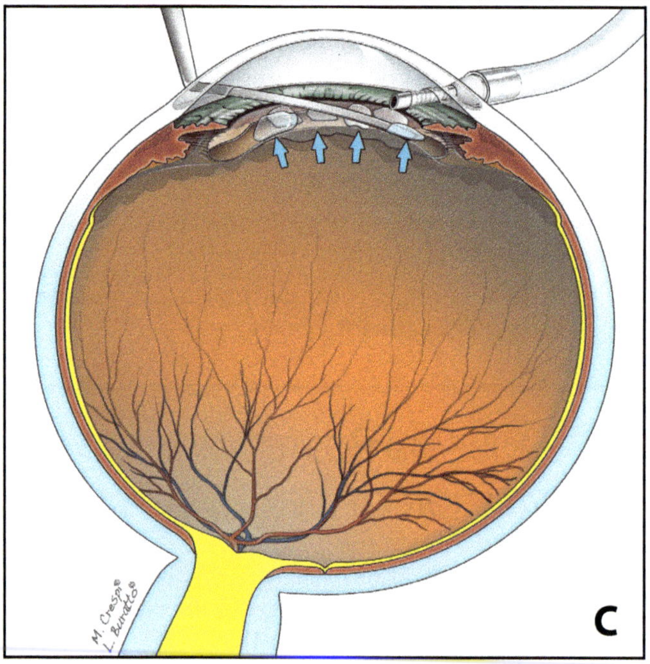

Figure 10-4. Technique of posterior-assisted levitation of lens material (PAL). If the nucleus is extremely dense, the vitreous cavity can be filled with PFCL to elevate the lens into the AC. The PFCL is injected through a sclerotomy underneath the fragments; its density is high, allowing the lens fragments to float on the anterior surface of the bubble. (A) Progressive injection of PFCL fills the vitreous chamber, pushing the fragments toward the iris diaphragm. (B) The fragments can be emulsified and aspirated in the vitreous chamber; (C) alternately, the surgeon can fill the chamber with PFCL beyond the iris diaphragm, expressing the lens fragments through a limbal incision. After filling the chamber with PFCL, the lens fragments may disappear underneath the iris diaphragm (as they are displaced on the meniscus of the bubble) and disappear from view; in this case, the surgeon proceeds with appropriate filling of the chamber with PFCL continuing with mechanical displacement of the fragments to the center of the pupil with a blunt spatula.

Prognosis

The most common cases of visual acuity loss are corneal edema (15%), cystoid macular edema (23% to 29%), retinal detachment (9% to 13%), increased IOP (5%), and formation of epiretinal membranes (4%).[6,12] The incidence of these complications do not appear to be correlated with the timing of the vitrectomy following the cataract operation.[6,12] A significant correlation has been seen with retinal detachment and waiting more than 30 days between the cataract surgery and the vitrectomy (P = 0.00047) and a further correlation exists with retinal detachment and capsule tears in young patients (P = 0.007).[6] Visual recovery better than 20/40 occurs in 50% to 70% of patients.[6,12]

References

1. Pande M, Dabbs TR. Incidence of lens matter dislocation during phacoemulsification. *J Cataract Refract Surg.* 1996;22(6):737-742.
2. Leaming DV. Practice styles and preferences of ASCRS members—1994 survey. *J Cataract Refract Surg.* 1995;21(4):378-385.
3. Chuang LH, Wu WC, Yang KJ, Tsao YP, Chen TL, Lai CC. Subtenon anesthesia for segmental scleral buckling and assessment of postoperative pain. *Chang Gung Med J.* 2002;25(1):16-22.
4. Ho LY, Doft BH, Wang L, Bunker CH. Clinical predictors and outcomes of pars plana vitrectomy for retained lens material after cataract extraction. *Am J Ophthalmol.* 2009;147(4):587-594, e1.

5. Androudi S, Brazitikos PD, Papadopoulos NT, Dereklis D, Symeon L, Stangos N. Posterior capsule rupture and vitreous loss during phacoemulsification with or without the use of an anterior chamber maintainer. *J Cataract Refract Surg.* 2004;30(2):449-452.
6. Merani R, Hunyor AP, Playfair TJ, et al. Pars plana vitrectomy for the management of retained lens material after cataract surgery. *Am J Ophthalmol.* 2007;144(3):364-370.
7. Hubschman JP, Bourges JL, Tsui I, Reddy S, Yu F, Schwartz SD. Effect of cutting phases on flow rate in 20-, 23-, and 25-gauge vitreous cutters. *Retina.* 2009;29(9):1289-1293.
8. Hubschman JP, Gupta A, Bourla DH, Culjat M, Yu F, Schwartz SD. 20-, 23-, and 25-gauge vitreous cutters: performance and characteristics evaluation. *Retina.* 2008;28(2):249-257.
9. Lifshitz T, Levy J. Posterior assisted levitation: long-term follow-up data. *J Cataract Refract Surg.* 2005;31(3):499-502.
10. Schutz JS, Mavrakanas NA. Posterior-assisted levitation in cataract surgery. *Curr Opin Ophthalmol.* 2010;21(1):50-54.
11. Morris RE, Shere JL, Witherspoon CD, et al. Intraoperative retinal detachment prophylaxis in vitrectomy for retained cataract fragments. *J Cataract Refract Surg.* 2009;35(3):491-495.
12. Scott IU, Flynn HW Jr, Smiddy WE, et al. Clinical features and outcomes of pars plana vitrectomy in patients with retained lens fragments. *Ophthalmology.* 2003;110(8):1567-1572.

11

Endophthalmitis Following Cataract Surgery

Lucio Buratto, MD; Stephen F. Brint, MD, FACS; and Mario R. Romano, MD, PhD

The term *endophthalmitis* is used to define any inflammation secondary to infective agents: bacterial, fungal, and more rarely viral and protozoan. It is the most devastating complication of intraocular procedures and can lead to permanent and complete loss of vision. Endophthalmitis, largely secondary to trauma or intraocular surgery, results from diffusion of external organisms into the eye. In this chapter, we will examine postoperative infective endophthalmitis.[1]

Endophthalmitis secondary to cataract surgery is classified on the basis of signs and symptoms: acute endophthalmitis (appearing within 5 days of surgery), chronic endophthalmitis, and late onset endophthalmitis (6 weeks from surgery).

The incidence of postoperative endophthalmitis is 0.265%,[2] ranging from 0.07%[3] to 0.40%.[4] Recently, improvements in microsurgical techniques, improvements in technology and surgical materials, prophylactic use of wide spectrum antibiotics, and better understanding of the causes of infection have led to a reduction in this complication.[2] Nevertheless, a number of risk factors associated with endophthalmitis have been identified.[5]

Intraoperative Risk Factors

Age

Advanced patient age is correlated with factors such as slower rate of healing or lower resistance to infection. The incidence of endophthalmitis in patients over 90 is 3.6 times greater.[6]

Race

There is considerable evidence in the literature that Black people have a greater incidence of postoperative endophthalmitis. The reason for this appears to be a greater incidence of comorbidity (ie, diabetes).[7]

Diabetes

The literature suggests diabetic retinopathy plays an important role in the development of endophthalmitis in the diabetic population.[8] Gram-positive coagulase negative organisms have greater growth inside eyes of diabetic patients (58.6%) as compared to nondiabetic patients (45.0%).

Buratto L, Brint SF, Romano MR.
Cataract Surgery Complications (pp 89-96).
© 2013 Taylor & Francis Group.

Wound Leak

In the early postoperative period, there may be intraocular contamination due to passage of contaminated tears or conjunctival organisms into the AC. This will cause an inflammatory reaction with the release of proteases and bacterial endotoxins, causing direct cell damage. If there is any doubt, the surgeon should use a single 10-0 nylon suture.

Silicone Intraocular Lenses

The risk of endophthalmitis is 3.13 times greater with silicone intraocular lenses (IOLs) as compared to acrylic IOLs. This is due to the hydrophobic nature of silicone that increases bacterial adhesion to the implant.[9]

Surgeon Experience

No association between the experience of the surgeon and the incidence of endophthalmitis has been demonstrated. However, the incidence appears to be greater for expert surgeons as they are more likely to perform the more complex cases, including those that may lead to endophthalmitis.[9]

Intraoperative Complications

Rupture of the posterior capsule, retained lens material, iris prolapse, and vitreous loss are correlated with the development of endophthalmitis because of inflammation and exposure of the vitreous, an excellent culture medium for potential growth of the infective agents.[10]

Etiology

The Endophthalmitis Vitrectomy Study (EVS) demonstrated that the pathogenic agents responsible for endophthalmitis are part of the normal flora of the surface and surrounding mucosa.[11]

The most frequently isolated organisms (94, 2%) are gram positives (*Staphylococcus epidermidis* and *Staphylococcus aureus*, the former being less virulent). More rare are the gram negatives (*Serratia*, *Proteus*, and *Pseudomonas*), *Propionibacterium acnes*, and fungal infections, which are commonly considered to lead to late onset endophthalmitis.[12] Species such as *Bacillus* are rarely associated with postoperative endophthalmitis.[13] A rare cause of endophthalmitis may be the *Enterobacter*, an environmental pathogen that normally creates infection only when inoculated in high doses.[14]

The most serious intraocular infections are caused by *S aureus*, *Enterococci*, *Bacillus*, or untreatable gram-negative strains.[15] Epidemic clusters of different strains are a rare occurrence and may contaminate instruments, surgeon, and staff in the operating room.[16]

Micro-organisms isolated from chronic endophthalmitis are often less virulent pathogens or fungal spores. The incidence of these is 63% for *Propionibacterium*, 16% for *S epidermidis*, 16% for *Parapsilosis candida*, and 5% for *Corynebacterium* 5%. *Actinomyces, Nocardia, Achromobacter, Cephalosporium, Acremonium, Paecilomyces,* and species of *Aspergillus* are involved less frequently.[17]

Diagnosis

Clinical Diagnosis

Ninety-eight percent of patients with endophthalmitis will have at least one of the following 4 symptoms: blurred vision (93%), red eyes (81%), pain (75%), and swollen eyelids (33%).[11]

White hypopyon is seen in 85% of cases; it has a mean elevation of 1.5 mm (range 0.1 to 12 mm), and is formed by stratification of leukocytes.[18] The combination of hypopyon and vitreous that is echographically empty may indicate an infection by a coagulase-negative *Staphylococcus*. Ophthalmic echography is a useful tool in the diagnosis and management of infective endophthalmitis. It can provide useful details in the density of the vitreous, detachment of the posterior vitreous, vitreous trapping, retinal detachment, choroidal detachment, and edema of the optic nerve. Dacey et al demonstrated that choroidal detachment is the main visual outcome predictor in these eyes.[19] The presence of any vitreo-retinal involvement probably indicates the need for more involved surgery.

Signs and Symptoms of Acute Endophthalmitis

- Blurred vision (93%)
- Red eye (81%)
- Pain (75%)
- Swollen eyelids (33%)
- Hypopyon in the AC and ocular fundus that is difficult or impossible to see (85%)

Late onset endophthalmitis has more uncertain and insidious symptoms with signs of granulomatous uveitis, endothelial or iris precipitates, and cells in the vitreous. Sometimes late onset forms may be secondary to an Nd:YAG capsulotomy because of the release of low virulent material trapped in the capsular bag.[20]

White "pearls-on-a-string" infiltrates close to the capsular bag are characteristic of a fungal infection.[21,22] With infection by *P acnes*, a white intracapsular plate is observed,

Recognition and Treatment of Endophthalmitis

1. Suspected endophthalmitis includes the following:
   - The eye will be painful and inflammation will be seen in the AC from the first day.
   - Following initial improvement, there will be a marked deterioration with a reduction in visual acuity and pain, and the fundus cannot be seen easily.
   - NB: Pain is absent in 25% of cases; an ocular fundus that cannot be visualized is extremely suspicious (but this may be due to something else).
2. The clinical diagnosis of endophthalmitis must be confirmed by the following:
   - The simultaneous presence of hypopyon in the AC and exudate in the vitreous confirms the diagnosis.
   - Inflammation in the AC (no hypopyon) and exudate in the vitreous may confirm the diagnosis.
   - Absence of hypopyon and exudate in the vitreous—suspected sterile inflammation.
   - NB: the presence of exudate in the vitreous is highly suspicious for endophthalmitis
3. To confirm the microbiological diagnosis of endophthalmitis:
   - Obtain vitreous using the vitrectomy (25 gauge if possible). Insert 3 trocars pars plana and perform an initial dry vitrectomy (with infusion inactive) of 0.1 to 0.5 mL. Then open the infusion line and acquire a larger amount of vitreous (2 mL). The biopsy sample is injected onto a blood and chocolate agar dish, thioglycollate broth (at 37°C) and Sabouraud's medium (25°C) to detect bacteria (aerobic and anaerobic) and fungal spores.
4. Treatment
   - Intravitreal injection of vancomycin (1 mg/0.1 mL) and ceftazidime (2.25 mg/0.1 mL) with separate 1-mL syringes.
   - Topical treatment with steroids, antibiotics (fourth-generation fluoroquinolones), and cycloplegics.
   - Systemic treatment with imipenem (intravenously) + steroids (oral 30 mg prednisone 2 times daily for 5 to 10 days with taper).
5. Surgery
   - Observe the evolution of the clinical picture in terms of anterior inflammation and visibility of the ocular fundus. If there is no improvement in 24 to 36 hours, the surgeon should proceed with a vitrectomy.
   - NB: A vitrectomy is considered to be the initial approach with marked posterior exudation.

often being associated with retention of lens material and responsible for recurrent endophthalmitis.

Microbiological Diagnosis

A sample of undiluted vitreous will have greater sensitivity than a sample of aqueous (30% to 55% of positive vitreous samples will have a negative aqueous).[23] In eyes with infective keratitis, intraocular samples should include a sample of the corneal epithelium.

The vitreous is sampled via a pars plana approach with a 25-gauge vitrectomy (0.1 to 0.5 mL); the aqueous is sampled with a paracentesis of the AC using a 27- or 30-gauge needle.

The sample of aqueous and vitreous are injected onto a blood and chocolate agar dish, thioglycollate broth (at 37°C), and Sabouraud's medium (25°C) to detect bacteria (aerobic and anaerobic) and fungal spores.

Grading of the Opacity of the Media for Examination of the Fundus

- Grade 1: Good visibility
- Grade 2: Visualization of second order branches of the retinal vessels
- Grade 3: Visualization of some retinal vessels
- Grade 4: Vessels not visible, red reflex not present
- Grade 5: Absence of red reflex
- NB: The red reflex is absent because of the inveterate retinal detachment, vitreous hemorrhage, nucleus dislocation in the vitreous chamber, and severe posterior uveitis.

The chain reaction of the polymerase may provide a better method of specific diagnosis, allowing the detection of DNA from infective micro-organisms. The results are generally available within 48 hours. Anaerobic cultures must be kept for at least 14 days to detect species with low growth rates (ie, *P acnes*). Fungal cultures must be stored for several weeks. The EVS reported an incidence of positive samples in 68.2% of cases of endophthalmitis.[23] A lack of a positive culture may be the result of organisms such as *P acnes*, which is difficult to isolate, or *S epidermidis*, which can become sterile spontaneously.[24]

Differential Diagnosis

Differential diagnosis of endophthalmitis should include retained lens material, a sterile inflammation of the AC postoperatively, or infections of adjacent structures such as conjunctival blebs or keratitis (Table 11-1).

Toxic anterior segment syndrome (TASS) can lead to a marked sterile inflammation caused by detergents, preservatives, and intraocular solutions that have a chemical composition that is inadequate for the pH and intraocular osmolarity.[25] Even an ointment applied at the end of surgery has been associated with this syndrome.[26] TASS is usually accompanied by a predominantly anterior inflammation.

Table 11-1

Differential Diagnosis Between Infection and Sterile Inflammation

	Inflammation	Infection
Onset	Within 24 hours	48 to 72 hours
Blurred vision	Moderate	Severe
Pain	Moderate	Severe
Anterior reaction	Severe	Moderate-severe
Focal infiltrates	Rare	Present
Exudate	Milky white	Yellow
Intraocular pressure	Normal to high	Low
Course	Tends to improve	Deteriorates

Medical Treatment

Treatment has not been coded by evidence-based medicine because it is not supported by randomized clinical studies, given the pathology under examination. The only study with limitations that could provide guidelines is the EVS published in 1995.[11]

Intravitreal Injection

Intravitreal injection is the most direct method for administering adequate concentration of a drug to the infected tissues. Antibacterial therapy must cover gram positives that have shown sensitivity to vancomycin, including methicillin resistant *S aureus* (MRSA).[11] Ceftazidime appears to provide adequate cover for the gram negatives and does not possess the retinal toxicity of the aminoglycosides, amikacin and gentamicin[27] (Table 11-2). The current recommendations for empirical therapy are vancomycin (1 mg/0.1 mL) and ceftazidime (2.25 mg/0.1 mL). Amikacin (0.4 mg/0.1 mL) can be used as a replacement of ceftazidime in patients sensitive to the lactamics.

The role of the fourth-generation fluoroquinolones in intravitreal therapy is still unclear. These drugs have a broad spectrum and may prove useful in the treatment of endophthalmitis particularly when caused by gram-negative bacteria. The optimal dosage for the eye is not known. Experimental rabbit data suggest that doses of 400 µg/0.1 mL gatifloxacin or moxifloxacin may be adequate.[28] The coagulase-negative *Staphylococcus* have shown greater resistance to cefazolin. The resistance of gram-positive bacteria to vancomycin is rare but is a serious threat for the future. Antifungal treatment is rarely necessary and involves intravitreal injection of amphotericin B (5 µg/0.1 mL). The most frequently isolated fungals are *Aspergillus* and *Candida albicans*.

Toxicity of Intravitreal Antibiotics

Potential complications associated with intravitreal antimicrobial therapy range from corneal opacity to retinal toxicity. The risk of toxicity with therapeutic doses of vancomycin and ceftazidime is very low.[29,30]

Intravitreal ceftazidime can cause retinal toxicity if administered in higher doses than recommended (2.25 mg/0.1 mL). Toxicity of the retina with severe sight loss has been reported following therapy with aminoglycosides, gentamicin in particular.[31] The toxicity of aminoglycosides, gentamicin in particular, involves the neurons, with consequent retinal hypoxia and macular infarction. The

Table 11-2

Antibiotics Commonly Used in Intravitreal Injections

Drug	Dose to Be Injected	Spectrum Covered	Notes
Vancomycin	1 mg/0.1 mL	Gram positive	Do not use in combination with other drugs as it can precipitate
Ceftazidime	2.25 mg/0.1 mL	Gram negative (including *Pseudomonas*)	
Cefazolin	2.25 mg/0.1 mL	Gram positive (active on *Staphylococcus*)	
Amikacin	0.4 mg/0.1 mL	Gram negative (active on *Staphylococcus*)	Retinal toxicity (even though it is 4 times less than gentamicin)
Amphotericin B	5 µg/0.1 mL	Antifungal	

fourth-generation fluoroquinolones moxifloxacin,[32] gatifloxacin,[28] and voriconazole (an antimycotic agent) do not appear to induce any toxicity in animals. Findings from prospective studies on human eyes are still not available.

Systemic Antibiotics

Systemic antibiotics do not achieve therapeutically adequate intraocular concentrations. Systemic treatment is advocated as an accessory treatment for postoperative endophthalmitis. The objective of systemic treatment is the possibility of prolonging the action of intravitreal therapy, reducing the need for repeated intravitreal injections. The results of EVS did not indicate any significance in the use of systemic therapy for acute endophthalmitis.[11]

The fluoroquinolones gatifloxacin and moxifloxacin appear to be more promising, and following oral administration, have a vitreous concentration above the minimal quantities of inhibition. Nevertheless, neither gatifloxacin nor moxifloxacin achieve MIC 90 vitreous levels for *Pseudomonas aeruginosa, Enterococcus,* and *Bacteroides fragilis.*

Imipenem is also recommended for IV administration in combination with the administration of intraocular antibiotics.[35]

Corticosteroids

The treatment objective of corticosteroids is to modulate the inflammatory response from the infective agent to minimize ocular damage induced by the inflammatory process.

The use of intravitreal corticosteroids is still controversial.

In EVS, patients were administered oral 30 mg prednisone twice a day for 5 to 10 days, with treatment starting on the first day postoperative and then tapered over the following days.[11] The benefit of oral corticosteroids was not examined by EVS, and no prospective study has been done. Chronic inflammation may initially respond to steroids, but there may be a relapse when treatment is suspended. With some of the fungal infections, however, the inflammation may paradoxically worsen with the steroids.[36] Consequently, the surgeon must pay attention to systemic administration of steroids in patients with contraindications such as diabetes, mellitus, or ulcers.

Surgical Treatment

The potential advantages associated with vitrectomy include reduction of the pathogenic load, injection of the antibiotic directly into the vitreous, the liberation of the rhegmatogenic adhesions, and direct sampling of the vitreous. A 0.2- to 0.5-mL sample of vitreous obtained at the beginning of vitrectomy without infusion may assist the microbiological analysis.

The findings involving vitrectomy are contradictory. The determining factor is the presence of posterior vitreous to avoid the formation of macular hypopyon and improvement with a "wash out" and retinal oxygenation. A study published in 2006 reported functional recovery with a final visual acuity of 20/40 in 47 eyes treated with vitrectomy, and creation of posterior vitreous detachment in 91% of eyes as opposed to 53% reported in EVS.[11,37,38]

Medical therapy is generally effective for late onset inflammation. If recurrent inflammation persists or is caused by virulent germs, it is advisable to proceed with IOL removal with the capsular bag, delaying secondary implantation until the recurring inflammation has been eliminated.

Chronic forms are not always caused by low virulence organisms. We have described cases of recurrent hypopyon caused by MRSA treated by removing the IOL and capsular bag.

The clinical situation of recurrent inflammation was caused by an extremely virulent pathogen. Once the IOL/capsular bag had been removed, results were positive with complete resolution of the hypopyon and recurrent inflammation.[39]

The use of silicone oil is not recommended in every case; it is suitable only in the presence of retinal tears induced by the surgeon during the vitrectomy.

Prophylaxis

Ciulla et al presented a meta-analysis of 88 peer-reviewed articles. Iodopovidone has been considered to be the most efficacious means of achieving an aseptic state.[40]

The fourth-generation fluoroquinolones, namely gatifloxacin and moxifloxacin, offer a number of advantages over levofloxacin in prophylactic treatment.[41]

Advantages include a broad spectrum of antibacterial activity, greater effect against the gram-positive pathogens, superior characteristics of ocular penetration for moxifloxacin, and reduced sensitivity to development of resistance.

Of the 2 fourth-generation fluoroquinolones, when required, moxifloxacin should be considered to be superior for treatment in terms of efficacy and penetration.

The conclusions of a study by the European Society of Cataract and Refractive Surgeons suggested the use of cefuroxime as the gold standard administered intracamerally at the end of modern phacoemulsification. Nevertheless, an optimal regime of antibiotics to prevent postoperative endophthalmitis has still not been defined.[9,42,43] Moreover, a handful of studies have examined potential intraocular toxicity of cefuroxime.[44,45] There are some gaps in the use of cefuroxime as an antimicrobial prophylactic; these include gram-negative pathogens and *Enterococcus*.[46,47] Finally, Wallin et al suggest a statistical relationship between the use of an ocular bandage and reduced probability of postoperative endophthalmitis even though reports in the literature are inconclusive.[48]

References

1. Mamalis N, Kearsley L, Brinton E. Postoperative endophthalmitis. *Curr Opin Ophthalmol.* 2002;13(1):14-18.
2. Taban M, Behrens A, Newcomb RL, et al. Acute endophthalmitis following cataract surgery: a systematic review of the literature. *Arch Ophthalmol.* 2005;123(5):613-620.
3. Das T, Kunimoto DY, Sharma S, et al. Relationship between clinical presentation and visual outcome in postoperative and posttraumatic endophthalmitis in south central India. *Indian J Ophthalmol.* 2005;53(1):5-16.
4. Rosha DS, Ng JQ, Morlet N, et al. Cataract surgery practice and endophthalmitis prevention by Australian and New Zealand ophthalmologists. *Clin Experiment Ophthalmol.* 2006;34(6):535-544.
5. Sandvig KU, Dannevig L. Postoperative endophthalmitis: establishment and results of a national registry. *J Cataract Refract Surg.* 2003;29(7):1273-1280.
6. Norregaard JC, Thoning H, Bernth-Petersen P, Andersen TF, Javitt JC, Anderson GF. Risk of endophthalmitis after cataract extraction: results from the International Cataract Surgery Outcomes study. *Br J Ophthalmol.* 1997;81(2):102-106.
7. West ES, Behrens A, McDonnell PJ, Tielsch JM, Schein OD. The incidence of endophthalmitis after cataract surgery among the U.S. Medicare population increased between 1994 and 2001. *Ophthalmology.* 2005;112(8):1388-1394.
8. Enzenauer RW. Diabetes and the EVS: a different interpretation of the results. *Arch Ophthalmol.* 2002;120(2):231-233.
9. Endophthalmitis Study Group, European Society of Cataract & Refractive Surgeons. Prophylaxis of postoperative endophthalmitis following cataract surgery: results of the ESCRS multicenter study and identification of risk factors. *J Cataract Refract Surg.* 2007;33(6):978-988.
10. Kamalarajah S, Ling R, Silvestri G, et al. Presumed infectious endophthalmitis following cataract surgery in the UK: a case-control study of risk factors. *Eye (Lond).* 2007;21(5):580-586.
11. Results of the Endophthalmitis Vitrectomy Study. A randomized trial of immediate vitrectomy and of intravenous antibiotics for the treatment of postoperative bacterial endophthalmitis. Endophthalmitis Vitrectomy Study Group. *Arch Ophthalmol.* 1995;113(12):1479-1496.
12. Stern GA, Engel HM, Driebe WT Jr. The treatment of postoperative endophthalmitis. Results of differing approaches to treatment. *Ophthalmology.* 1989;96(1):62-67.
13. Roy M, Chen JC, Miller M, Boyaner D, Kasner O, Edelstein E. Epidemic *Bacillus* endophthalmitis after cataract surgery I: acute presentation and outcome. *Ophthalmology.* 1997;104:1768-1772.
14. Barza M, Pavan PR, Doft BH, et al. Evaluation of microbiological diagnostic techniques in postoperative endophthalmitis in the Endophthalmitis Vitrectomy Study. *Arch Ophthalmol.* 1997;115(9):1142-1150.
15. Callegan MC, Gilmore MS, Gregory M, et al. Bacterial endophthalmitis: therapeutic challenges and host-pathogen interactions. *Prog Retin Eye Res.* 2007;26(2):189-203.
16. Kodjikian L, Burillon C, Freney J. Endophthalmitis and biomaterials. *Acta Ophthalmol Scand.* 2005;83(5):633; author reply 633-634.
17. Pflugfelder SC, Flynn HW Jr, Zwickey TA, et al. Exogenous fungal endophthalmitis. *Ophthalmology.* 1988;95(1):19-30.
18. Weber DJ, Hoffman KL, Thoft RA, Baker AS. Endophthalmitis following intraocular lens implantation: report of 30 cases and review of the literature. *Rev Infect Dis.* 1986;8(1):12-20.
19. Dacey MP, Valencia M, Lee MB, et al. Echographic findings in infectious endophthalmitis. *Arch Ophthalmol.* 1994;112(10):1325-1333.
20. Carlson AN, Stewart WC, Tso PC. Intraocular lens complications requiring removal or exchange. *Surv Ophthalmol.* 1998;42(5):417-440.

21. Fox GM, Joondeph BC, Flynn HW Jr, Pflugfelder SC, Roussel TJ. Delayed-onset pseudophakic endophthalmitis. *Am J Ophthalmol.* 1991;111(2):163-173.
22. Samson CM, Foster CS. Chronic postoperative endophthalmitis. *Int Ophthalmol Clin.* 2000;40(1):57-67.
23. Wisniewski SR, Capone A, Kelsey SF, Groer-Fitzgerald S, Lambert HM, Doft BH. Characteristics after cataract extraction or secondary lens implantation among patients screened for the Endophthalmitis Vitrectomy Study. *Ophthalmology.* 2000;107(7):1274-1282.
24. Meredith TA, Trabelsi A, Miller MJ, Aguilar E, Wilson LA. Spontaneous sterilization in experimental *Staphylococcus epidermidis* endophthalmitis. *Invest Ophthalmol Vis Sci.* 1990;31(1):181-186.
25. McCray E, Rampell N, Solomon SL, Bond WW, Martone WJ, O'Day D. Outbreak of *Candida parapsilosis* endophthalmitis after cataract extraction and intraocular lens implantation. *J Clin Microbiol.* 1986;24(4):625-628.
26. Werner L, Sher JH, Taylor JR, et al. Toxic anterior segment syndrome and possible association with ointment in the anterior chamber following cataract surgery. *J Cataract Refract Surg.* 2006;32(2):227-235.
27. Irvine WD, Flynn HW Jr, Miller D, Pflugfelder SC. Endophthalmitis caused by gram-negative organisms. *Arch Ophthalmol.* 1992;110(10):1450-1454.
28. Kazi AA, Jermak CM, Peyman GA, Aydin E, Riazi-Esfahani M. Intravitreal toxicity of levofloxacin and gatifloxacin. *Ophthalmic Surg Lasers Imaging.* 2006;37(3):224-229.
29. Homer P, Peyman GA, Koziol J, Sanders D. Intravitreal injection of vancomycin in experimental *Staphylococcal* endophthalmitis. *Acta Ophthalmol (Copenh).* 1975;53(3):311-320.
30. Pflugfelder SC, Hernandez E, Fliesler SJ, Alvarez J, Pflugfelder ME, Forster RK. Intravitreal vancomycin. Retinal toxicity, clearance, and interaction with gentamicin. *Arch Ophthalmol.* 1987;105(6):831-837.
31. Campochiaro PA, Conway BP. Aminoglycoside toxicity—a survey of retinal specialists. Implications for ocular use. *Arch Ophthalmol.* 1991;109(7):946-950.
32. Gao H, Pennesi ME, Qiao X, et al. Intravitreal moxifloxacin: retinal safety study with electroretinography and histopathology in animal models. *Invest Ophthalmol Vis Sci.* 2006;47(4):1606-1611.
33. Hariprasad SM, Mieler WF, Holz ER. Vitreous and aqueous penetration of orally administered gatifloxacin in humans. *Arch Ophthalmol.* 2003;121(3):345-350.
34. Hariprasad SM, Shah GK, Mieler WF, et al. Vitreous and aqueous penetration of orally administered moxifloxacin in humans. *Arch Ophthalmol.* 2006;124(2):178-182.
35. Engelbert M, Mino de Kaspar H, Thiel M, et al. Intravitreal vancomycin and amikacin versus intravenous imipenem in the treatment of experimental *Staphylococcus aureus* endophthalmitis. *Graefes Arch Clin Exp Ophthalmol.* 2004;242(4):313-320.
36. Zambrano W, Flynn HW Jr, Pflugfelder SC, et al. Management options for *Propionibacterium acnes* endophthalmitis. *Ophthalmology.* 1989;96(7):1100-1105.
37. Kuhn F, Gini G. Vitrectomy for endophthalmitis. *Ophthalmology.* 2006;113(4):714.
38. Kuhn F, Gini G. Ten years after... are findings of the Endophthalmitis Vitrectomy Study still relevant today? *Graefes Arch Clin Exp Ophthalmol.* 2005;243(12):1197-1199.
39. Khan JM, Romano MR, Groenewald C. Recurrent hypopyon due to methicillin-resistant *Staphylococcus aureus* after cataract surgery. *Eye (Lond).* 2009;23(5):1235.
40. Ciulla TA, Starr MB, Masket S. Bacterial endophthalmitis prophylaxis for cataract surgery: an evidence-based update. *Ophthalmology.* 2002;109(1):13-24.
41. Mah FS. Fourth-generation fluoroquinolones: new topical agents in the war on ocular bacterial infections. *Curr Opin Ophthalmol.* 2004;15(4):316-320.
42. Seal DV, Barry P, Gettinby G, et al. ESCRS study of prophylaxis of postoperative endophthalmitis after cataract surgery: case for a European multicenter study. *J Cataract Refract Surg.* 2006;32(3):396-406.
43. Barry P, Seal DV, Gettinby G, Lees F, Peterson M, Revie CW. ESCRS study of prophylaxis of postoperative endophthalmitis after cataract surgery: preliminary report of principal results from a European multicenter study. *J Cataract Refract Surg.* 2006;32(3):407-410.
44. Montan PG, Wejde G, Koranyi G, Rylander M. Prophylactic intracameral cefuroxime. Efficacy in preventing endophthalmitis after cataract surgery. *J Cataract Refract Surg.* 2002;28(6):977-981.
45. Gupta MS, McKee HD, Saldana M, Stewart OG. Macular thickness after cataract surgery with intracameral cefuroxime. *J Cataract Refract Surg.* 2005;31(6):1163-1166.
46. Noviello S, Ianniello F, Leone S, Esposito S. Comparative activity of garenoxacin and other agents by susceptibility and time-kill testing against *Staphylococcus aureus, Streptococcus pyogenes,* and respiratory pathogens. *J Antimicrob Chemother.* 2003;52(5):869-872.
47. von Eiff C, Friedrich AW, Becker K, Peters G. Comparative in vitro activity of ceftobiprole against staphylococci displaying normal and small-colony variant phenotypes. *Antimicrob Agents Chemother.* 2005;49(10):4372-4374.
48. Wallin T, Parker J, Jin Y, Kefalopoulos G, Olson RJ. Cohort study of 27 cases of endophthalmitis at a single institution. *J Cataract Refract Surg.* 2005;31(4):735-741.

12

Cystoid Macular Edema Following Cataract Surgery

Lucio Buratto, MD; Stephen F. Brint, MD, FACS; and Mario R. Romano, MD, PhD

Postoperative cystoid macular edema (CME) is one of the most frequent complications following cataract surgery. It is sometimes associated with complications during surgery as well. It was first described by Irvine in 1953 as "vitreous syndrome following cataract surgery."[1] We have seen a reduction in its frequency as techniques have improved with less invasive surgery. Currently, angiographic or optical coherence tomography (OCT) incidence of postoperative intraretinal edema is approximately 20%, with a functional incidence of 1%.[2-4]

Pathogenesis

Phacoemulsification and intraocular lens (IOL) implantation induce an inflammatory response caused by mechanical stimuli (eg, ultrasound, fluid turbulence, surgical manipulations) or chemical stimuli (eg, viscoelastic substances, intraocular antibiotics, detergents) to the iris or other intraocular structures. These stimuli induce production of prostaglandins (mostly PGF2) and other cytokines that can reach the vitreous and retina. Recently, using an animal model, it was seen that cataract surgery induces activation of pro-inflammatory genes coding for IL1-beta, CCL2, and complement (C3, C5b-9, CFB) produced directly by the retina and choroid.[5] These mediators bind to receptors present on endothelial cells, modulating the permeability of the blood retina barrier (BRB). The internal BRB is formed by endothelial cells and tight junctions regulating vascular permeability, toward the intraretinal space. The mediators increase the permeability of the internal BRB, with accumulation of intraretinal fluid, normally compensated by adequate reabsorption by the retinal pigmented epithelium ([RPE], forming the external BRB). If the inflammatory stimulus persists, CME develops because of fluid accumulation in the extracellular matrix. The accumulation of extracellular fluid has vasogenic origins. Intracellular edema results from a cytotoxic effect of cell swelling and may lead to irreversible damage.

This inflammatory stimulus may also develop without intraoperative surgical complications.

Risk Factors

Microincision Surgery

These maneuvers may lead to increased macular edema seen with OCT. It is related to more rapid liquid flow as opposed to traditional techniques.[10] OCT changes just 5 weeks after surgery are statistically significant as compared to a control group.[10]

Buratto L, Brint SF, Romano MR.
Cataract Surgery Complications (pp 97-102).
© 2013 Taylor & Francis Group.

Intraoperative Complications

The following are associated with a 4-fold increased risk of developing macular edema.[11,12] Intraoperative iris trauma, vitreous prolapse into the anterior chamber (AC), and vitreous inceration in the wound are the most common risk factors associated with clinically significant macular edema, with an incidence of 20% in eyes after the following complications.[13]

- Secondary implants: Posterior capsule rupture may require a secondary implant. AC lenses (angle supported or with iris fixation) may induce macular edema more frequently than IOLs implanted in the sulcus. Another good alternative for secondary implantation are iris-sutured lenses, which induce macular edema in 12% of cases.[14]
- The use of intraocular antibiotics (vancomycin and cefuroxime) placed in the infusion fluid or intracamerally at the end of the procedure have an increased incidence of macular edema. Angiography demonstrates an incidence of 55% in patients treated with intraocular antibiotics versus 19% in the control group.[15] It also showed a clinically significant incidence of edema in 23% versus 7% of the control group.[15] Cases of macular infarction also have been reported, resulting from intraocular administration of incorrect concentrations of antibiotic.[16,17]
- Diabetes: This is an important risk factor for postoperative macular edema. Eighty-one percent of diabetic patients develop macular edema following cataract surgery and in 25% of cases, the edema persisted for 12 months.[18] In moderate diabetic retinopathy, macular OCT changes may be seen, tending to improve spontaneously with time, but not statistically significant long term compared to a control group.[19] Macular edema induced by surgery does not appear to be correlated with progressive diabetic retinopathy.
- Another risk factor is chronic anterior or posterior uveitis, which can reactivate following cataract surgery. In 56% of cases, this leads to macular edema becoming chronic after the first week postsurgery.[20]

Diagnosis

The patient reports reduction in contrast sensitivity sometimes associated with metamorphopsia. Symptoms may increase between the 4th and 12th weeks with a peak between weeks 4 and 6. The diagnosis is confirmed with tomography (SD-OCT). Postoperatively, in addition to variation of retinal thickness, this allows evaluation of the external retinal layers (external limiting membrane and junction of the internal/external segment), variations in thickness, and position of the intraretinal cysts. Retinal angiography confirms the diagnosis and excludes neovascular complications potentially increasing the edema.

Diagnosis of Macular Edema

Edema can be diagnosed using angiograpy, tomography, and clinical symptoms.

Angiography in postoperative macular edema is characterized by leakage of dye from the perifoveal capillaries in later stages of the angiogram, with intraretinal pooling having a petaloid appearance when the edema also involves the external plexiform layer. Angiographic signs of macular edema are seen 4 to 6 weeks after surgery, very rarely in the first week postsurgery.[6]

Tomography with SD-OCT reveals hyporeflective cysts in the internal nuclear layer. Using OCT, macular edema is defined as an increase of 40% of retinal thickness from baseline.[7] Tomography is used to exclude the concomitant presence of vitreous traction or tractional membranes, not only in the macular region, that can cause recurrent chronic inflammation associated with edema.[8] This OCT is also important as it provides a possible surgical approach to resolve the edema.

Macular edema is considered clinically significant if visual acuity is worse than 0.5 (20/40) in association with ophthalmologic and angiographic findings. The incidence varies between 0.4% and 2.3%.[9]

Angiography and tomography are not strictly correlated with reduction in visual acuity that may be good despite the fact that the angiography and OCT show macular edema.

Prognosis

Eighty percent of the time, the natural course is progressive improvement over 2 to 12 months. Functional improvement is related to the length of time the edema has persisted following surgery. With capsular rupture and vitreous loss, 83% of patients will have visual acuity better than 0.5; in cases in which macular edema lasts more than 6 months, only 29% of patients will recover visual acuity better than 0.5 (20/40).[11,21]

Treatment of Macular Edema

With nontractional postoperative macular edema: A combination of acetazolamide (250 mg bid) and nepafenac (1 drop tid) or bromfenac (1 drop bid) for the first 6 weeks is recommended.

If there is no symptomatic improvement, the surgeon should continue with sub-Tenon's injections of triamcinolone every 3 weeks.

If the edema persists for more than 6 weeks, the surgeon should plan an injection of Ozurdex (Allergan Inc, Irvine, CA).

Medical Treatment

The objective of medical treatment is to block the production of cytokines that change the permeability of the internal BRB using steroids and nonsteroidal anti-inflammatory drugs (NSAIDs). No standardized approaches exist. We will now explore the most popular medical and surgical approaches.[9]

Corticosteroids inhibit the production of phospholipase A2, an enzyme that transforms phospholipids into arachidonic acid, inhibiting formation of prostaglandins and leukotrienes.

The administration of oral steroids, normally 1 to 1.5 mg/kg/day prednisone, is recommended with a gradual tapering of the dose after the first 2 weeks.

The use of high-dose topical steroids (1% prednisolone or 1% dexamethasone every hour) is recommended, particularly in cases of iridocyclitis or direct mechanical trauma to the iris.

A sub-Tenon's injection of steroids will allow good penetration of the steroids to the posterior pole, similar to retrobulbar. Twenty milligrams of triamcinolone is injected every 3 to 6 weeks or alternately, 4 mg of betamethasone injected every week[22] (Figure 12-1).

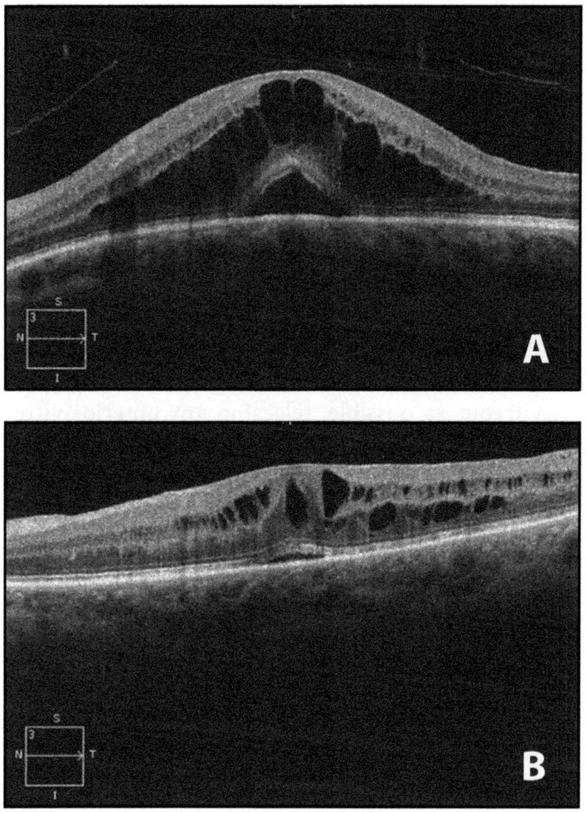

Figure 12-1. (A) Sub-Tenon's injection of betamethasone. CME following uncomplicated phacoemulsification. Detachment of the neuroepithelium is seen with large intraretinal cysts localized in the external plexiform layer. (B) Following 30 days of weekly sub-Tenon's injections of triamcinolone, progressive decreased size of the intraretinal cysts and detachment of the neuroepithelium in the macula.

Intravitreal injection of triamcinolone, between 2 and 25 mg, has produced good anatomical and functional results tending to regress 4 to 6 weeks after treatment[23] with an IOP increase in 40% of cases.[24]

Finally, there is a lot of interest in Ozurdex, a slow release implant of dexamethasone into the vitreous chamber. An improvement of 3 lines of visual acuity occurs in 53% of patients 6 months following injection.[25]

The most important side effect of this implant is increased IOP ≥10 mm Hg in 38% of cases.[25]

Anti-Vascular Endothelial Growth Factor Drugs

Intravitreal injection in patients with chronic macular edema demonstrated functional efficacy (an improvement of 2 lines in 72% of cases) and tomography efficacy (reduction of approximately 200 μm in retinal thickness) after 12 months, with a mean number of 2.7 injections administered at a mean interval of 15 weeks.[26] There are contradictory findings for this treatment, and no functional results have been reported.[27]

NSAIDs have been effective in reducing and preventing postoperative CME. An Italian study of diclofenac demonstrated an incidence of macular edema in patients treated with 0.1% diclofenac 3 times less frequent than the control group, with complete elimination of edema after approximately 13 months.[28] 0.1% nepafenac and 0.09% bromfenac, instilled 2 to 3 times daily, are well absorbed at the posterior pole with good functional results that were comparable to those treated with topical steroids.[29,30]

Other anti-inflammatories such as valdecoxib, a COX-2 inhibitor, are currently being studied and results appear to be promising.[31]

Finally, interferon alpha-2a was used in 3 patients who did not respond to other treatments for chronic Irvine-Gass syndrome. The dose was 3 million IU per day for 4 weeks. The results were good and no side effects were reported.[32]

Carbonic anhydrase inhibitors (acetazolamide) at doses of 500 mg/day are often combined with topical treatment initially.[33] The evidence has not been supported by prospective studies.

Surgical Treatment

When postoperative edema persists 3 months after surgery with a visual acuity less than 0.25, despite prolonged medical treatment, surgical treatment should be considered. Surgical treatment involves a vitrectomy with removal of as much vitreous as possible, releasing any anterior vitreous traction forces. The removal of the internal barrier is also recommended to remove tangential tractional components (vitreo-scission of the posterior hyaloid or contraction of the ILM) and stimulating a reduction in edema through contraction of the Müller cells. A vitrectomy should also be performed in the presence of exudative macular edema associated with traction forces induced by the posterior hyaloid or epiretinal membrane.[34-36]

References

1. Irvine SR. A newly defined vitreous syndrome following cataract surgery. *Am J Ophthalmol.* 1953;36(5):499-619.
2. Peterson M, Yoshizumi MO, Hepler R, Mondino B, Kreiger A. Topical indomethacin in the treatment of chronic cystoid macular edema. *Graefes Arch Clin Exp Ophthalmol.* 1992;230(5):401-405.
3. Hollick EJ, Spalton DJ, Ursell PG, et al. The effect of polymethylmethacrylate, silicone, and polyacrylic intraocular lenses on posterior capsular opacification 3 years after cataract surgery. *Ophthalmology.* 1999;106(1):49-54; discussion 54-45.
4. Stark WJ Jr, Maumenee AE, Fagadau W, et al. Cystoid macular edema in pseudophakia. *Surv Ophthalmol.* 1984;28(suppl):442-451.
5. Xu H, Chen M, Forrester JV, Lois N. Cataract surgery induces retinal pro-inflammatory gene expression and protein secretion. *Invest Ophthalmol Vis Sci.* 2011;52(1):249-255.
6. Klein RM, Yannuzzi L. Cystoid macular edema in the first week after cataract extraction. *Am J Ophthalmol.* 1976;81(5):614-615.
7. Kim SJ, Bressler NM. Optical coherence tomography and cataract surgery. *Curr Opin Ophthalmol.* 2009;20:46-51.
8. Martinez MR, Ophir A. Pseudophakic cystoid macular edema associated with extrafoveal vitreo-retinal traction. *Open Ophthalmol J.* 2011;5:35-41.
9. Zur D, Fischer N, Tufail A, Mones J, Loewenstein A. Postsurgical cystoid macular edema. *Eur J Ophthalmol.* 2010;21:62-68.
10. Ghosh S, Roy I, Biswas PN, et al. Prospective randomized comparative study of macular thickness following phacoemulsification and manual small incision cataract surgery. *Acta Ophthalmol.* 2010;88(4):e102-e106.
11. Nikica G, Ljerka HP, Jelena P, Metez-Soldo K, MLaden B. Cystoid macular edema in anterior chamber lens implantation following posterior capsule rupture. *Doc Ophthalmol.* 1992;81(3):309-315.
12. Bergman M, Laatikainen L. Cystoid macular edema after complicated cataract surgery and implantation of an anterior chamber lens. *Acta Ophthalmol (Copenh).* 1994;72(2):178-180.
13. Frost NA, Sparrow JM, Strong NP, Rosenthal AR. Vitreous loss in planned extracapsular cataract extraction does lead to a poorer visual outcome. *Eye (Lond).* 1995;9(pt 4):446-451.
14. Güell JL, Velasco F, Malecaze F, Vazquez M, Gris O, Manero F. Secondary Artisan-Verysise aphakic lens implantation. *J Cataract Refract Surg.* 2005;31(12):2266-2271.
15. Axer-Siegel R, Stiebel-Kalish H, Rosenblatt I, Strassmann E, Yassur Y, Weinberger D. Cystoid macular edema after cataract surgery with intraocular vancomycin. *Ophthalmology.* 1999;106(9):1660-1664.
16. Qureshi F, Clark D. Macular infarction after inadvertent intracameral cefuroxime. *J Cataract Refract Surg.* 2011;37:1168-1169.
17. Delyfer MN, Rougier MB, Leoni S, et al. Ocular toxicity after intracameral injection of very high doses of cefuroxime during cataract surgery. *J Cataract Refract Surg.* 2011;37(2):271-278.
18. Pollack A, Leiba H, Bukelman A, Abrahami S, Oliver M. The course of diabetic retinopathy following cataract surgery in eyes previously treated by laser photocoagulation. *Br J Ophthalmol.* 1992(4);76:228-231.
19. Eriksson U, Alm A, Bjarnhall G, Granstam E, Matsson AW. Macular edema and visual outcome following cataract surgery in patients with diabetic retinopathy and controls. *Graefes Arch Clin Exp Ophthalmol.* 2011;249:349-359.
20. Kirwan C, O'Keeffe M. Cystoid macular edema in pediatric aphakia and pseudophakia. *Br J Ophthalmol.* 2006;90(3):37-39.
21. Ruiz RS, Saatci OA. Visual outcome in pseudophakic eyes with clinical cystoid macular edema. *Ophthalmic Surg.* 1991;22(4):190-193.
22. Randazzo A, Vinciguerra P. Chronic macular edema medical treatment in Irvine-Gass syndrome: case report. *Eur J Ophthalmol.* 2010;20(2):462-465.
23. Antcliff RJ, Spalton DJ, Stanford MR, Graham EM, Ffytche TJ, Marshall J. Intravitreal triamcinolone for uveitic cystoid macular edema: an optical coherence tomography study. *Ophthalmology.* 2001;108(4):765-772.
24. Tao Y, Jonas JB. Intravitreal triamcinolone. *Ophthalmologica.* 2011;225:1-20.
25. Williams GA, Haller JA, Kuppermann BD, et al. Dexamethasone posterior-segment drug delivery system in the treatment of macular edema resulting from uveitis or Irvine-Gass syndrome. *Am J Ophthalmol.* 2009;147(6):1048-1054, e1041-e1042.
26. Arevalo JF, Maia M, Garcia-Amaris RA, et al. Intravitreal bevacizumab for refractory pseudophakic cystoid macular edema: the Pan-American Collaborative Retina Study Group results. *Ophthalmology.* 2009;116(8):1481-1487, e1481.
27. Spitzer MS, Ziemssen F, Yoeruek E, Petermeier K, Aisenbrey S, Szurman P. Efficacy of intravitreal bevacizumab in treating postoperative pseudophakic cystoid macular edema. *J Cataract Refract Surg.* 2008;34(1):70-75.
28. Efficacy of diclofenac eyedrops in preventing postoperative inflammation and long-term cystoid macular edema. Italian Diclofenac Study Group. *J Cataract Refract Surg.* 1997;23(8):1183-1189.
29. Mathys KC, Cohen KL. Impact of nepafenac 0.1% on macular thickness and postoperative visual acuity after cataract surgery in patients at low risk for cystoid macular oedema. *Eye (Lond).* 2010;24(1):90-96.
30. Endo N, Kato S, Haruyama K, Shoji M, Kitano S. Efficacy of bromfenac sodium ophthalmic solution in preventing cystoid macular oedema after cataract surgery in patients with diabetes. *Acta Ophthalmol.* 2010;88(8):896-900.
31. Reis A, Birnbaum F, Hansen LL, Reinhard T. Successful treatment of cystoid macular edema with valdecoxib. *J Cataract Refract Surg.* 2007;33(4):682-685.

32. Deuter CM, Gelisken F, Stubiger N, Zierhut M, Doycheva D. Successful treatment of chronic pseudophakic macular edema (Irvine-Gass syndrome) with interferon alpha: a report of three cases. *Ocul Immunol Inflamm.* 2011;19(3):216-218.
33. Ismail RA, Sallam A, Zambarakji HJ. Pseudophakic macular edema and oral acetazolamide: an optical coherence tomography measurable, dose-related response. *Eur J Ophthalmol.* 2008;18(6):1011-1013.
34. Johnson MW. Tractional cystoid macular edema: a subtle variant of the vitreomacular traction syndrome. *Am J Ophthalmol.* 2005;140(2):184-192.
35. Radetzky S, Walter P, Fauser S, Koizumi K, Kirchhof B, Joussen AM. Visual outcome of patients with macular edema after pars plana vitrectomy and indocyanine green-assisted peeling of the internal limiting membrane. *Graefes Arch Clin Exp Ophthalmol.* 2004;242(4):273-278.
36. Scarpa G. Bilateral cystoid macular edema after cataract surgery resolved by vitrectomy. *Eur J Ophthalmol.* 2011;21(5):677-679.

13

Complications in Cataract Surgery With Femtosecond Laser

Lucio Buratto, MD; Stephen F. Brint, MD, FACS; and Mario R. Romano, MD, PhD

The recent adoption of femtosecond laser-assisted refractive cataract surgery represents a significant advancement in cataract surgery. Valid alternatives to ultrasound emulsification are still being sought. As with all new technologies, the use of the femtosecond laser in cataract surgery has a learning curve, with the objective of optimizing "pre-phaco" treatment, making the surgeon's work easier. Like all procedures, this has its own unique potential complications. They are primarily intraoperative. Also, with this technique, it has been reported that the complication rate decreases significantly with the learning curve and as the surgeon performs more cases. First, the surgeon must learn docking of the eye and alignment with the laser optics, interpretation of the optical coherence tomography (OCT) images, and correctly adjust laser parameters. If performed incorrectly, these steps may create complications for which even expert cataract surgeons may not be prepared.

In addition, the surgeon faces new situations during the surgery, different from those previously encountered with more "traditional" phacoemulsification. Situations that, unless correctly understood or interpreted, may cause minor or major complications.

Incorrect Eye Alignment

The first step, new to the cataract surgeon, is obtaining proper docking, ensuring that the laser suction ring is well centered on the cornea, activating suction, then, using OCT, obtaining precise intraocular measurements.

Correct docking also requires that the applanation is parallel to the front and back surface of the lens, so that the laser treatment is performed in the correct planned orientation to the structures that the laser is treating, first of all the anterior capsule. Thus, it is extremely important to ensure stability of the eye and its alignment with the optical system of the laser. If the optics of the laser are misaligned by even a fraction of a millimeter, the energy will diminish at least partially, and will be misdirected with less performance and less precise results. Possible complications include incomplete capsulorrhexis, incorrect corneal incisions, incomplete nuclear incisions, and allowing laser treatment at an incorrect plane, which in extremely rare cases may cause a posterior capsule rupture. Good docking can be achieved by ensuring correct patient positioning, avoiding the nose, and ensuring that the patient is looking at the fixation light. However, this is not all; good exposure of the eye is also required, with tight conjunctiva, a dry conjunctival sac, and good cooperation from the patient when fixating.

Buratto L, Brint SF, Romano MR.
Cataract Surgery Complications (pp 103-108).
© 2013 Taylor & Francis Group.

Last but not least, a stable surgical bed capable of fine movements that are controlled by the surgeon, for optimal bed/patient/laser alignment.

During the femto-assisted laser procedure, a suction ring is applied to prevent eye movement, but more importantly to allow the integrated OCT to obtain exact measurements and emit laser energy at the correct depth, thus avoiding laser cutting errors.

Experimental and clinical studies have shown that the use of the suction ring causes fluctuations, although small, of the intraocular pressure.[1] This may cause iatrogenic damage, varying from changes to the conjunctival goblet cells to retinal damage.[2] In spite of the relatively long suction times, docking is normally well tolerated by most patients. However, it often creates subconjunctival hemorrhage, particularly in patients taking systemic anticoagulants. Although of little importance, this complication occurs rarely in traditional phacoemulsification.

Some articles regarding microkeratome use in LASIK procedures have shown that during suction, from the microkeratome suction ring, there is a reduction of lens thickness and increased anterior-posterior vitreous traction.[3] These changes may occur similarly during suction in femtosecond laser treatment, causing vitreous detachment, temporary choroidal circulation changes,[4,5] macular hemorrhage,[6] and optic atrophy.[7]

Another suction-related complication is loss of suction during the laser application. Youth; small, tight lids; and flat corneas have been identified as risk factors. The incidence of suction loss with femtosecond lasers in LASIK procedures has been shown to have an occurrence from 0.06% to 0.27%.[9-11] Today, there are no data regarding the incidence of suction loss with the femtosecond laser in cataract surgery. Nevertheless, this does occur.

Suction loss during the use of the laser in cataract surgery must be detected immediately. The appearance of a meniscus, or redundant conjunctiva, may indicate an imminent suction loss. Even with this, treatment can often continue, at least as far as intraocular pretreatment procedures are concerned. However, during corneal incision creation using the laser it should always be interrupted, and completed with traditional keratomes.

Energy Dissipation

Energy emission in the anterior chamber (AC) stimulates miosis directly or through prostaglandin release. This can be partially treated by instilling one drop of 10% phenylephrine after the laser procedure.[12] In extreme cases, this induced miosis may cause difficulty for the surgeon. A useful solution to prevent laser-induced miosis is the preoperative use of 1% atropine and intraoperative use of preservative-free epinephrine in the irrigation bottle.

The infrared laser beam may theoretically be focused on any intraocular tissue, and the energy must be able to properly cut the tissue. With insufficient energy, or incorrect distance between laser spots, the laser cannot achieve the surgeon's objective. The laser effect is based on the creation of microscopic water and carbon dioxide bubbles, the expansion of which creates the sectioning of the tissue.

With a corneal opacity, use of the femtosecond laser may prove inappropriate. Laser energy may be unable to fully overcome, or may only partially be able to overcome, a media opacity, therefore failing to achieve the desired result. This may result in incomplete incisions of the anterior capsule or incomplete nucleus fracture.

Incomplete Incisions of the Anterior Capsule

Palanker et al reported the presence of microtears at the edge of the anterior capsulorrhexis,[13] with the formation of small folds that can lead to tears of the capsule.[12,14] Therefore, in these cases it is important for the capsulorrhexis to be completed manually with forceps to prevent equatorial and posterior extensions of these microtears at the anterior capsule margin.

The presence of "capsular bridges," or small portions of the capsule not cut by the laser, is relatively frequent. The surgeon must be diligent in recognizing them, using increased magnification with the microscope if necessary, and increased light; otherwise, removal of the capsule using forceps may allow rhexis escape and its associated dangerous effects on the completion of the procedure.

One must also remember that while performing the anterior capsulorrhexis, the laser is also cutting the anterior cortical layer of the lens. This limits visibility of the anterior capsule, sometimes even making the aqueous slightly cloudy, limiting the surgeon's intraocular acute visibility.

Besides, the incision of the anterior cortex also causes more difficulties during its removal using irrigation/aspiration (I/A) cannulas. Here, the surgeon may sometimes need to use alternative techniques. A very useful one is the Buratto bimanual I/A technique. The use of a rounded spatula passed along the posterior surface of the anterior capsule has also been suggested to create cortical "tags" that facilitate engagement and complete aspiration of the cortex. The basic issue is that with the laser's perfect capsulorrhexis comes an underlying cortical rhexis, which makes traditional I/A maneuvers not work as well, as the cortical margin is sharp and more difficult to grasp and aspirate than the ragged cortex we are used to (see Figures A1 to A6).

Incomplete Nucleus Fracture

Before proceeding with laser lens fragmentation, the surgeon must plan the depth and pattern of laser treatment to be delivered to the lens. It is recommended that a safe distance is maintained from the posterior capsule as identified by the intralaser OCT.

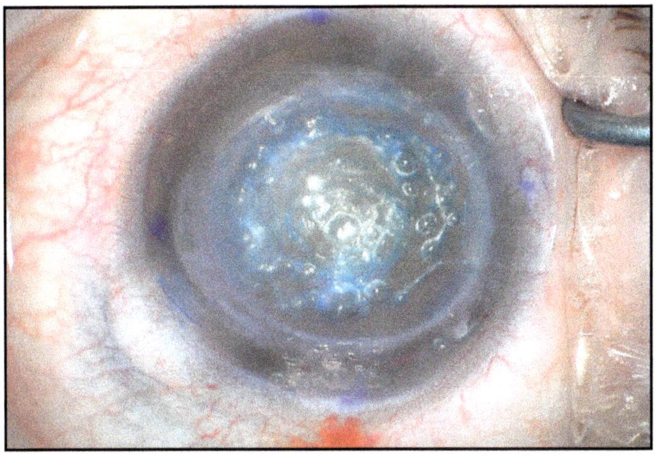

Figure A1. In cataracts secondary to penetrating keratoplasty, the femtosecond laser can be a source of problems because the presence of corneal scarring does not allow a perfect cut of the anterior capsulorrhexis.

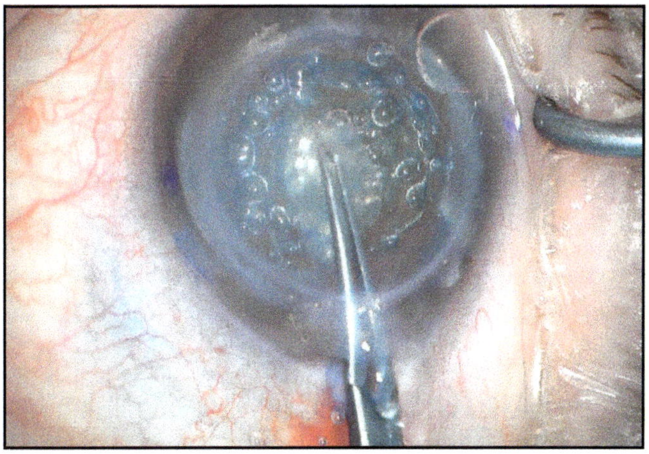

Figure A2. The capsule is stained with trypan blue and then the residual capsular bridges are opened slowly and gradually removed.

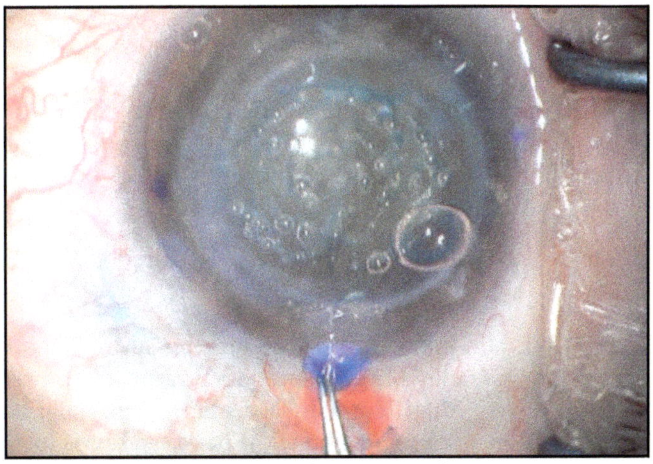

Figure A3. The anterior capsule is removed.

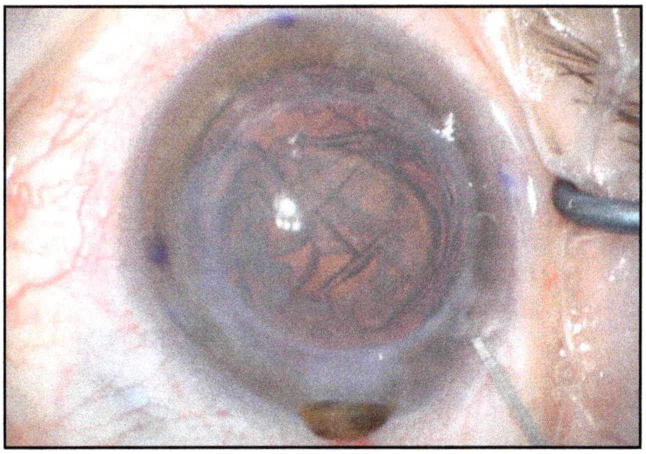

Figure A4. Presence of iris prolapse through the corneal incision at the time of ultrasound probe removal.

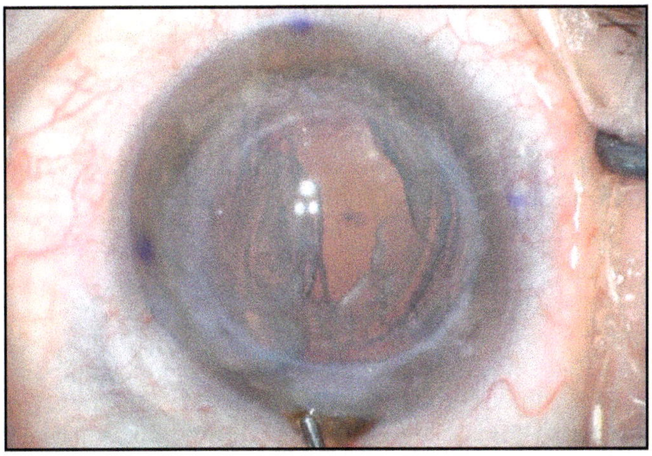

Figure A5. The iris is repositioned and the incision is closed with sutures.

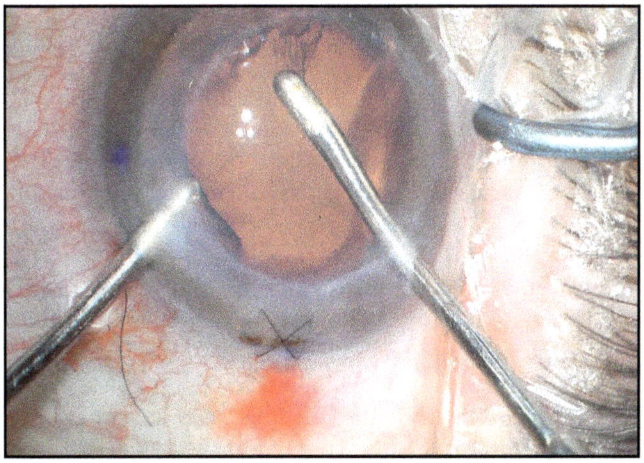

Figure A6. I/A is then performed.

With very dense nuclei, the effect of the laser is not yet sufficient, thus resulting in incomplete ablation with shallow or absent grooves. Thus other nuclear fracture instruments are required in a more traditional manner.

Nevertheless, the surgeon must be capable of managing a shallowly divided nucleus, resulting in a residual nuclear plate, uncut because of its proximity to the posterior capsule. It is recommended to flip the nuclear plate, or, if a larger quantity of lens is still present, try to sculpt, inducing complete separation of the nucleus.

Rupture of the Capsule

The most dreaded complication, also with femtosecond laser treatment, is rupture of the posterior capsule.

The formation of large gas bubbles in the AC, smaller around the edge of the capsulorrhexis, and gas inclusions inside the nucleus of the lens, can cause hydration damage. The gas produced by the laser increases the intracapsular volume. When not correctly managed, this causes a rupture of the posterior capsule resulting in dislocation of the lens into the vitreous chamber. This is partially due to an increase of intracapsular pressure, but mostly to improper hydrodissection, which can cause a further increase of intracapsular pressure.

Predisposing factors include polar posterior cataracts, mature cataracts, long axial length, and overly rapid and aggressive hydrodissection.[15]

In order to avoid this complication, the following are recommended[12]:

- Try not to over-fill the AC with viscoelastic material before the removal of the anterior capsule.
- Decompress the AC before and after hydrodissection by putting pressure on the back lip of the corneal incision.
- During hydrodissection, lift the edge of the anterior capsule.
- Inject the hydrodissection fluid slowly, using the visible wave expansion as a reference. This is the most common mistake by the beginning femtolaser surgeon, who wants to perform traditional hydrodissection. Because of the perfect capsulorrhexis and tight cortical adhesions, also with trapped gas posterior to the lens, the room for egress of the hydrodissection fluid is less than the surgeon is used to, creating the set-up for potentially blowing out the posterior capsule as reported by Lawless et al. This immediately stops after the first occurrence as the learning curve suggests gentle smaller injections allowing fluid/gas escape as you go.
- The most effective method is undoubtedly the use of a prechopper or chopper, or even a cannula, to divide the nucleus of the lens to allow the gas and/or liquid to escape, performing hydrodissection only after this happens.

According to the small number of papers published regarding cataract surgery using the femtolaser, rupture of the posterior capsule and dislocation of lens fragments into the vitreous chamber are more likely to occur than when using the standard phacoemulsification technique. Rupture of the posterior capsule has been reported as having an incidence of 0.53% to 1.9%, while the incidence of the posterior dislocation of the nucleus into the vitreous chamber is 0.1% to 0.12%.[18,19]

The main cause of posterior capsule rupture and lens dislocation is the extension of radial tears of the anterior capsule. It is imperative that microtears at the margin of the capsulotomy are recognized and managed with care. These are either due to an incomplete laser incision of the capsule, the inability of the surgeon to see possible postlaser capsule microbridges, or other factors (lens tilt, corneal opacity, thickening of the capsule).

It is imperative that microincisions at the margin of the capsulotomy are recognized and managed with care by the surgeon.

After the learning curve of the first 50 cases, complications of posterior capsule rupture or dislocation of lens material into the vitreous are significantly reduced.

Cortical Aspiration

It is common knowledge for all surgeons using femtophaco that aspiration of the cortex is much more complex and time-consuming than standard phaco. This may be associated with less progression of the balanced saline solution (BSS) fluid wave during hydrodissection. The surgeon fears, due to the presence of intracapsular air bubbles, that this may cause excessive intracapsular pressure.

However, it might also be due to the fact that the air bubbles released during the creation of nuclear incisions may cause greater adhesion of the cortex to the anterior and equatorial posterior capsule.

In any case, cortical removal is much easier when using the Buratto bimanual technique, which offers better access to the entire 360 degrees of the capsular bag.

Complications of Incisions

It is not always easy for the surgeon to correctly predict the outer limit of the corneal incision and its location. An incision that is placed too peripheral in the limbus may not lead to the desired effect, and therefore may not allow the opening of the incision itself.

Sometimes, the incision is too anterior in the cornea, causing difficulties for the surgeon during the various intraocular maneuvers. Sometimes it may be oblique, creating difficulties for the surgeon and inducing slight irregular astigmatism.

Lastly, relaxing incisions for astigmatic correction must originate from nomograms, initially unreliable but now rapidly evolving, that provide predictable and repeatable results.

References

1. Vetter JM, Holzer MP, Teping C, et al. Intraocular pressure during corneal flap preparation: comparison among four femtosecond lasers in porcine eyes. *J Refract Surg.* 2011;27(6):427-433.
2. Davis RM, Evangelista JA. Ocular structure changes during vacuum by the Hansatome microkeratome suction ring. *J Refract Surg.* 2007;23(6):563-566.
3. Mirshahi A, Kohnen T. Effect of microkeratome suction during LASIK on ocular structures. *Ophthalmology.* 2005;112(4):645-649.
4. Luna JD, Artal MN, Reviglio VE, Pelizzari M, Diaz H, Juarez CP. Vitreo-retinal alterations following laser in situ keratomileusis: clinical and experimental studies. *Graefes Arch Clin Exp Ophthalmol.* 2001;239(6):416-423.
5. Smith RJ, Yadarola MB, Pelizzari MF, Luna JD, Juarez CP, Reviglio VE. Complete bilateral vitreous detachment after LASIK retreatment. *J Cataract Refract Surg.* 2004;30(6):1382-1384.
6. Moshfeghi AA, Harrison SA, Reinstein DZ, Ferrone PJ. Valsalva-like retinopathy following hyperopic laser in situ keratomileusis. *Ophthalmic Surg Lasers Imaging.* 2006;37(6):486-488.
7. Conway ML, Wevill M, Benavente-Perez A, Hosking SL. Ocular blood-flow hemodynamics before and after application of a laser in situ keratomileusis ring. *J Cataract Refract Surg.* 2010;36(2): 268-272.
8. Asano-Kato N, Toda I, Hori-Komai Y, Takano Y, Tsubota K. Risk factors for insufficient fixation of microkeratome during laser in situ keratomileusis. *J Refract Surg.* 2002;18(1):47-50.
9. Haft P, Yoo SH, Kymionis GD, Ide T, O'Brien TP, Culbertson WW. Complications of LASIK flaps made by the IntraLase 15- and 30-kHz femtosecond lasers. *J Refract Surg.* 2009;25(11): 979-984.
10. Davison JA, Johnson SC. Intraoperative complications of LASIK flaps using the IntraLase femtosecond laser in 3009 cases. *J Refract Surg.* 2010;26(11):851-857.
11. Binder PS. One thousand consecutive IntraLase laser in situ keratomileusis flaps. J Cataract Refract Surg. 2006;32(6):962-969.
12. Bali SJ, Hodge C, Lawless M, Roberts TV, Sutton G. Early experience with the femtosecond laser for cataract surgery. *Ophthalmology.* 2012;119(5):891-899.
13. Palanker DV, Blumenkranz MS, Andersen D, et al. Femtosecond laser-assisted cataract surgery with integrated optical coherence tomography. *Sci Transl Med.* 2010;2(58):58ra85.
14. Marques FF, Marques DM, Osher RH, Osher JM. Fate of anterior capsule tears during cataract surgery. *J Cataract Refract Surg.* 2006;32(10):1638-1642.
15. Miyake K, Ota I, Ichihashi S, Miyake S, Tanaka Y, Terasaki H. New classification of capsular block syndrome. *J Cataract Refract Surg.* 1998;24(9):1230-1234.
16. Jaycock P, Johnston RL, Taylor H, et al. The Cataract National Dataset electronic multi-centre audit of 55,567 operations: updating benchmark standards of care in the United Kingdom and internationally. *Eye (Lond).* 2009;23(1):38-49.
17. Zaidi FH, Corbett MC, Burton BJ, Bloom PA. Raising the benchmark for the 21st century--the 1000 cataract operations audit and survey: outcomes, consultant-supervised training and sourcing NHS choice. *Br J Ophthalmol.* 2007;91(6):731-736.
18. Misra A, Burton RL. Incidence of intraoperative complications during phacoemulsification in vitrectomized and non-vitrectomized eyes: prospective study. *J Cataract Refract Surg.* 2005;31(5):1011-1014.
19. Clark A, Morlet N, Ng JQ, Preen DB, Semmens JB. Whole population trends in complications of cataract surgery over 22 years in Western Australia. *Ophthalmology.* 2011;118(6):1055-1061.

Section II

14

Complications of Capsulorrhexis

Michael E. Snyder, MD and Mauricio A. Perez, MD

Since the anterior capsule cannot be mended once a complication has occurred, management must be prompt and principles of prevention are paramount.

The mathematical finite element method teaches us how the capsule behaves under stress with varying configurations. The smooth edge of the continuous capsulorrhexis has maximal strength due to the low and uniform stress distribution across the entire rhexis margin with a higher resistance to tears. In contradistinction, the point of maximum stress is located exactly at the leading edge of a capsular tear.[1] This understanding guides our recognition of potential dangers and management options once a problem occurs.

Errant Peripheral Deviation of a Capsulorrhexis

We divide the errant tear into 3 categories:

1. **Partial tear not reaching the equator or zonules**

   Prompt recognition is required when the control of the direction of the capsule tear is lost and it starts deviating peripherally. This typically occurs as a result of shallowing of the anterior chamber (AC), posterior pressure, or both, causing an increase in equatorial zonular tension. The first step in management is to immediately overpressurize the AC to negate the inciting physical forces. The peripheral forces can also be mitigated by "dry" aspiration of underlying cortical material with a 27-gauge cannula or by reducing vitreous volume with intravenous hyperosmotics. Next, a couple of options are available. Dr. Brian Little's rescue maneuver uses mathematical addition of forces to allow a tear-out to return to the circular desired path.[2] This maneuver requires unfolding the capsule and applying traction retrograde from the initial path in order to deviate the tear centrally and allow the surgeon to safely complete the capsulorrhexis. This technique is extremely useful in the presence of an intact zonular apparatus with uniform force distribution across the capsular plane. When zonular integrity is compromised, however, this maneuver may behave unpredictably. Our technique of choice in such settings requires the use of microforceps through a paracentesis to fold over the loose edge capsule and redirect the tear centrally using shearing forces. This technique may also be used when the tear approaches the equator of the capsule.

2. **Full tear reaching to but not through the equator and the zonules**

   In these cases, any attempt to retrieve the capsular tear has high chances of extending it posteriorly;

Buratto L, Brint SF, Romano MR.
Cataract Surgery Complications (pp 111-114).
© 2013 Taylor & Francis Group.

therefore, our recommendation is to first complete the capsulorrhexis from the opposite side, avoiding contact with the highest stress point during the procedure. Consideration of primary posterior continuous curvilinear capsulorrhexis (PCCC) with optic capture will guarantee long-term intraocular lens (IOL) centration.[3]

3. **Full tear that goes beyond the equator and loops to the posterior capsule**

   This is a critical situation that more commonly occurs during phaco or later steps. If it happens during the initial capsulorrhexis maneuver, it is likely to be unrecognized and often results in loss of support and, perhaps, posterior luxation of nuclear material. With tears beyond the equator (Figure 14-1, orange arrows), options are limited and risks are high. Continuation of the tear all the way around may result in a "hemi-bag" with a lack of structural support for the IOL. When visualized, we prefer to transform this situation with one high stress point located at the end of the tear (see Figure 14-1) to a balanced force distribution by converting this point into a continuous tear that circles back to the initial radial extension (Figure 14-2). This will allow uniform distribution of the forces, with no single high stress point, and will increase capsular resistance, as described by the finite element method (Figure 14-3).

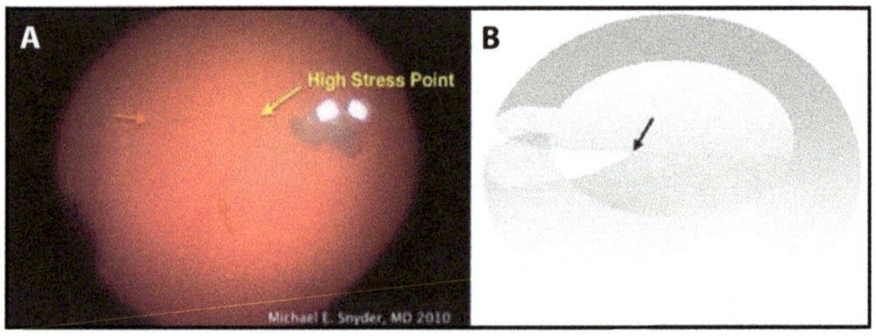

Figure 14-1. Extension of capsulorrhexis tear to posterior capsule. Highest stress point indicated by arrow. (A) Operative image. (B) Scheme.

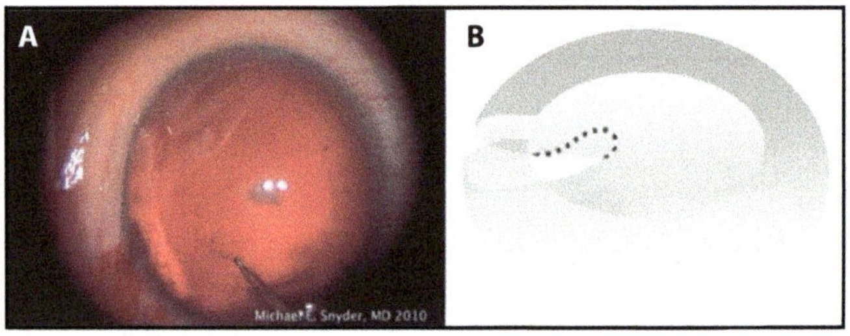

Figure 14-2. Dotted line indicates path of conversion from one high stress point to continuous tear, preventing the likelihood of extension.

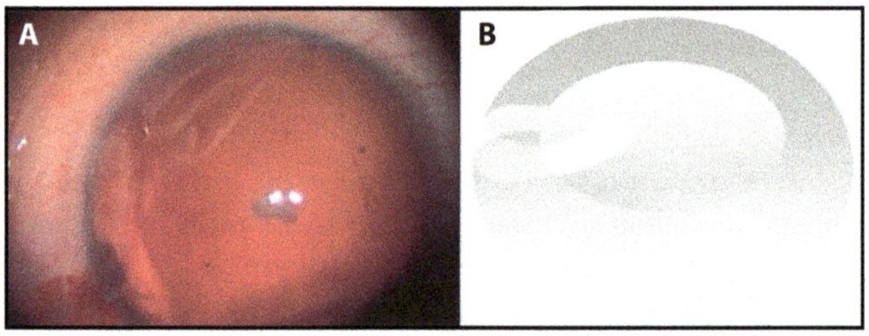

Figure 14-3. Appearance of continuous tear capsular margin after salvage maneuver.

Capsulorrhexis Is Too Small

When the continuous curvilinear capsulorrhexis (CCC) is too small, the surgeon can carefully enlarge it by making a small tangential snip in the CCC and peeling the desired amount off the margin in a spiral. This maneuver can be repeated until the desired CCC size is achieved, remembering that although enlarging the opening is a bit challenging, reducing its size is impossible. We recommend waiting until after posterior IOL implantation before enlarging a CCC.

Capsulorrhexis Is Too Big

Considering that a capsule cannot be resutured to attempt decreasing a CCC diameter, the surgeon can consider one of the following alternatives to manage this complication:

1. **Changing the dioptric power of the IOL**

   If the CCC does not fully cover the optic, the IOL will shift forward, with the zonular plane at the posterior IOL surface rather than splitting the IOL optic, thereby increasing its effective power and achieving a more myopic result. A similar IOL with a weaker dioptric power can be used to counteract this phenomenon.

2. **Choosing an IOL with a larger optic**

   Selecting an IOL with a larger optic than the CCC will mitigate the change in power shift.

3. **PCCC with optic capture**

   One could choose to create a PCCC smaller than the desired optic size, place the haptics in the bag, and capture the IOL optic into Berger's space, using the original power calculation formula.

Capsule Will Not Pierce With Cystotome

This problem is encountered both in the elastic juvenile capsule and in the normal elasticity adult capsule when there is inadequate zonular countertraction. Clinically, a "pin cushion" effect is seen on attempted anterior capsule puncture.

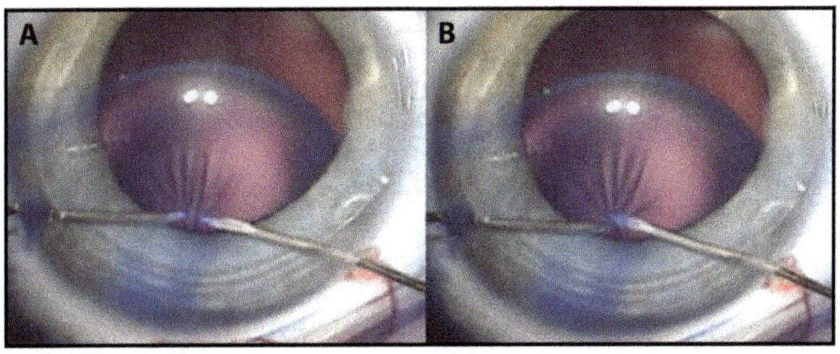

Figure 14-4. (A) The anterior capsule is pinched between 2 30-gauge needles. (B) As the needle tips are advanced toward each other, one or both (the right one in this image) will penetrate the capsule.

We can modulate the biomechanical properties of the highly elastic capsule using trypan blue stain, which reduces capsular elasticity both in clinical and experimental settings.[4,5]

Several techniques can manage this difficulty. Our technique of choice is the crossed-swords, capsule-pinch technique[6] (Figure 14-4), which utilizes opposing forces from the tips of 2 30-gauge needles directed toward each other, pinching a fold of anterior capsule between them with one tip acting as countertraction to the other, thereby penetrating the membrane. This avoids stress on the zonules and prevents anteroposterior displacement of the loose lens. Continuing the CCC can be a struggle due to the lack of zonular countertraction. Iris hooks or a temporary capsular tension segment can supplement the reduced or lacking centrifugal forces required to counteract the centripetal force applied by the surgeon (Figure 14-5). A few new devices, the MST Capsule Retractors (MicroSurgical Technology, Redmond, WA)[7] and the AssiAnchor (Hanita Lenses, Kibbutz Hanita, Israel),[8] both use the capsular equator to apply this countertraction. These devices can be moved or added sequentially during CCC completion.

Capsulorrhexis Is Too Fragile

This condition is specifically encountered when attempting a CCC on a congenital aniridia patient or glassblower's cataract, whose anterior capsules are thinner and more friable.[9]

In these patients, we avoid the use of trypan blue for capsular staining because we do not desire to decrease elasticity of the already-fragile capsule. If capsular staining is required (eg, to differentiate the capsule and an opaque prosthesis), we recommend the use of indocyanine green, which allows an adequate staining without the effect on the biomechanical properties of the capsule.[10-12]

On these thin capsule cases, similarly to when we are creating a PCCC, tactile feedback from the capsule is limited, and we need to rely on visual feedback during the capsular tear.

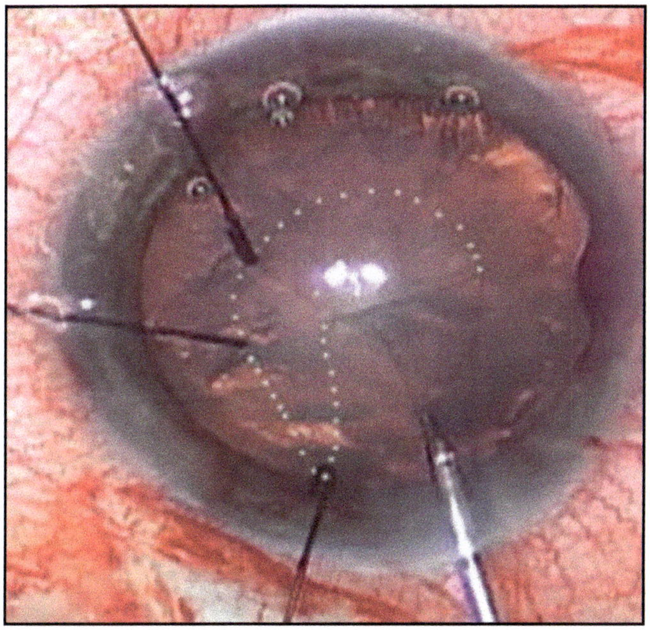

Figure 14-5. Iris hooks help support a very loose lens during capsulorrhexis. The dotted line indicates the path of the capsulorrhexis, which has already been torn. The leading flap is grasped with a 25-gauge microforceps.

Postoperative Complications of the Continuous Curvilinear Capsulorrhexis

Sometimes the capsulorrhexis can create problems postoperatively with CCC phimosis. In some instances, this can limit vision through the pupillary aperture, requiring laser or operative "rhexisotomy." When highly flexible lenses are used, it can even cause a hyperopic shift in the refraction.[13]

Conclusion

While capsulorrhexis complications are infrequent, attentiveness and awareness to these special techniques can rescue the challenged capsulorrhexis.

References

1. Krag S, Corydon L, Kyster B. Biomechanical aspects of the anterior capsulotomy. *J Cataract Refract Surg*. 1994;20:410-416.
2. Little BC, Smith JH, Packer M. Little capsulorrhexis tear-out rescue. *J Cataract Refract Surg*. 2006;32:1420-1422.
3. Gimbel HV, DeBroff BM. Intraocular lens optic capture. *J Cataract Refract Surg*. 2004;30(1):200-206.
4. Wollensak G, Spörl E, Pham D-T. Biomechanical changes in the anterior lens capsule after trypan blue staining. *J Cataract Refract Surg*. 2004;30:1526-1530.

5. Dick HB, Aliyeva SE, Hengerer F. Effect of trypan blue on the elasticity of the human anterior lens capsule. *J Cataract Refract Surg.* 2008;34:1367-1373.
6. Snyder ME, Lindsell LB. Crossed-swords, capsule-pinch technique for capsulotomy in pediatric and/or loose lens cataract extractions. *J Cataract Refract Surg.* 2010;36:197-199.
7. MST Capsular Support System. *MicroSurgical Technology Web site.* http://www.mst-surgical.com/home.
8. Assia EI, Ton Y, Michaeli A. Capsule anchor to manage subluxated lenses: initial clinical experience. *J Cataract Refract Surg.* 2009;35(8):1372-1379.
9. Schneider S, Osher RH, Burk SE, Lutz TB, Montione R. Thinning of the anterior capsule associated with congenital aniridia. *J Cataract Refract Surg.* 2003;29(3):523-525.
10. Snyder ME. Staining the capsule in congenital aniridic eyes. *J Cataract Refract Surg.* 2012;38(2):373-374.
11. Khng C, Snyder ME. Indocyanine green-emitted fluorescence as an aid to anterior capsule visualization. *J Cataract Refract Surg.* 2005;31:1454-1455; errata, 1857.
12. Snyder ME, Osher RH. Evaluation of trypan-blue and indocyanine-green staining of iris prostheses. *J Cataract Refract Surg.* 2011;37:206-207.
13. Ozturk F, Snyder ME, Osher RH, Bishop JR III. Hyperopic shift with posterior bowing of a Collamer posterior chamber intraocular lens. *J Cataract Refract Surg.* 2007;33:159-161.

15

Complications of Phacoemulsification

Ozana Moraru, MD

Modern sutureless cataract surgery, using sophisticated phaco devices, together with advanced intraocular lens (IOL) technologies, has made phacoemulsification one of the safest medical procedures. Still, phacoemulsification has potential complications. One critical complication is rupture of the posterior capsule, with or without vitreous prolapse, with or without retained nuclear fragments (Figure 15-1).

How to handle this complication? It depends on the time during the procedure when the rupture occurred. If it happens at the beginning (eg, rupture of the anterior continuous curvilinear capsulorrhexis [CCC], extending to the equator and to the posterior capsule, or perforation of the posterior capsule with the phaco tip at the beginning of sculpting/chopping/splitting of the nucleus), converting to planned extracapsular extraction is advisable because the threat of a dropped nucleus at this phase of the surgery is great and it is better to avoid that.

Ophthalmic viscoelastic devices (OVDs) injected posterior to the nucleus, to prevent its posterior displacement, and anterior to the nucleus, to protect the endothelium, should be the first step. With the OVDs injected posterior to the nucleus, the surgeon tries gently to push the nucleus from posterior to anterior in the anterior chamber (AC), anterior to the iris plane, followed by enlargement of the limbal incision and extracapsular extraction, aided by a loop. Of course, vitrectomy is mandatory because vitreous prolapse is almost always present when the posterior capsule breaks early in phacoemulsification. Triamcinolone injected in the AC is of great help for visualization of the vitreous in the AC, even small vitreous strands, thus helping us to perform a complete anterior vitrectomy.

If the rupture occurs later, during phaco aspiration of the divided pieces of nucleus, the surgeon can continue the phaco procedure. The first step is to lower the infusion bottle and then, before taking the hand piece out of the AC, inject a large amount of OVD through a lateral paracentesis, but from posterior to anterior, making a sort of "cushion" underneath, trying to avoid dropping nuclear pieces into the vitreous. Dry vitrectomy, with low aspiration rate and 600 to 800 cutter frequency, is mandatory, in order to avoid vitreous traction. Another cushion-like support for the nuclear pieces can be made by a Sheath glide (Beaver Visitec, Waltham, MA) inserted under the nucleus on the anterior CCC, or by a 3-piece IOL injected under the pieces of nucleus onto the iris (Agarwal technique) after having brought the pieces into the AC.

The phacoemulsification continues in the AC, and care should be taken to protect the endothelium. The following phacoemulsification must be done with low vacuum/aspiration settings: 20 to 25 cc/min, vacuum of 200 to 250, slowly, to avoid turbulence in the AC with possible further dropping of nuclear fragments.

Buratto L, Brint SF, Romano MR.
Cataract Surgery Complications (pp 115-118).
© 2013 Taylor & Francis Group.

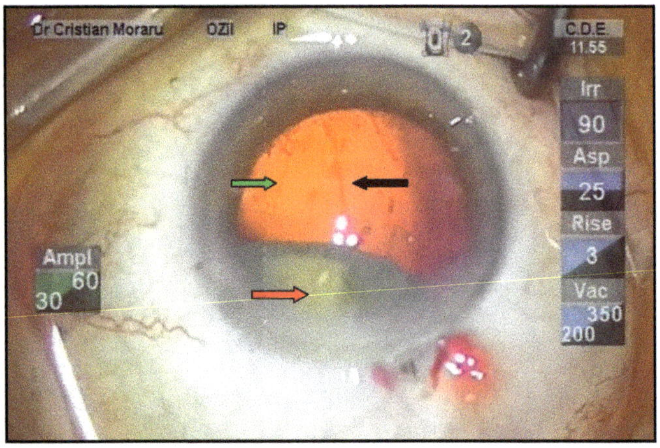

Figure 15-1. Posterior capsule rupture (black arrow). Anterior CCC (green arrow). Remaining nucleus to be emulsified (red arrow).

If the tear in the posterior capsule is not very large, or with a radially-oriented tear, a posterior CCC under OVD should be done, with local dry vitrectomy, thus preventing further enlargement of the tear remaining phacoemulsification or during the IOL insertion.

One way or another, the goal is to avoid vitreous remnants in the AC, vitreous traction, and to emulsify and aspirate all the nuclear pieces, epinucleus, and cortex. Total cleaning of the capsular bag and AC and preservation of as much as possible of the posterior capsule, or at least of an intact anterior CCC, must be attempted in order to facilitate correct IOL implantation and position and to minimize the postoperative inflammatory reaction. The vitrectomy can be done either through the limbal incisions or through pars plana, depending on the size of the tear and location, and the surgeon's experience.

The Dropped Nucleus

Losing the nucleus or parts of it in the vitreous because of a break in the posterior capsule is one of the most unwanted complications of cataract surgery because of its potential complications and difficulties of management. Once this happens, the surgeon has to make a decision:

- Proceed with vitrectomy and phacofragmentation of the fallen pieces (this can be done at the time of the surgery, sometimes by the cataract surgeon him- or herself if he or she has experience in posterior segment surgery, or later [ie, after 1 or 2 days] by the vitreoretinal surgeon).
- Or, if the dropped pieces are small and the surgeon has not had much experience, he or she can leave the pieces, continue the surgery with anterior vitrectomy via the AC, complete cleaning of the bag, and implant a suitable IOL, depending on the available posterior or anterior capsule support. During the next few days, if there is no further complication (intraocular pressure [IOP] rise, inflammatory reaction, impaired visual acuity), a second surgery may not be needed, just close observation of the patient. If there are any of these complications, the retinal surgeon must proceed with posterior vitrectomy and phacoaspiration of the fallen pieces.

Other Possible Complications During Phacoemulsification

Descemet's detachment can occur when entering with the phaco tip at the main incision site. To avoid this, a proper incision is required, with injection of OVD in the AC and in the incision, followed by careful insertion of the tip and sleeve in the AC, usually by a rotation of 90 degrees of the tip when entering the AC.

Iris root detachment (iridodialysis) can occur when entering the AC with the phaco tip, especially in a shallow AC, and can lead to pupil distortion, posterior synechia, and even iris atrophy, if it is combined also with persistent iris prolapse.

Endothelial touch can occur with the phaco tip or the chopper/nucleus rotator, especially in a flat AC. A large quantity of dispersive protective OVD, given repeatedly during phacoemulsification, can diminish its damage to the cornea (eg, edema, Descemet's folds).

When pinching or catching of the iris in the phaco tip occurs, especially with small pupils and/or in floppy iris syndrome, deepening the AC with a good cohesive OVD and lowering the infusion bottle and the vacuum/aspiration rate parameters are recommended. Sometimes it is necessary to engage the pupil margins temporarily with devices (eg, Malyugin ring [MicroSurgical Technology, Redmond, WA] or iris hooks) that will keep the pupil margin from the aspirating phaco tip.

Iris prolapse through the lateral paracentesis (Figure 15-2), quite common in floppy iris syndrome, can be avoided or minimized by lowering the infusion bottle and the aspiration rate/vacuum parameters and by initially performing a smaller paracentesis, through which the chopper or rotator must be very carefully introduced and withdrawn. When withdrawing it, the surgeon stops infusion first, presses a little bit on the iris at the paracentesis site, keeping the iris inside, decompresses the AC, and only after this maneuver can he or she withdraw carefully the instrument, thus avoiding further damage of the prolapsed iris at the paracentesis site.

Another complication can arise, although it is very rare with modern microincisional cataract surgery and sophisticated phaco machines—intraocular hemorrhage. Sometimes blood can come from iris vessels because of

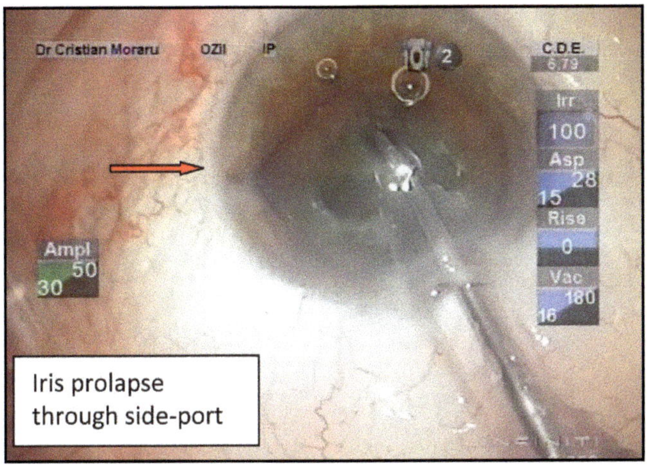

Figure 15-2. Iris prolapse through side port.

poor surgical technique with the phaco tip hitting the iris. Once blood is in the AC, a temporary IOP rise by injecting a balanced salt solution (with or without adrenaline 1:5,000) or OVD in the AC can solve the problem. Sometimes, if the iris vessel is quite big and the hemorrhage cannot be stopped, an adequate cautery probe (needle tipped) can be used to stop the iris bleeding. Choroidal effusion or hemorrhage is quite rare in phacoemulsification, due to the small incisions into the eye, but it is not impossible. The surgeon should stop the surgery temporarily. Usually, this occurs in patients with arterial hypertension or in myopic, glaucomatous, or nanophthalmic eyes. The intraoperative signs are sudden IOP elevation, followed immediately by a shallow AC, which cannot be deepened by any means. If the red reflex of the retina becomes darker, a choroidal hemorrhage must be suspected. In the worst situation, this may proceed to an expulsive hemorrhage (very rare in microincisional phaco surgery). This is an intraoperative emergency; the incision must be quickly closed (sutured), a hyperosmotic solution (eg, mannitol) administered intravenously, and OVD in the AC in order to achieve a deeper AC. In severe cases, a sclerotomy might be needed. The cataract surgery can be completed at a later date, days or even weeks later.

Suggested Readings

Chang DF. Use of Malyugin pupil expansion device for intraoperative floppy-iris syndrome: results in 30 consecutive cases. *J Cataract Refract Surg.* 2008;34(5):835-841.

Hyams M, Mathalone N, Herskovitz M, Hod Y, Israeli D, Geyer O. Intraoperative complications of phaco emulsification in eyes with and without pseudo exfoliation. *J Cataract Refract Surg.* 2005;31(5):1002-1005.

Khng C, Osher RH. Surgical options in the face of positive pressure. *J Cataract Refract Surg.* 2006;32(9):1423-1425.

Kohnen T, Wang L, Friedman NJ, Koch DD. Complications of cataract surgery. In: Yanoff M, Duker JS, eds. *Ophthalmology.* 2nd ed. Maryland Heights, MO: Mosby; 2004:381-390.

Little BC, Smith JH, Packer M. Little capsulorrhexis tear-out rescue. *J Cataract Refract Surg.* 2006;32(9):1420-1422.

Masket S. Consultation section. Cataract surgical problem. *J Cataract Refract Surg.* 2009;35(10):1836-1843.

Safar AN, Afshari NA, Assi A. The Sheath glide maneuver. In: Melki SA, Azar DT, eds. *101 Pearls in Cataract, Corneal, and Refractive Surgery.* 2nd ed. Thorofare, NJ: SLACK Incorporated; 2006: 113-114.

Safar AN, Afshari NA, Assi A. Posterior-assisted levitation. In: Melki SA, Azar DT, eds. *101 Pearls in Cataract, Corneal, and Refractive Surgery.* 2nd ed. Thorofare, NJ: SLACK Incorporated; 2006: 111-112.

Shingleton BJ, Marvin AC, Heier JS, et al. Pseudoexfoliation: high risk factors for zonule weakness and concurrent vitrectomy during phacoemulsification. *J Cataract Refract Surg.* 2010;36(8): 1261-1269.

Tint NL, Yeung AM, Alexander P. Management of intraoperative floppy-iris syndrome-associated iris prolapse using a single iris retractor. *J Cataract Refract Surg.* 2009;35(11):1849-1852.

Wagoner MD, Cox TA, Ariyasu RG, Jacobs DS, Karp CL. Intraocular lens implantation in the absence of capsular support. *Ophthalmology.* 2003;840-859.

16

Complications
Phaco Device Related

Roger F. Steinert, MD

Barring a catastrophic malfunction of the machine, most complications related to machines and tubing are due to fluidics. Understanding the normal behavior of the fluidics, and the ability to recognize and diagnose fluidic problems, will allow a surgeon to minimize complications related to the machine and tubing. This chapter will briefly outline the key issues.

Surge and Posterior Capsule Rupture

Clinical presentation: Sudden shallowing of the anterior chamber (AC) may lead to contact of the posterior capsule (PC) and the phaco tip with PC rupture and vitreous prolapse.

Cause: Surge is the result of the release of potential energy inside the tubing. When the phaco tip is occluded and vacuum builds, a subtle but critical contraction of the flexible tubing occurs. When the occlusion clears, the tubing rapidly expands back to its original diameter. AC fluid is aspirated into that space, leading to AC shallowing.

Prevention:

- Sophisticated computer-driven fluidic control found in current-generation, high-quality phaco machines
- Tightly wound construction minimizing leakage
- Adequate infusion bottle height
- Conservative vacuum settings (peristaltic pumps) or aspiration limits (venturi pumps)
- Low compliance (relatively rigid) tubing on the aspiration side

Surgeon maneuvers: Since surge can never be fully avoided, toward the completion of nucleus and epinucleus removal, keep a flat spatula-shaped instrument between the phaco tip and the PC.

Obstructed Fluid Flow

Clinical presentation: Depending on the location of the obstruction, the AC may shallow or the removal of lens material may slow or halt. The appearance of "lens milk" during nuclear phaco, lack of material engagement in the tip, and lack of disappearance of lens material are all signs of obstructed aspiration. In cases where the ultrasound energy continues to be delivered, in the absence of adequate fluid cooling, wound burn may occur (see subsequent section).

Buratto L, Brint SF, Romano MR.
Cataract Surgery Complications (pp 119-120).
© 2013 Taylor & Francis Group.

Causes: Lack of fluid inflow is due to the following:

- Bottle height is set too low
- Allowing the fluid to be depleted from the infusion bottle
- A crimp in the infusion line
- Obstructed aspiration can be located within the hand piece or in the tubing leading back to the machine, usually due to accumulated hard lens material or inadequately cleaned hand pieces and tips, where autoclaving then solidifies the material inside the hand piece and tip.

Prevention:

- Train operating room personnel to be observant about fluid levels in the infusion
- Avoid awkward tubing pathways that can lead to crimping
- Maintain clean tips and hand pieces
- Replace obsolete phaco machines where tubing has narrow zones that trap lens material

Surgeon maneuvers: Obstructed outflow is apparent by both lack of followability of the lens fragments and an audible signal from the machine indicating high vacuum. The surgeon must recognize these signs and stop. Removing the hand piece and connecting the infusion line to the aspiration line determines the location of the obstruction. If the vacuum level builds when the surgeon steps on the pedal, the obstruction is in the line, usually at a tubing connection.

If the fluid flows freely with the 2 ends of the tubing directly connected to each other, then the obstruction is in the hand piece. The surgeon must flush the hand piece and tip with balanced salt solution in a syringe, or use a new hand piece if the obstruction cannot be cleared.

Wound Burn

Clinical presentation: Whitening of the incision stroma, with stromal contraction and wound gaping in severe cases.

Causes: The fundamental cause of wound burn is lack of flow of cooling fluid when ultrasound energy is being applied. This can be due to lack of inflow around the irrigating sleeve so that the phaco tip is not cooled externally (lack of infusion fluid or excessively tight incision), obstruction of outflow so that the phaco tip is not cooled internally (obstructed outflow [see previous section] or inadequate aspiration and vacuum, especially if using low settings for "sculpting" and/or in the presence of dispersive viscoelastics), or a combination of both.

Prevention:

- Match incision size to the sleeve and phaco tip
- Be alert to signs of outflow obstruction
- Be cautious with low flow and vacuum settings

Surgeon maneuvers: Maintain alert observation of phaco parameters and the behavior of the fluidics. Unexpected chamber shallowing, poor followability of lens fragments, and unexpected high vacuum alerts are all warning signs of fluidic mismatch that may lead to wound burn.

References

1. Fishkind WJ, Neuhann TF, Steinert RF. The phaco machine: the physical principles guiding its operation. In: Steinert RF, ed. *Cataract Surgery*. 3rd ed. London, England: Elsevier; 2010:75-92.
2. Seibel BS. *Phacodynamics: Mastering the Tools and Techniques of Phacoemulsification Surgery*. 3rd ed. Thorofare, NJ: SLACK Incorporated; 2004.

17

Intraocular Lens as a Scaffold to Prevent Dropped Nuclei

Athiya Agarwal, MD, DO

Intraocular Lens Scaffold

A foldable intraocular lens (IOL) is used as a scaffold to prevent nuclear fragments from dropping into the vitreous in cases of posterior capsule rupture. After anterior vitrectomy, a 3-piece foldable IOL is injected using the existing corneal incision with one haptic above the iris and the other haptic extending outside the incision (Figure 17-1). The IOL can alternately be placed into the sulcus, or, if the iris is not floppy, both haptics can be implanted above the iris. The nucleus is emulsified with the phaco above the IOL optic. Cortical cleaning is done, and the IOL is then placed over the remnants of the capsule in the ciliary sulcus (Figure 17-2). This can be performed in eyes with moderate to soft cataracts. It avoids corneal incision extension and thus limits induced astigmatism. This technique was conceived by Professor Amar Agarwal.

Scaffold

The word *scaffold* comes from Medieval Latin *scaffaldus*, which means "a temporary platform." In the IOL scaffold technique, the 3-piece IOL acts as a temporary platform and prevents the nuclear fragments from falling into the vitreous cavity.

Surgical Technique

When there is a posterior capsule rupture[1-3] (Figure 17-3), an anterior chamber (AC) maintainer is introduced through a 1.2-mm stab incision using a microvitreo-retinal blade. The position of the AC maintainer should be away from the posterior capsule rupture, and flow should be kept low. Anterior vitrectomy is done with the vitrectomy cutter to remove the vitreous in the AC. An Agarwal globe stabilization rod (Katena, Denville, NJ) passed through the side port helps to push the fragment away from the rupture. The fragments are brought into the AC. A foldable IOL is then injected using the existing corneal wound and is maneuvered below the nucleus. The leading haptic of the IOL is positioned above the iris, and the trailing haptic is placed just outside the incision. Using a dialer in the nondominant hand, the junction of the optic-haptic junction on the trailing side is maneuvered so that the IOL occludes the pupil. Thus, the IOL acts now as a scaffold, preventing fragments from falling into the vitreous. The nuclear fragment is then removed with phaco (low flow and vacuum). Cortex is removed with low aspiration using a vitrectomy probe. The nondominant hand adjusts the trailing optic-haptic junction so that the IOL is well centered over the pupil, acting as a scaffold while emulsifying the nucleus. Once cortical cleaning is done, the IOL is placed over the capsular

Buratto L, Brint SF, Romano MR.
Cataract Surgery Complications (pp 121-124).
© 2013 Taylor & Francis Group.

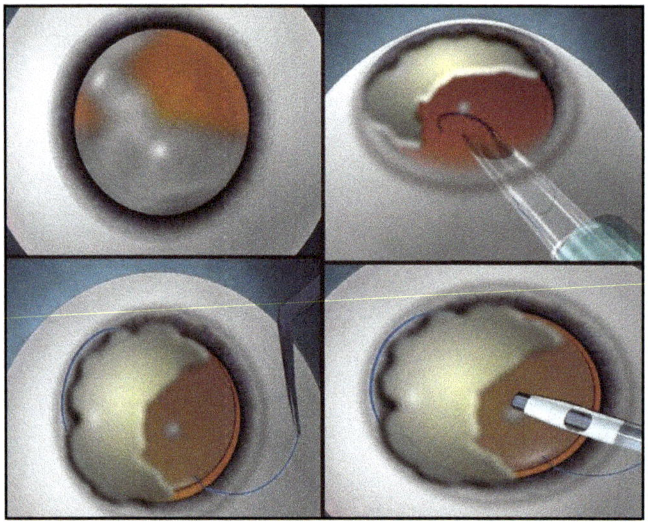

Figure 17-1. Illustrations depicting the IOL scaffold technique.

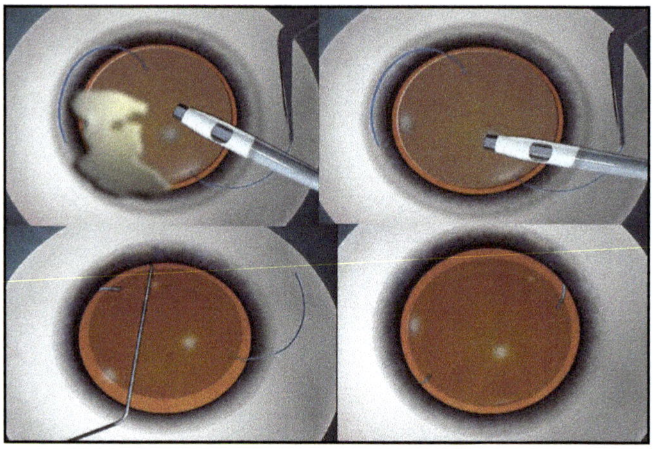

Figure 17-2. Illustrations depicting repositioning of the posterior chamber IOL into the sulcus.

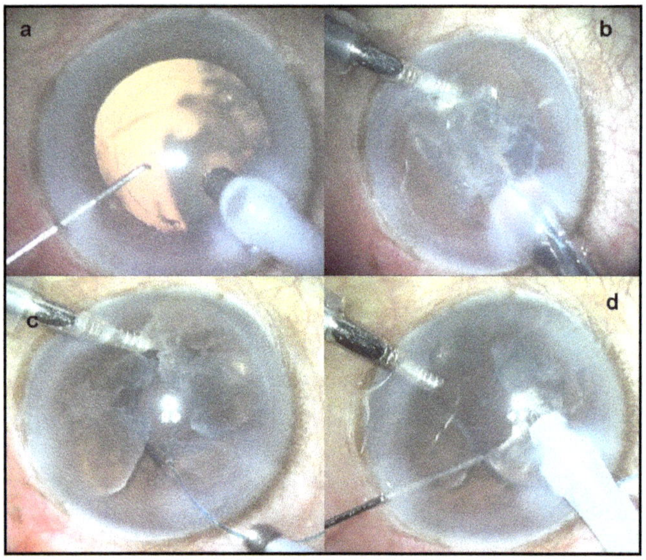

Figure 17-3. IOL scaffold technique. (A) Posterior capsule rupture during epinucleus removal. (B) AC maintainer placed. Foldable IOL is injected through the clear corneal wound. (C) One haptic is placed over the iris and the other outside the incision. (D) Epinucleus removed with phaco probe.

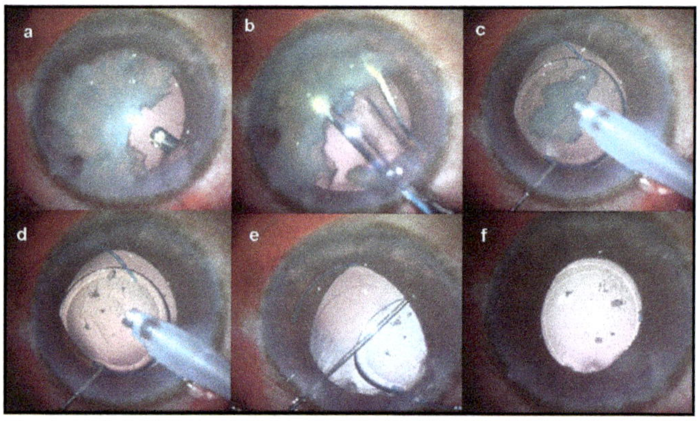

Figure 17-4. IOL scaffold technique with 23-gauge trocar infusion and moderately soft nucleus. (A) Posterior capsule rupture during nucleus removal. (B) Foldable IOL is injected through the clear corneal wound. (C) Nucleus removed with phaco probe above the IOL optic. (D) Cortical aspiration done. (E) IOL positioned into the ciliary sulcus. (F) IOL well centered at the end of surgery.

remnants in the ciliary sulcus. The AC maintainer is then removed and wound hydration performed. Postoperatively, topical ofloxacin and corticosteroid eye drops are used 4 times daily for 2 weeks. A short-acting mydriatic drop twice daily is used for 3 days. Postoperative AC flare is graded by slit-lamp examination.

Instead of an AC maintainer, one can use a sutureless trocar cannula also. This technique can be easily done in moderately soft nuclei (Figure 17-4). In very hard cataracts, it might be better to extend the incision and remove the nucleus to avoid corneal damage.

Intraocular Lens Scaffold Technique

Though there have been techniques performed to prevent nucleus fragments from dropping into the vitreous after intraoperative posterior capsule rupture, this method of using the IOL as a scaffold has not been previously reported. The IOL scaffold technique comes into play once the nuclear pieces have been brought into the AC. Conversion of phacoemulsification to extracapsular cataract extraction is done when a large nucleus is still left. Some surgeons prefer to use the Sheets lens glide to deliver the nucleus. In both methods, corneal wound extension is required, and this can increase the risk of postoperative suture-induced astigmatism.

Another technique used is nuclear removal by the phaco sandwich method, where a vectis and a spatula are used. However, the incision in a phaco sandwich is sclerocorneal and requires enlargement. In eyes with the nucleus dropped into the anterior vitreous, Viscoat (sodium chondroitin sulphate and sodium hyaluronate) posterior-assisted levitation is done followed by nucleus emulsification with phaco above a trimmed Sheets glide after wound extension. With the Sheets glide (Beaver Visitec, Waltham, MA), the problem is one has to enlarge the incision. Then, after the nucleus is removed, one obviously still has to do vitrectomy and cortical removal in which, once again, the wound has to be sutured.

Another technique one can use is Keiki Mehta's HEMA life boat. In this method, a contact lens is injected between the iris and the nucleus to prevent the nucleus from falling back. After emulsification, the contact lens is removed. The difference between this and the IOL scaffold is that in the IOL scaffold the IOL need not be removed. Also the fear of the IOL falling into the vitreous, unlike the contact lens, is less, as one haptic is still outside the eye. In the IOL scaffold technique, the wound remains clear corneal, and there is no wound enlargement. Since there is no wound enlargement, there is no need for suturing and less chance of induced astigmatism. The foldable IOL acts as a barrier to nuclear pieces dropping into the vitreous and works like an artificial posterior capsule. The method is termed as *scaffold* since the IOL optic acts as a temporary platform over which emulsification is performed. Since one haptic is kept out of the incision, the IOL position can be readily adjusted if the nucleus rotates in the AC, and the chances of IOL drop are also decreased as the haptic is controlled from the incision. The presence of the IOL also serves to compartmentalize the eye, which in turn decreases hydration of the vitreous from the AC maintainer as well as prevents vitreous prolapse into the AC. Once the nucleus is removed, the same posterior chamber IOL is repositioned into the sulcus.

When compared to an open wound (after extension), posterior capsule rupture during phacoemulsification is associated with a relatively low incidence of vitreous loss because the self-sealing, small, clear-corneal incision provides control of ocular integrity. This maintains the AC and intraocular pressure and discourages forward movement of the vitreous, which would occur in the presence of an "open globe" as in extracapsular cataract extraction.

Glued Intraocular Lens Scaffold

The problem with IOL scaffolds occurs in cases in which iris support is not sufficient with no capsular support. In such cases, we cannot implant the IOL to support the nuclear pieces as the IOL may sink. This can happen in cases like an iris coloboma in which a posterior capsular rupture has occurred and there is no capsular support at all. This can also happen in the case of floppy iris where the iris is not taut enough to support the IOL, or the pupil is very dilated and not constricting due to trauma. In such cases, we combine the glued IOL with IOL scaffold (glued IOL scaffold) by implanting an intrascleral fixated PC IOL under the nucleus, emulsifying the nucleus, and finally gluing the haptics of the IOL to the scleral flaps.

References

1. Thatte S, Raju VK. Phaco sandwich technique. *J Cataract Refract Surg.* 1999;25(8):1039-1040.
2. Chang DF, Packard RB. Posterior assisted levitation for nucleus retrieval using Viscoat after posterior capsule rupture. *J Cataract Refract Surg.* 2003;29(10):1860-1865.
3. Michelson MA. Use of a Sheets glide as a pseudo posterior capsule in phacoemulsification complicated by posterior capsule rupture. *Eur J Implant Refract Surg.* 1993;5:70-72.

Suggested Reading

Agarwal A, Kumar DA, Jacob S, Baid C, Agarwal A, Srinivasan S. Fibrin glue–assisted sutureless posterior chamber intraocular lens implantation in eyes with deficient posterior capsules. *J Cataract Refract Surg.* 2008;34(9):1433-1438.

Kumar DA, Agarwal A, Prakash G, Jacob S, Agarwal A, Sivagnanam S. IOL scaffold technique for posterior capsular rupture. *J Refract Surg.* 2012;28(5):314-315.

18

Complications of Intraocular Lens Implantation

Šárka Pitrová, MD and Eva Vlková, MD

To achieve optimal positioning of the intraocular lens (IOL) into the bag, some rules are proven.

The Size of the Incision Should Be Adjusted to the Size of the Cartridge Tip

For safe implantation, it is recommended to insert just the tip of the beveled part of the cartridge into the wound, slightly elevate and, just after that, insert the lens into the eye. The implantation of the lens should be continuous, without interruption. During implantation, it is advisable to stabilize the eyeball with a second instrument.

Complication #1

If the wound is too tight and the surgeon has to use force during implantation, the lens may inject uncontrolled into the eye, causing injury to the ciliary body on the opposite side of the incision. The problem may be even more dramatic if implantation is performed with only one hand. Almost immediately, massive bleeding appears between the iris and the anterior lens capsule or directly into the bag beneath the IOL or into the vitreous.

Solution to #1

A large air bubble is placed into the anterior chamber (AC) until the bleeding stops. After that we use an irrigation/aspiration cannula for AC irrigation.

Complication #2

More complicated and time consuming is the irrigation of blood from the bag behind the IOL. In this case, the surgeon performs the implantation not continuously, with interruption, and the folded lens may lodge in the wound (Figure 18-1).

Solution to #2

The solution depends on the size of the lens segment that remains outside the eye or inside the AC. In the first case, we may try to carefully pull the captured lens out of the wound using implantation forceps (mostly without damage to the lens). In the second case, we try to push the lens with the implantation forceps into the AC with positioning into the bag. In most cases, we are successful without having to enlarge the wound. But, on the other hand, we may damage the lens (ie, tear the haptic off) while pulling it out of the eye or enlarging the incision. Because of that, if we expect an unusual implantation (ie, in hypotonic myopic eyes), it is better to enlarge the incision slightly in advance. Enlarged incisions may not be tight enough at the end of the surgery, so a suture may be required.

Buratto L, Brint SF, Romano MR.
Cataract Surgery Complications (pp 125-128).
© 2013 Taylor & Francis Group.

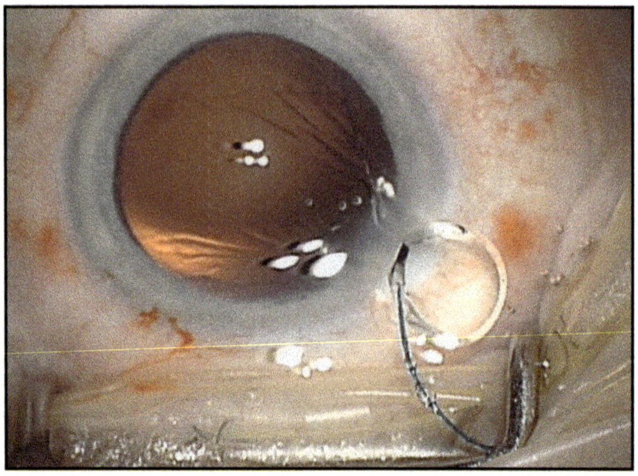

Figure 18-1. The folded 3-piece IOL is squeezed into a clear-corneal incision. (Reprinted with permission of Dr. Šárka Pitrová and Dr. Eva Vlková.)

Perform a Careful Continual Anterior Capsulorrhexis

The surgeon needs to perform a careful continual anterior capsulorrhexis that will ensure safe implantation of the IOL and proper positioning in the bag (Figure 18-2). The diameter of the capsulorrhexis depends on the diameter of the optic of the IOL. In special types of cataracts (eg, congenital cataracts, ectopic lens in Marfan's syndrome), we enlarge the originally smaller capsulorrhexis before implantation.

Complication #1

Tear of the anterior capsulorrhexis to the equator forms a so-called keyhole (Figure 18-3), which usually is related to an interruption during performing the capsulorrhexis (eg, poor visualization of the operation field, uncooperative patient). The tear may occur during phacoemulsification if we touch the phaco tip to the edge of the capsule, mostly the lower part.

Solution to #1

If the capsulorrhexis is torn to the equator only, the IOL may be implanted into the bag without problems, but the axis of the haptics should be oriented perpendicularly to the axis of the tear.

Complication #2

The tear of the anterior capsulorrhexis will spread behind the equator to the posterior capsule with or without loss of vitreous.

Solution to #2

With an intact vitreous face and small rupture of the posterior capsule from the equator, an experienced surgeon may implant, with caution, the IOL into the remnants of the bag on both sides of the tear, placing cohesive viscoelastic between the anterior and posterior capsules. It is also advantageous to protect the intact anterior vitreous face from rupture using a dispersive viscoelastic (eg, Viscoat). For a less experienced surgeon, it would be safer to implant the IOL into the sulcus.

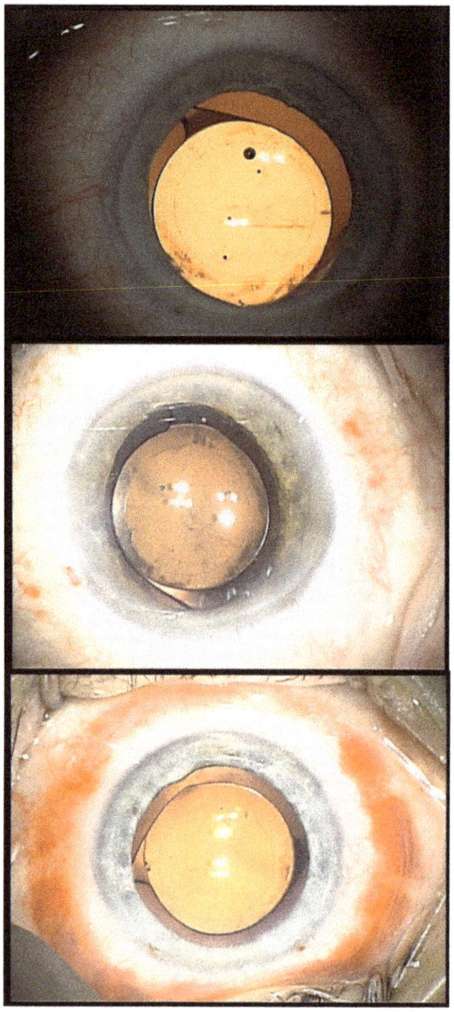

Figure 18-2. Optimal centration of the IOL in the capsular bag. (Reprinted with permission of Dr. Šárka Pitrová and Dr. Eva Vlková.)

If the rupture of the posterior capsule is large and accompanied by vitreous prolapse, which strategy to use depends on the surgeon. First, it is necessary to perform an anterior vitrectomy to clean space for implantation and then to decide on appropriate positioning for the IOL. With a bit of luck, it is possible to implant the IOL into the ciliary sulcus. Personally we choose a polymethylmethacrylate (PMMA) lens with large optic (7 mm) and haptic (13 mm) diameters, which has a good chance to stay well positioned. There is a risk that the surgeon will be not able to determine precisely if the IOL will stay in its proper place or if its position may change (from lying to sitting and remain stable). A good clue to determine IOL stability is irrigation/aspiration of the viscoelastic after the implantation, which may show decentration of the IOL. If, in such a case, we correct the IOL position (ie, a small rotation), we are surprised on the

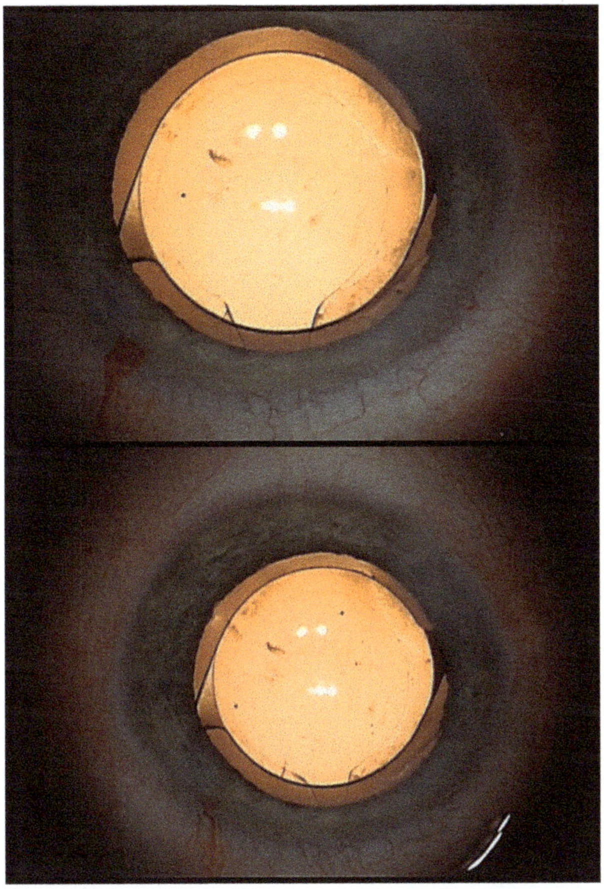

Figure 18-3. Rupture of the anterior capsulorrhexis to the equator (keyhole). (Reprinted with permission of Dr. Šárka Pitrová and Dr. Eva Vlková.)

first postoperative day (or later) if the IOL is in the vitreous. The other possibility is to suture the lens to the iris or to the sulcus.

The final decision is not to implant at all, if we are not able to perform a good anterior vitrectomy or other complications appear (eg, bleeding). We suture the wound, perform an iridectomy, wait at least 3 months, and then implant a secondary IOL.

Complication #3

Zonulysis may begin in the initial stages of implantation when we inject the leading haptic into the bag, and with more pressure and pulling (with a smaller capsulorrhexis) we try to place the trailing haptic into the bag as well. Zonulysis then appears typically under the incision (vitreous prolapse or into the AC is possible). Zonulysis may occur anywhere in the circumference with inadequate IOL rotation (Figure 18-4).

Solution to #3

It is necessary to manage zonulysis by capsular ring implantation. If the zonulysis occurs after the entire IOL is already placed in the bag, it is sufficient to remove one haptic out of the bag, implant the capsular ring, and replace the haptic back into the bag. If vitreous appears in the wound

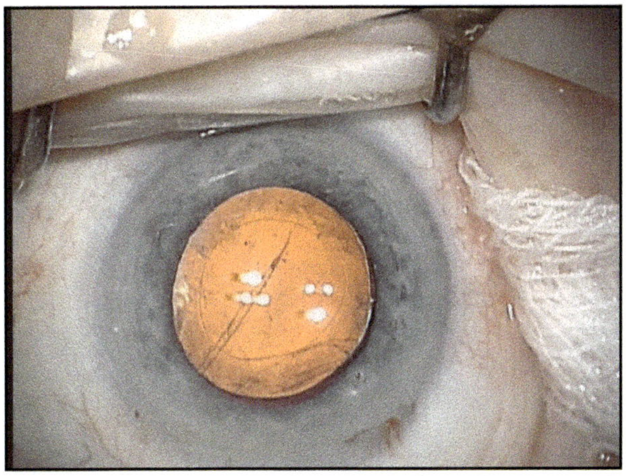

Figure 18-4. A torn posterior capsule from the equator is visible in front of anterior capsule in place under the incision, the anterior capsulorrhexis is intact, and an IOL is implanted in the capsular bag. (Reprinted with permission of Dr. Šárka Pitrová and Dr. Eva Vlková.)

at the beginning of implantation, it is better to close this wound with suture after performing an anterior vitrectomy and implant the IOL from another location.

Check if Both Haptics Are Correctly Unfolded and in the Bag

In some cases (small pupils, vitreous pressure) incomplete unfolding of the haptics and incorrect positioning in the bag is seen.

Complication #1

Decentration (dislocation) of the IOL, diplopia (double vision), and tilt of the IOL.

Solution to #1

The solution to this complication is mostly surgical and depends on the situation. We usually cut the haptic from the optic and reposition the lens, sometimes exchanging the IOL if the haptic is deformed.

References

1. Arbisser LB. Radial rhexis tear or sulcus implantation. *Cataract & Refractive Surgery Today.* 2004;4:55-57.
2. Bhogal MS, Angunawela RI, Allan BDS. Haptic misfolding during aspheric IOL insertion. *J Cataract Refract Surg.* 2011;37:208-209.
3. Braga-Mele R. Sulcus implantation of IOL's do's & don'ts. In: Spotlight on Cataracts: Clinical Decision-Making With IOL Complications. AAO Symposium, October 18, 2010, Chicago, IL.
4. Chang DF, Masket S, Miller KM, et al. Complications of sulcus placement of single piece acrylic intraocular lenses: recommendations for backup IOL implantation following posterior capsule rupture. *J Cataract Refract Surg.* 2009;35:1445-1458.

5. Chen CK, Tseng VL, WuW-C, Greenberg PB. A survey of the current role of manual extracapsular cataracta extraction. *J Cataract Refract Surg.* 2012;36:692-693.
6. Condon GP. Simplified small incision peripheral iris fixation of an Acrysof intraocular lens in the absence of capsular support. *J Cataract Refract Surg.* 2003;29:1663-1667.
7. Gimbel H, Sun R, Heston J. Management of zonular dialysis in phacoemulsification and IOL implantation using the capsular tension ring. *Ophthalmic Surg Lasers.* 1997;28:273-281.
8. Lin CP, Tseng HY. Suture fixation technique for posterior chamber intraocular lenses. *Ophthalmic Surg.* 1993;24:375-381.
9. Mackool RJ, Nicolich S, Mackool R Jr. Effect of viscodissection on posterior capsule rupture during phacoemulsification. *J Cataract Refract Surg.* 2007;33:553.
10. Menapace RM. Cataract surgical problem. *J Cataract Refract Surg.* 2012;38:724.
11. Mercieca K, Brahma AK, Patton N, McKee HD. Intraoperative conversion from phacoemulsification to manual extracapsular cataract extraction. *J Cataract Refract Surg.* 2011;37:787-788.
12. vanVreeswijk H. Safe and easy way to release sticking haptic of a single piece AcrySof intraocular lens. *J Cataract Refract Surg.* 2008;34:1611.

19

Posterior Capsule Rupture

Šárka Pitrová, MD and Eva Vlková, MD

Posterior capsule rupture may occur at any step of surgery after hydrodissection. Sudden deepening of the anterior chamber (AC), hypotony, and difficult manipulation with lens contents are undoubtedly symptoms of rupture. The surgeon should immediately stop. The next steps should be chosen according to the situation, the surgeon's experience, and his or her ability to solve the complications.

Posterior Capsule Rupture During Hydrodissection

The most common causes of posterior capsule rupture during hydrodissection are posterior polar cataract and intraoperative capsular block syndrome. Each of them has been documented in several articles, presentations, and videos.

Posterior Capsule Rupture During Phacoemulsification

Posterior capsule rupture during phacoemulsification may appear at any time.

Complication #1

At the beginning of hard nucleus phaco, a less-experienced surgeon may cause peripheral rupture of the posterior capsule opposite the incision by moving the fast-moving phaco tip on the nucleus surface to the lens periphery and then stopping it behind the posterior capsule. In cases where the nucleus is softer and thinner, and the surgeon does not consider this, he or she may widely open the posterior capsule in the center, with the Kelman bent phaco tip, just at the beginning of phacoemulsification.

Solution to #1

In the case of a large hard nucleus, which is not divided at all, or only just a little bit, and the operation field is not clear enough, and the site of the rupture and its extent are hard to establish, the safest solution is to convert to extracapsular extraction. As the first step, the nucleus has to be luxated into the AC. We use cohesive viscoelastic material and perform viscoexpression, introducing the cannula as far as possible to the periphery and repeatedly inject small amounts of viscoelastic until the equator of the lens appears at the rim of the capsulorrhexis. Thereafter, we easily finish the nucleus luxation into the AC in front of the iris. The nucleus is then removed out of the AC through the sclerocorneal tunnel incision. The necessary precondition for viscoexpression is that the capsulorrhexis diameter is slightly smaller than the diameter of the lens nucleus.

Buratto L, Brint SF, Romano MR.
Cataract Surgery Complications (pp 129-134).
© 2013 Taylor & Francis Group.

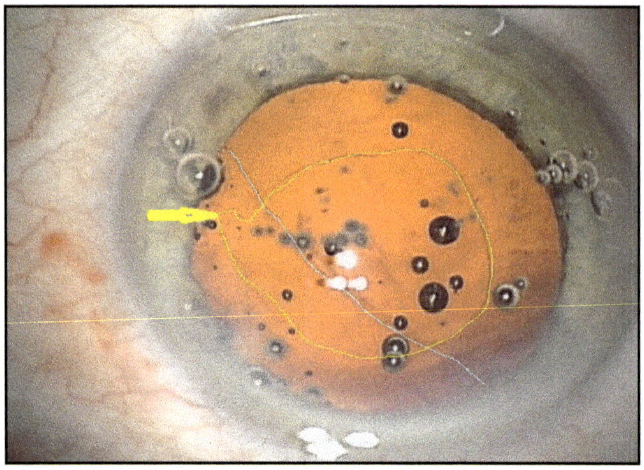

Figure 19-1. The eye after cataract removal. The intact anterior capsulorrhexis was damaged during anterior vitrectomy under the anterior capsule, large posterior capsule rupture (white = capsule rupture, yellow = continuous anterior capsulorrhexis was damaged during anterior vitrectomy = arrow). (Reprinted with permission of Dr. Šárka Pitrová and Dr. Eva Vlková.)

In the opposite case, the surgeon has to enlarge the capsulorrhexis either by cutting the anterior capsule obliquely and continuing in circular continuous capsulorrhexis or simply cuts the rim of the capsulorrhexis with scissors radial in 1 or 2 places. The rest of the cortex may be removed without extensive loss of vitreous with low settings of irrigation/aspiration.

With vitreous prolapse, it is always necessary to perform careful anterior vitrectomy, especially under the anterior capsule. We pay maximum attention to not damage it and preserve it as a support for the implanted lens (Figure 19-1).

Complication #2

During phacoemulsification, an unstable AC and its fluctuation, shallow AC, or vitreous pressure may contribute to this complication.

Solution to #2

If parts of the nucleus with cortex remain in the capsule or in the AC, the surgeon should use the glide (Figure 19-2), which is introduced through the corneal incision behind the iris, under the anterior capsule, to cover the posterior capsule rupture (Figure 19-3). Above the glide, it is possible to remove the rest of the nucleus with the phaco tip (Figure 19-4) and to perform cortex aspiration. We always use the low settings of the phaco machine. Before the glide removal out of the eye, visco should be gently applied into the AC to prevent vitreous prolapse and unwanted dropping of nucleus parts and cortex into the vitreous space. As a matter of course, a careful anterior vitrectomy should be performed. If there is very limited vitreous prolapse, we may cover the ruptured area with Viscoat (sodium chondroitin sulfate and sodium hyaluronate) and then aspirate with the cannula or use bimanual irrigation/aspiration to remove part of the cortical material trapped between the anterior

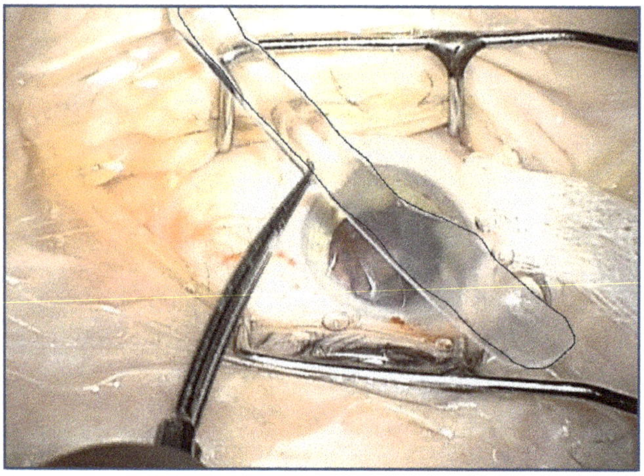

Figure 19-2. Glide is adapted for the small incision. (Reprinted with permission of Dr. Šárka Pitrová and Dr. Eva Vlková.)

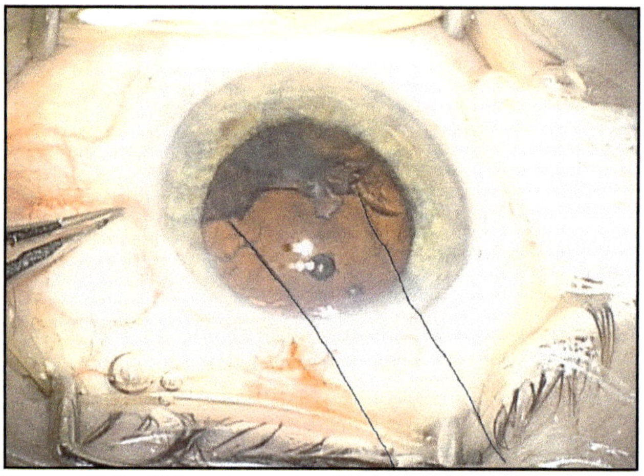

Figure 19-3. Glide is located behind the iris and anterior capsule. The cortex is located above the glide. (Reprinted with permission of Dr. Šárka Pitrová and Dr. Eva Vlková.)

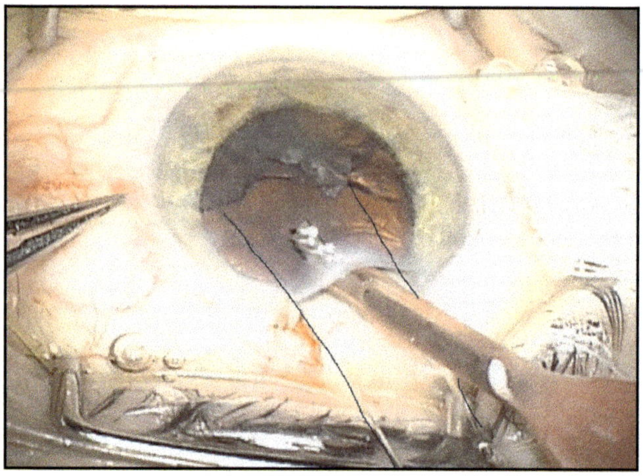

Figure 19-4. Phaco tip is located above the glide, protecting the posterior capsule rupture. (Reprinted with permission of Dr. Šárka Pitrová and Dr. Eva Vlková.)

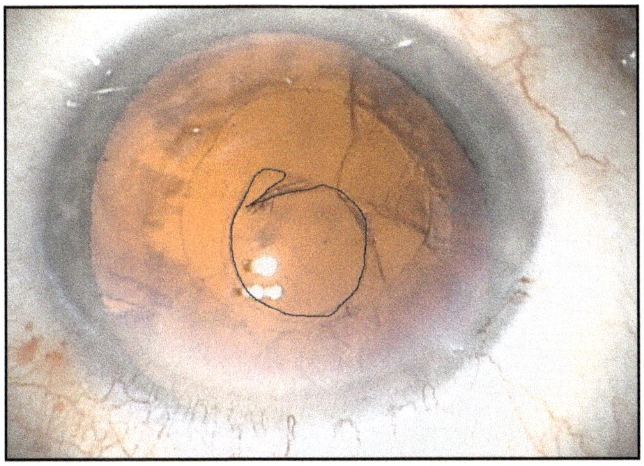

Figure 19-5. Posterior capsule opening after irrigation/aspiration. (Reprinted with permission of Dr. Šárka Pitrová and Dr. Eva Vlková.)

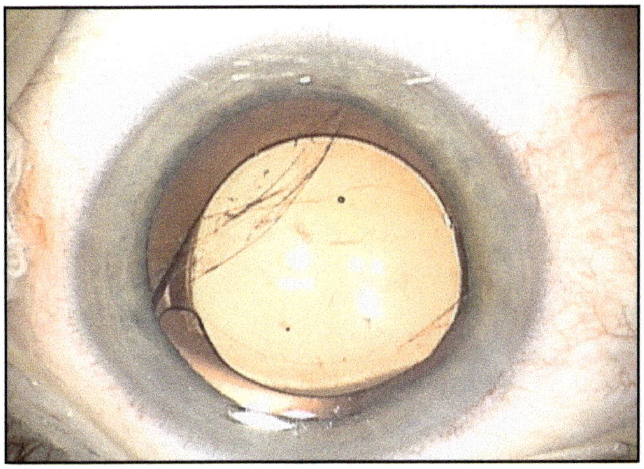

Figure 19-6. IOL is implanted by sandwich technique. The torn capsule is visible in the temporal lower part. (Reprinted with permission of Dr. Šárka Pitrová and Dr. Eva Vlková.)

and posterior capsules. We use a low level of infusion, the irrigating cannula is introduced into the anterior chamber filled with cohesive material at the 0 position, and its opening should be situated as far as possible (preferably to the equator area) between the anterior and posterior capsule to the place from where we would like to aspirate the residual cortex. We then step on the foot pedal, go to position 2, and perform aspiration. With this maneuver we can manage to remove a fair amount of cortex without aspirating vitreous. After lens removal and pupil dilatation, it is necessary to perform indirect ophthalmoscopy. If nucleus fragments dropped into the vitreous and the vitreo-retinal surgeon is not available, the cataract surgeon should carefully clean the anterior segment, implant the intraocular lens (IOL), and refer the patient to the vitreo-retinal specialist the next day. The optimal solution in this complication is to perform a 23-gauge pars plana vitrectomy.

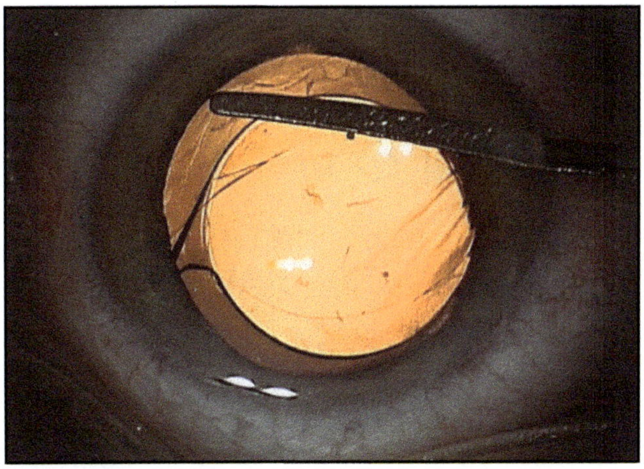

Figure 19-7. Repositioning of the torn capsule toward the equator. (Reprinted with permission of Dr. Šárka Pitrová and Dr. Eva Vlková.)

Posterior Capsule Rupture May Occur Anywhere During Irrigation/Aspiration

If vitreous prolapse is not present, finishing of the posterior capsulorrhexis should treat the rupture (Figure 19-5), and the IOL may be implanted into the bag. Be careful during irrigation of the visco that the irrigation fluid does not open the anterior vitreous membrane at the end. If there is prolapsing vitreous present, the rupture may easily spread to the periphery and then anterior vitrectomy is necessary (dry or wet vitrectomy). If the anterior capsule is intact and the anterior capsulorrhexis is not damaged, it is possible to perform the sandwich implantation technique using the IOL, in which the haptics are located in the ciliary sulcus and the optic is enclavated behind the capsulorrhexis (Figures 19-6 through 19-8). The other possible ways of

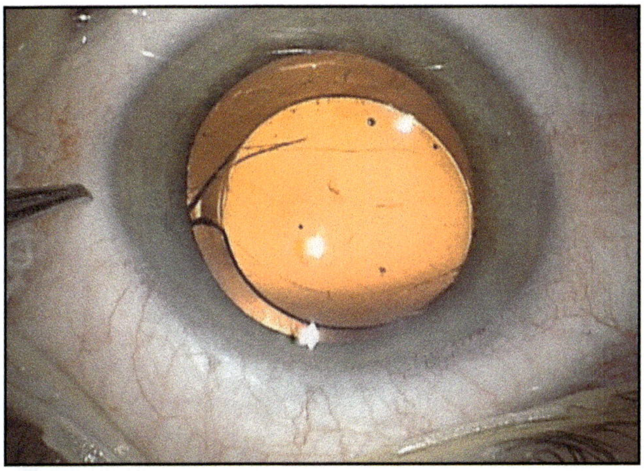

Figure 19-8. Final result after repositioning of the torn capsule. (Reprinted with permission of Dr. Šárka Pitrová and Dr. Eva Vlková.)

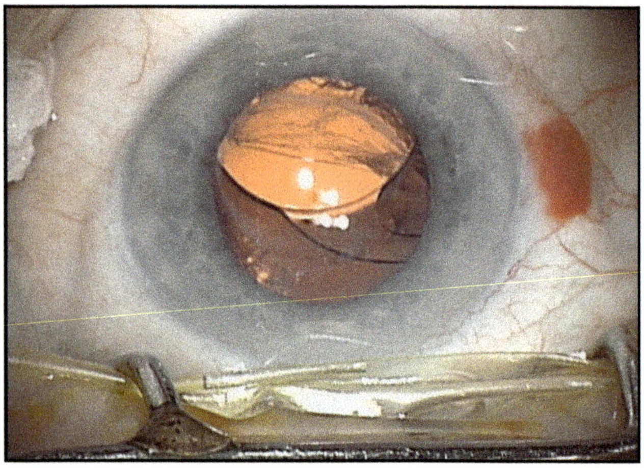

Figure 19-9. A large portion of the IOL was implanted through the posterior capsule rupture into the vitreous cavity. (Reprinted with permission of Dr. Šárka Pitrová and Dr. Eva Vlková.)

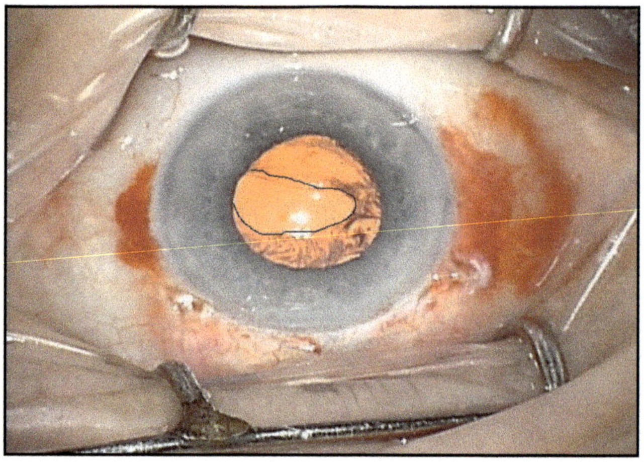

Figure 19-10. The eye after IOL exchange. The new lens is located in the sulcus ciliaris. In the smaller pupil, posterior capsule rupture is visible behind the lens (black = posterior capsule rupture). (Reprinted with permission of Dr. Šárka Pitrová and Dr. Eva Vlková.)

implantation are discussed in Chapter 6 "Complications With Intraocular Lens Implantation."

Rupture of the Posterior Capsule During Implantation of the Intraocular Lens

Rupture of the posterior capsule during implantation of the IOL may occur for several reasons, such as a too-tight tunnel for implantation and too much power to push the IOL into the eye, and at the same time the cartridge tip is oriented too perpendicularly. The IOL instead may end up through the capsule, directly in the vitreous (Figures 19-9 and 19-10). Sometimes it manages to catch the upper haptic by the forceps and lift the IOL into the AC.

After vitrectomy of the vitreous prolapse, the surgeon, using viscoelastic material, may implant the IOL in the bag or in the ciliary sulcus or suture the lens. If the AC is shallow and the vitreous is pushing the posterior capsule forward, it may be the haptic of the even-carefully implanted IOL that rolls the capsule away. In this situation, it is better to implant the IOL primarily in the AC and then rotate it into the bag.

References

1. Akura J, Hatta S, Kaneda S, Ishihara M, Matsuura K, Tamai A. Management of posterior capsule rupture during phacoemulsification using the dry technique. *J Cataract Refract Surg.* 2001;27:982-989.
2. Allen D, Wood C. Minimizing risk to the capsular during surgery for posterior polar cataract. *J Cataract Refract Surg.* 2002;28:742-744.
3. Arbisser LB. Radial rhexis tear or sulcus implantation. *Cataract & Refractive Surgery Today.* 2004;4:55-57.
4. Buratto L, Packard R. Complications in cataract surgery in complicated cases. In: Buratto L, Osher R, Masket S, eds. *Cataract Surgery in Complicated Cases.* Thorofare, NJ: SLACK Incorporated; 2000:311-350.
5. Carifi G. Capsulorrhexis optic intraocular lens capture technique. *J Cataract Refract Surg.* 2011;37:427.
6. Chalm KV, Shah VA. Succesful management of cataract surgery associated vitreous loss with sutereless small gauge pars plana vitrectomy. *Am J Ophthalmol.* 2004;138:79-87.
7. Fine IH, Packer M, Hoffman RS. Management of posterior polar cataract. *J Cataract Refract Surg.* 2003;29:16-19.
8. Gimbel HV, DeBroff BM. Intraocular lens optic capture. *J Cataract Refract Surg.* 2004;30:200-206.
9. Gimbel HV, Sun R, Ferensowicz M, Anderson Penno E, Kamal A. Intraoperative management of posterior capsule rupture tears in phacoemulsification and intraoperative lens implantation. *Ophthalmology.* 2001;108:2186-2189.
10. Hayashi K, Hayashi H, Nakao F, Hayashi F. Outcomes of surgery for posterior polar cataract. *J Cataract Refract Surg.* 2003;29:45-49.
11. Jones JJ, Jin GJC. Intraoperative complications. In: Olson RJ, Jin GJC, Ahmed IIK, et al, eds. *Cataract Surgery from Routine to Complex.* Thorofare, NJ: SLACK Incorporated; 2011:149-161.
12. Jones JJ, Jin GCJ. Posterior polar cataract. In: Olson RJ, Jin GJC, Ahmed IIK, et al, eds. *Cataract Surgery from Routine to Complex.* Thorofare, NJ: SLACK Incorporated; 2011:111-113.
13. Mackool RJ, Nicolich S, Mackool R Jr. Effect of viscodissection on posterior capsule rupture during phacoemulsification. *J Cataract Refract Surg.* 2007;33:553.
14. Merani R, Hunyor AP, Playfair TJ, et al. Pars plana vitrectomy for the management of retained lens material after cataract surgery. *Am J Ophthalmology.* 2007;144:364-370.
15. Miyake K. Intraoperative capsular block syndrome. *Cataract & Refractive Surgery Today.* 2005;5:53-54.
16. Miyake K. Intraoperative capsular block syndrome. In: Spotlight on Cataract Surgery 2005: New Pearls on Managing Complicated Cases and Complications. American Academy of Ophthalmology, October 17th, Chicago, IL.
17. Miyake K, Ota I, Ichihashi S, Miyake S, Tanaka Y, Terasaki H. New classification of capsular block syndrome. *J Cataract Refract Surg.* 1998;24:1230-1234.

18. Moyer OD, Osher RH. Posterior polar cataract. In: Buratto L, Osher R, Masket S, eds. *Cataract Surgery in Complicated Cases.* Thorofare, NJ: SLACK Incorporated; 2000:25-27.
19. Osher RH, Yu BCY, Koch DD. Posterior polar cataracts: a predisposition to intraoperative posterior capsule rupture. *J Cataract Refract Surg.* 1990;16:157-162.
20. Singh K, Mittal V, Kaur H. Oval capsulorrhexis for phacoemulsification in posterior polar cataract with preexisting posterior capsule rupture. *J Cataract Refract Surg.* 2011;37:1183-1188.
21. Tjia KF. Iatrogenic zonular disaster. *Cataract & Refract Surgery Today.* 2010;5(3):51-52.
22. Valsavada A, Singh R. Phacoemulsification in eyes with posterior polar cataract. *J Cataract Refract Surg.* 1999;25:238-245.
23. Vasavada AR, Singh R. Phacoemulsification in posterior polar developmental cataracts. In: Lu LW, Fine IH, eds. *Phacoemulsification in Difficult and Challenging Cases.* New York, NY: Thieme Medical Publishers; 1999:121-128.

20

Cystoid Macular Edema Following Cataract Surgery

Nikica Gabric, MD, PhD and Iva Dekaris, MD, PhD

Cystoid macular edema (CME) is the accumulation of extracellular fluid in the outer plexiform and inner nuclear layers of the macula that occurs as the result of the breakdown of the blood-retinal barrier. The exact cause of CME is still unclear; the release of inflammatory mediators seems to be the most probable causing factor. It is characterized by cystoid fluid-filled spaces.

Early detection of CME has become easier with modern equipment, such as optical coherence tomography (OCT), which became a standard addition to biomicroscopy and fluorescein angiography. Fluorescein angiography shows perifoveal petaloid pattern of leakage and late leakage of the optic nerve. OCT shows cystic spaces in the outer nuclear layer.

CME has been classified either as angiographic or clinically significant. Clinically significant CME is defined as a Snellen visual acuity of 20/40 or worse. Common symptoms include decreased visual acuity and contrast sensitivity as well as metamorphopsia.

CME is the most common cause of poor visual outcome following cataract surgery when it is called pseudophakic CME (PCME). Although its incidence has declined with the advancement of modern cataract surgery, it still remains a significant problem that may cause lasting visual impairment. Any complication during phacoemulsification, especially posterior capsule rupture with vitreous loss or iris touch during surgery, or even just prolonged surgical times, may increase the chance for PCME , mainly due to increased secretion of proinflammatory mediators (eg, prostaglandins), which contribute to the inflammatory reaction in the macular region. Thus, PCME is much more common after complicated cataract surgery; however, it may unfortunately develop even after uneventful surgery for yet unclear reasons.

Over time, there has been a decrease in the incidence of PCME, which is attributed to improvements in surgical technique, reduced surgical time, and better intraocular lenses. The incidence of CME following phaco in uncomplicated, low-risk patients can vary from 2% to 12%. The peak incidence is 4 to 6 weeks after cataract surgery (Figure 20-1). If macular edema lasts less than 4 months, it is considered to be acute CME, which often resolves spontaneously. PCME that lasts more than 4 months is considered to be chronic and may cause severe vision problems.

Treatment options for PCME are several; however, there is a lack of well-designed randomized clinical trials to guide treatment of PCME. First-line treatment of postsurgical CME should include topical nonsteroidal anti-inflammatory drugs (NSAIDs) and corticosteroids (Figures 20-2 to 20-4). One of the first NSAIDs in use for acute, visually significant PCME was ketorolac; patients treated with combination therapy responded more quickly than patients

Buratto L, Brint SF, Romano MR.
Cataract Surgery Complications (pp 135-138).
© 2013 Taylor & Francis Group.

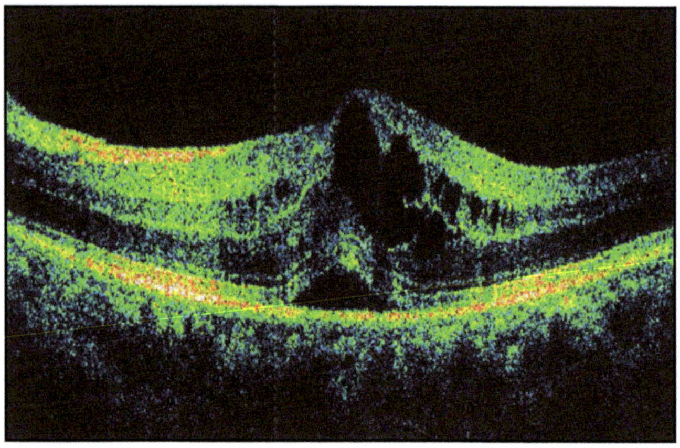

Figure 20-1. Foveal thickening and cystic changes specific for cystoid macular edema 6 weeks after the cataract surgery.

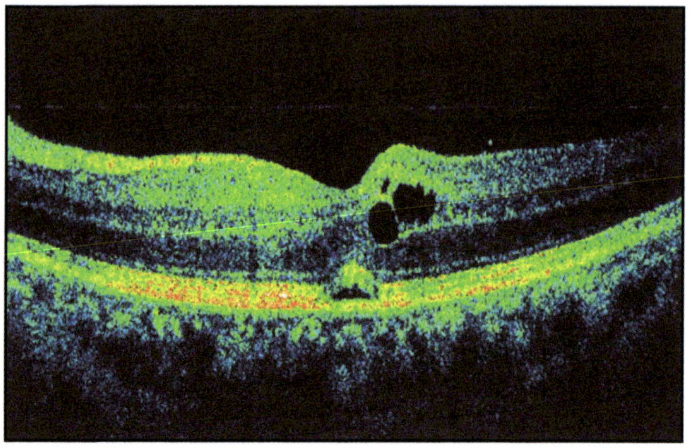

Figure 20-2. Decreased macular thickness after 2 weeks of treatment with combination of corticosteroid and NSAID.

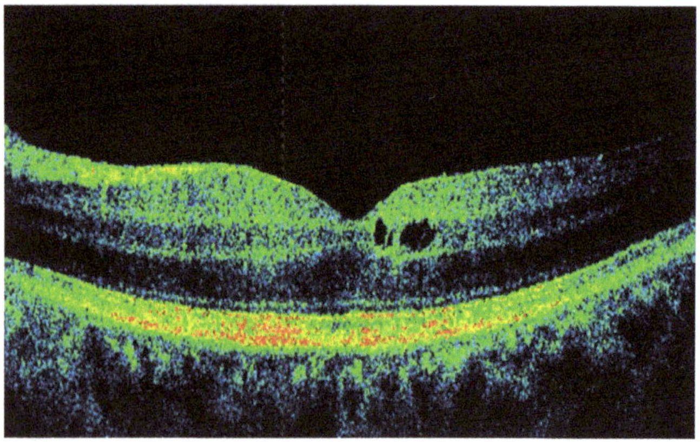

Figure 20-3. Significant reduction in retinal thickness after 1 month of treatment with combination of corticosteroid and NSAID.

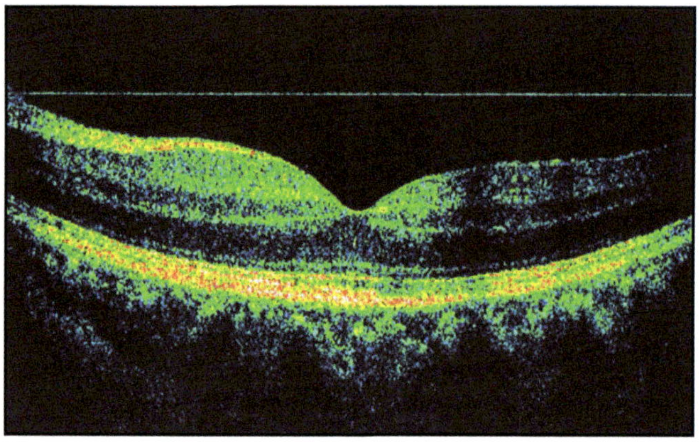

Figure 20-4. Complete resolution of foveal thickening and cystic changes after 2 months of treatment with combination of corticosteroid and NSAID.

treated with either prednisolone or ketorolac alone. There are several NSAIDs that are used in treatment of PCME, such as diclofenac, bromfenac, and ketorolac. There are conflicting clinical trials regarding the use of NSAIDs; 2 trials showed that 0.5% ketorolac tromethamine ophthalmic solution has a positive effect on chronic CME, and 2 trials found no positive effect of the same drug.

Those who advocate the use of NSAIDs emphasize the role they might have not only in treatment but also in prevention of PCME. Since NSAIDs have a positive effect in obtaining maximal pupil dilatation during surgery, they enhance faster surgery and thus lower the chance of PCME development. Oral carbonic anhydrase inhibitors can be considered complementary. In cases of resistant PCME, periocular and intraocular corticosteroids present an option. Intravitreal administration of triamcinolone has shown to be safe and effective in recalcitrant cases of PCME with a beneficial effect on the macular edema and visual acuity. However, a prospective randomized study is needed to confirm the efficacy, safety, and exact timing of intravitreal steroid applications.

The disadvantage of this approach is the need for repeated injections, so the development of a sustained-release intravitreal drug-delivery system would be beneficial. Therefore, an intravitreal dexamethasone 0.7-mg implant has been tried in resistant CME resulting in visual acuity improvement with a single intravitreal injection. Intravitreal antivascular endothelial growth factor (anti-vascular endothelial growth factor [VEGF]) should be considered for nonresponsive persistent PCME. There is a relatively low number of reported patients with refractory PCME who have been treated with intravitreal anti-VEGF (bevacizumab); short-term results suggest that this treatment is well tolerated and that it leads to a significant improvement in visual acuity and decrease in macular thickness.

Another novel treatment option that might be beneficial is the intravitreal use of infliximab (monoclonal antibody against proinflammatory cytokine—tumor necrosis factor alpha). Surgical options should be reserved for special indications.

References

1. Arevalo JF, Maia M, Garcia-Amaris RA, et al. Intravitreal bevacizumab for refractory pseudophakic cystoid macular edema: the Pan-American Collaborative Retina Study Group results. *Ophthalmology.* 2009; 116(8):1481-1487.
2. Bertelmann T, Witteborn M, Mennel S. Pseudophakic cystoid macular oedema [in German]. *Klin Monbl Augenheilkd.* 2012 Mar 15. [Epub ahead of print]
3. Conway MD, Canakis C, Livir-Rallatos C, Peyman GA. Intravitreal triamcinolone acetonide for refractory chronic pseudophakic cystoid macular edema. *J Cataract Refract Surg.* 2003;29(1):27-33.
4. Meyer LM, Schönfeld CL. Cystoid macular edema after complicated cataract surgery resolved by an intravitreal dexamethasone 0.7-mg implant. *Case Report Ophthalmol.* 2011;2(3):319-322.
5. Miyake K, Ota I, Miyake G, Numaga J. Nepafenac 0.1% versus fluorometholone 0.1% for preventing cystoid macular edema after cataract surgery. *J Cataract Refractive Surg.* 2011;37(9):1581-1588.
6. Sivaprased S, Bunce C, Crosby-Nwaobi R. Non-steroidal anti-inflammatory agents for treating cystoid macular oedema following cataract surgery. *Cochrane Database Syst Rev.* 2012;15:2:CD004239.
7. Wu L, Fernando Arevalo J, Hernandez-Bogantes E, Roca JA. Intravitreal infliximab for refractory pseudophakic cystoid macular edema: results of the Pan-American Collaborative Retina Study Group. *Int Ophthalmol.* 2012; 32(3):235-243.
8. Yonekawa Y, Kim IK. Pseudophakic cystoid macular edema. *Curr Opin Ophthalmol.* 2012;23(1):26-32.

21

Preventing Postoperative Posterior Capsular Opacification With the Endocapsular Ring

Tsutomu Hara, MD

Development of posterior capsular opacification (PCO) after cataract surgery is a long-term unresolved issue. PCO originates from the metamorphosed lens epithelial cells that are under the anterior capsule after cataract surgery. The endocapsular equator ring (E-ring)[1-5] was developed to prevent posterior movement of the activated lens epithelial cells at the capsular equator. The results are described in this chapter.

Structure of the E-Ring

The width and thickness of the silicone E-ring (Figure 21-1) are both 1 mm. The edge is square. The inner surface of the ring has a groove where the loops of the intraocular lens (IOL) can be fixed. The outer diameter is 9.5 mm, which fits most adult eyes despite the closed circular design of the E-ring. The device can be implanted through a 3.2-mm incision, which facilitates sutureless surgery.

Results in Animal Eyes

Severe PCO developed in rabbit eyes in which an IOL alone was implanted. PCO was prevented and the circular contour of the equator was maintained in rabbit eyes in which an E-ring and an IOL were implanted (Figure 21-2).

Results in Human Eyes

Fourteen patients received an E-ring and IOL in one eye and only an IOL in the contralateral eye. The mean ± standard deviation (SD) patient age was 69.9 ± 14.90 years (range, 22 to 80 years). All surgeries were performed between February 2002 and February 2006. The follow-up periods ranged from 2 years to 7 years (average, 4.9 ± 1.84 years). PCO did not develop in the eyes with an E-ring, and no eye required a postoperative Nd:YAG posterior capsulotomy (Figures 21-3 through 21-5).

Features of the E-Ring

- Significantly prevented PCO development
- Facilitates sutureless surgery through a 3.2-mm incision
- Adaptable to all cases using the one size E-ring (9.5 mm in the outer diameter)

Buratto L, Brint SF, Romano MR.
Cataract Surgery Complications (pp 139-142).
© 2013 Taylor & Francis Group.

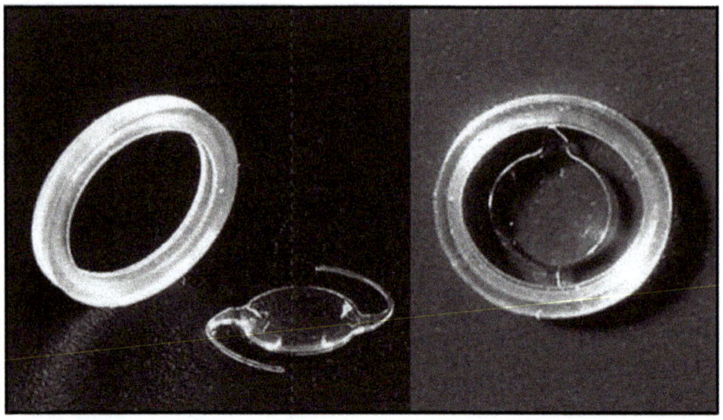

Figure 21-1. The E-ring is a closed silicone ring with a square edge, an outer diameter of 9.5 mm, and a width and thickness of 1.0 mm. A groove on the inner surface facilitates IOL loop fixation. (Reprinted with permission from the American Medical Association.)

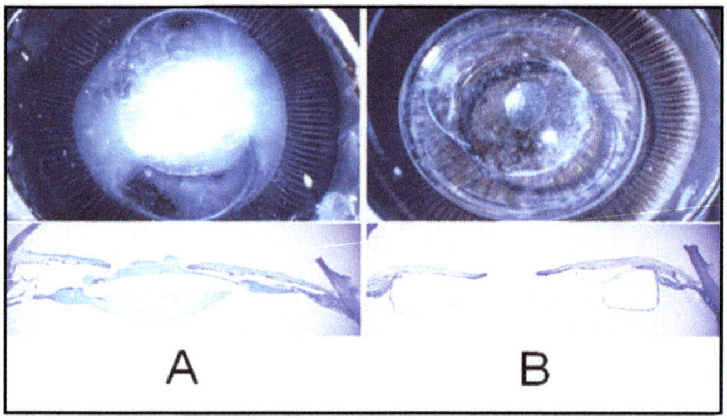

Figure 21-2. Postoperative findings in rabbit eyes. (A) A control eye 2.2 months postoperatively. (B) An E-ring eye 2.6 months postoperatively. (Reprinted with permission from the American Medical Association.)

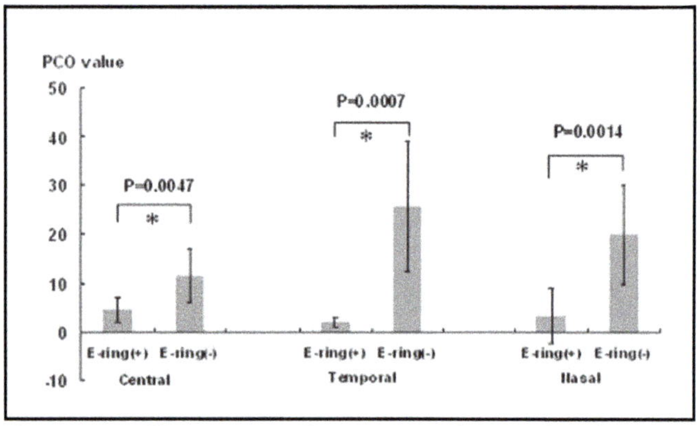

Figure 21-3. Human eyes. Comparison of PCO values between eyes with and without the E-ring using the Hayashi method.[6] (Reprinted with permission from the American Medical Association.)

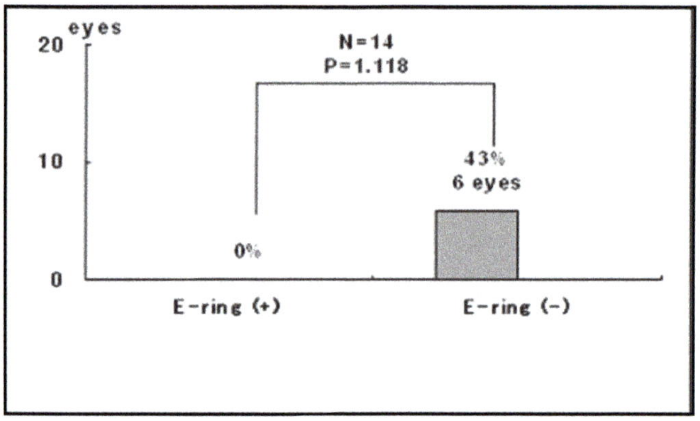

Figure 21-4. Human eyes. Comparison of the rates of Nd:YAG posterior capsulotomy (Fisher's exact test). (Reprinted with permission from the American Medical Association.)

Figure 21-5. Observation of a case 2 years and 6 months postoperatively. (Top) Retroillumination photographs. (Bottom) Scheimpflug slit images. (A) A control eye. Extensive PCO is observed in a control eye. The PCO value of the central area is 20.5. (B) An eye with an E-ring. The entire posterior capsule is clear. The PCO value of the central area is 1.5. There is no contact between the IOL optic and the posterior capsule. The E-ring has not caused elevation of the iris root. (Reprinted with permission from the American Medical Association.)

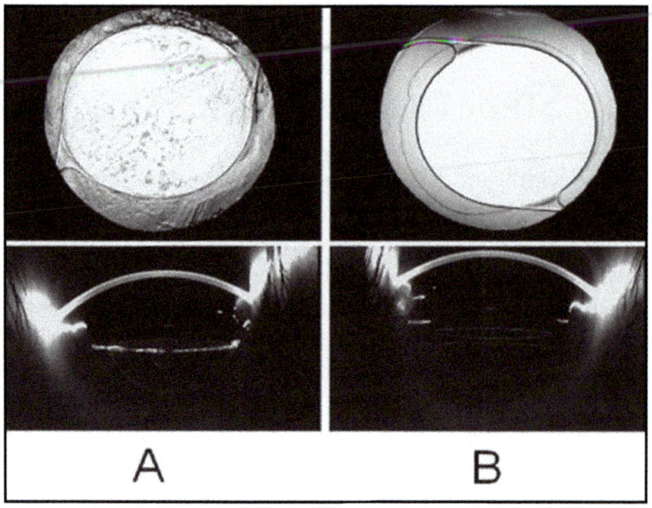

Application of the E-Ring

- Easy IOL exchange
- Pediatric eyes
- Power corrections
- Dissatisfied patients after multifocal IOL implantation
- Fixation on the exact axis of a toric IOL

References

1. Hara T, Hara T, Yamada Y. Equator ring for maintenance of the completely circular contour of the capsular bag equator after cataract removal. *Ophthalmic Surg.* 1991;22(6):358-359.
2. Hara T, Hara T, Sakanishi K, Yamada Y. Efficacy of equator rings in an experimental rabbit study. *Arch Ophthalmol.* 1995;113(8):1060-1065.
3. Hashizoe M, Hara T, Ogura Y, Sakanishi K, Honda T, Hara T. Equator ring efficacy in maintaining capsular bag integrity and transparency after cataract removal in monkey eyes. *Graefe's Arch Clin Exp Ophthalmol.* 1998;236(4):375-379.
4. Hara T, Hara T, Hara T. Preventing postoperative posterior capsule opacification with an endocapsular equator ring in a young human eye: 2-year follow-up. *Arch Ophthalmol.* 2007;125(4):483-486.
5. Hara T, Hara T, Narita M, Hashimoto T, Motoyama Y, Hara T. Long-term study of posterior capsular opacification prevention with endocapsular equator rings in humans. *Arch Ophthalmol.* 2011;129(7):844-863.
6. Hayashi H, Hayashi K, Nakao F, Hayashi F. Quantitative comparison of posterior capsule opacification after polymethylmethacrylate, silicone, and soft acrylic intraocular lens implantation. *Arch Ophthalmol.* 1998;116:1579-1582.

22

Clinical Management of Suspected Postsurgical Acute and Chronic Endophthalmitis

How to Proceed as an Initial Approach to Diagnosis and Treatment

Jorge L. Alió, MD, PhD and Felipe Soria, MD

Diagnosing acute endophthalmitis is one of the most challenging ophthalmic medical emergencies, and the initial treatment should not be postponed for more than 1 hour. It is mandatory to check visual acuity of the patient in both eyes separately for the important values of evolution and prognosis. Another important clinical practice is to follow the patient with clinical photographs whenever possible in order to illustrate the evolution of the condition.

The main cardinal signs and symptoms that a patient manifests will be an intense pain accompanied by blurring or vision loss, and marked intraocular inflammation with the formation of hypopyon. Other symptoms and signs, less specific but not less important, include swollen lids, chemotic conjunctivitis, corneal edema, afferent pupillary defect, vitritis, retinitis, and/or absent red reflex.

In the presence of the impossibility of correctly evaluating the fundus, ultrasonography should be assessed in order to evaluate vitritis and retinal detachment.

Depending on the evolution of endophthalmitis in terms of time, different micro-organisms will give particular signs that, by the terms of this chapter, are not going to be included.

After this essential approximation, the next step is to obtain an intraocular specimen for the definitive diagnosis of endophthalmitis. It is better to take a sample from the vitreous than from the aqueous. Because there is a greater percentage of positive culture and positive polymerase chain reaction (PCR) in the vitreous, the sample with syringes are mostly unreliable. So, every time possible, a vitreous sample with vitrectomy is preferred. In this chapter, we aim to offer a guideline for the surgeon and clinician about the steps to follow in the initial diagnosis and treatment of suspected postsurgical endophthalmitis based on the scientific evidence available.[1-14]

Buratto L, Brint SF, Romano MR.
Cataract Surgery Complications (pp 143-148).
© 2013 Taylor & Francis Group.

The following are 2 procedures to obtain a vitreous sample:

1. **Pars plana vitrectomy (gold standard)**

Previously anesthetize the patient (peribulbar, retrobulbar, or general anesthesia), and use a betadine preparation to clean the skin and the surface of the eye (10% and 5% dilution, respectively) and placement of a lid speculum. A conventional approximation is done for this procedure, and there are 2 considerations: the first one is in the use of a new cassette, and the second is that the aspiration of vitreous must be done in dry conditions; that is, not turning on infusion until aspiration is done with a syringe attached to the aspirating line. Once the procedure has been done, the syringe and the cassette should be put in a sterile recipient and be submitted to the laboratory for culture.

2. **Needle puncture**

Previously anesthetize the patient with peribulbar and use a betadine preparation to clean the skin and the surface of the eye (10% and 5% dilution, respectively) and the placement of a lid speculum; the syringe is inserted at the inferior temporal quadrant 3.5 mm from the limbus. Then aspirate approximately 0.1 mL.

Any sample must not be kept in the fridge because some microorganisms are not viable at a temperature of 4 degrees Celsius.

Previously anesthetize the patient with a peribulbar infiltration and use a betadine preparation to clean the skin and the surface of the eye (10% and 5% dilution, respectively) and the placement of a lid speculum. A 30-gauge needle bent 30 degrees (used for more comfortable access to the anterior chamber) is inserted in the corneal extreme periphery. Then proceed to aspirate at least 0.1 mL (Figure 22-1).

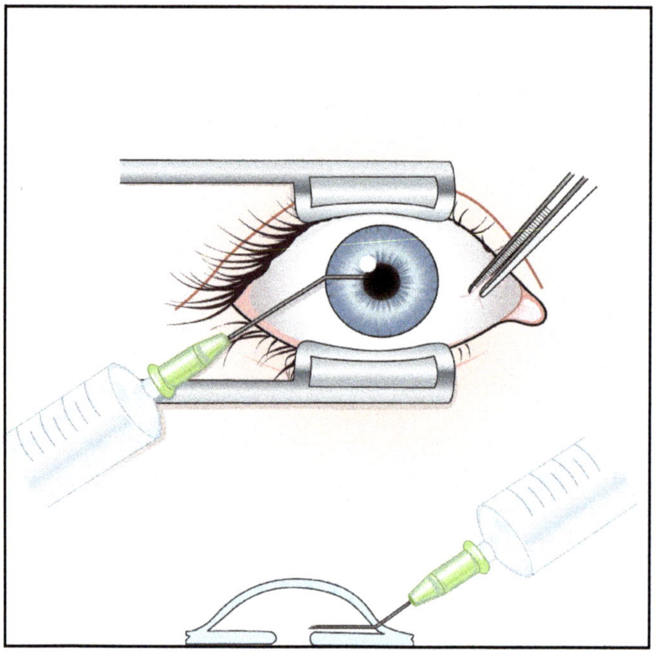

Figure 22-1. The syringe with the needle and its cap should be submitted to the laboratory immediately, leaving it at room temperature. If it is not possible to submit the sample, it should not be kept for more than 5 days.

Microbiological Laboratory Workout

Stainings:

- Gram (bacteria)
- Calcofluor (fungus)
- Giemsa (inflammatory cells)

Culture:

- Thioglycollate broth and Sabouraud's agar must be kept for 14 days in the case of positive *Propionibacterium acnes*.
- If there is a sufficient sample, a culture in blood agar and chocolate agar must be done.

PCR:

- Save a drop (50 µL) in a sterile tube for PCR at a temperature of 4°C in case it is necessary to repeat the PCR.

Initial Therapeutic Approach

Suspected Acute Bacterial Endophthalmitis Treatment

Intravitreal:

- Vancomycin 1 mg/0.1 mL
- Ceftazidime (2 mg/0.1 mL) or Amikacin (400 µg/0.1 mL)

Anti-inflammatory:

- Dexamethasone (0.4 mg/0.1 mL, preservative free)
- Systemic treatment
- Oral Moxifloxacin 400 mg/day

Topical treatment:

- Ciprofloxacin 3.5 mg/mL every 4 hours
- Dexamethasone 1 mg/mL every 4 hours
- Atropine 0.5% every 12 hours

After this initial treatment, the patient should be evaluated at 24 hours after the intravitreal injection (Figure 22-2). The clinical response and the pending outcomes of the culture will determine if antibiotic therapy should be modified.

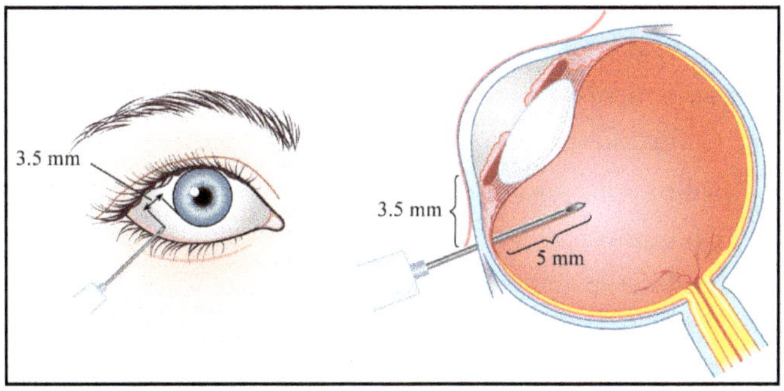

Figure 22-2. Each drug must be injected in a separate syringe with a 30-gauge needle through pars plana targeting the middle vitreous very slowly. In case of a vitrectomized patient, there should be a dilution of 50% of each medication.

Suspected Chronic Bacterial Endophthalmitis Treatment

After making the clinical diagnosis and obtaining samples of the intraocular specimen, treatment should be started.

Systemic treatment:

- Oral clarithromycin (500 mg/12 hours) for 2 weeks

The patient should be evaluated after 48 hours through a period of 2 weeks. According to clinical and microbiological results, the decision for more aggressive treatment will be assessed as the following:

Intravitreal treatment will be started with an injection of vancomycin (1 mg/0.1 mL). The evaluation will be at 1 week. In case the treatment is not successful, a pars plana vitrectomy, partial capsulectomy followed by another intravitreal injection of vancomycin will be the rule. If there is still no response to the treatment, a total capsulectomy and IOL extraction is indicated.

Suspected Fungal Endophthalmitis Treatment

The ophthalmologist should take into consideration this diagnosis principally in an immunodepressed patient and in a delayed-onset endophthalmitis, which the differential diagnosis should be made from a bacterial etiology. With an immunodepressed patient, an interdisciplinary treatment should be sought, trying to avoid systemic steroids whenever the clinical condition of the patient will allow it.

When microbiology and PCR results are positive for fungi specimen, the first choice treatment should be a combined therapy (intravitreal + systemic).

According to the species (ie, if it is yeast or filamentous fungi), drug treatment will differ.

Yeast

Intravitreal treatment:

- Amphotericin B (5 µg/0.05 mL)

Systemic treatment:

- Oral ketoconazol (20 to 400 mg/day)

Surgical treatment:

- Pars plana vitrectomy

Filamentous Fungi

Intravitreal treatment:

- Voriconazol (100 µg/0.1 mL)

Systemic treatment:

- Oral voriconazol (200 mg/12 hours)

Surgical treatment:

- Pars plana vitrectomy

If the anterior chamber is affected, the following treatment should be added:

- Intracameral treatment:
- Voriconazol (100 µg/0.1 mL)

Topical treatment:

- Yeast
    - Amphotericin (0.5 to 2%) every hour if necessary
- Filamentous fungi
    - Natamycin (5%) every hour if necessary

Immediately when the results of the causal agent or the fungal culture are received, the treatment should be modified.

According to the species, there are known resistances (ie, *Fusarium sp* is resistant to fluconazol, *Scedosporium apiospermum* is resistant to amphotericin B, and *Fusarium solani* is resistant to the majority of the azoles and poliens).

Tips for Antibiotic Preparation in Suspected Endophthalmitis

Antibiotics Drug Preparation

Preparations of medicines must be performed under strict sterile conditions and at an approved pharmacy for this purpose. Below are the preparations of the following drugs:

- Intravitreals
- Amikacin
- Amphotericin B
- Ceftazidime

- Dexamethasone
- Vancomycin
- Voriconazole
- Topical (drops)
- Amphotericin B

INTRAVITREALS

Intravitreal Amikacin (400 µg/0.1 mL)

Components:

- Amikacin solution 500 mg/2 mL
- Saline solution

Elaboration:

- Fill a 50-mL syringe with 40 mL of saline solution.
- In another syringe put 0.8 mL from the solution of amikacin.
- Place the solution of 0.8 mL of amikacin inside the syringe with the saline solution. Shake it and complete with saline solution.
- Fill a 0.5-mL syringe through a filter of 5 µ. Purge, seal, and label as a sterile product.

Expiration time from preparation: 24 hours

Conservation: Store protected away from the light and in the refrigerator.

Intravitreal Amphotericin B (5 µg / 0.05 mL)

Components:

- Amphotericin B vial 50 mg
- Water for injection

Elaboration:

- Reconstitute amphotericin B 50-mg vial with 10 mL of water for injection.
- Fill 1 mL from the reconstituted amphotericin B in a 1-mL syringe (syringe A).
- Fill 40 mL of water for injection in a 50-mL syringe (syringe B).
- Add the content of syringe A to syringe B. Complete the 50 mL with water for injection.
- Fill a syringe of 0.5 mL with the contents of syringe B. Purge until complete 50 µL.
- Seal and label as a sterile product.

Expiration time: 24 hours

Conservation: Store protected away from the light and in the refrigerator.

Intravitreal Ceftazidime (2 mg/0.1 mL)

Components:

- Ceftazidime 1 g vial
- Saline solution

Elaboration

- Add to the vial of ceftazidime 9.4 mL of water for injection.
- Shake and maintain the needle introduced in the vial in order to ventilate and to avoid the overpressure of carbon dioxide produced during the reconstitution. Maintain a negative pressure in the vial during the whole procedure.
- In a syringe of 10 mL, put 2 mL of the reconstituted vial. Complete the missing 8 mL with saline solution.
- Shake and fill a syringe of 0.5 mL through a filter of 5 µ. Purge, seal, and label as a sterile product.

Expiration time: 24 hours

Conservation: Store protected away from the light and in the refrigerator.

Intravitreal Dexamethasone (400 µg/0.1 mL)

Components:

- Dexamethasone 4-mg ampoule

Elaboration:

- Open the dexamethasone ampoule
- Fill a syringe with 0.5 mL through a filter of 5 µ (0.22 µ if not working in a horizontal flow bell).
- Purge, close the syringe, seal, and label as a sterile product.

Expiration time: 24 hours

Conservation: Store protected away from the light and in the refrigerator.

Intravitreal Vancomycin (1 mg/0.1 mL)

Components:

- Vancomycin 500-mg vial
- Saline solution

Elaboration:

- Reconstitute vancomycin 500-mg vial with 10 mL of saline solution.
- Fill a 2-mL syringe with the reconstituted vancomycin (syringe A).
- Inject 2 mL of syringe A into a sterile, empty vial (solution #1).

- Add 8 mL of saline solution to solution #1.
- Seal the vial. To withdraw the solution of vancomycin (1 mg/0.1 mL), a tuberculin syringe should be used with a needle different than the one for injection in the eye.

Expiration time: 96 hours, although the immediate utilization is recommended.

Conservation: Store protected away from the light and in the refrigerator.

Intravitreal or Intracameral Voriconazole (100 µg/0.1 mL)

Components:

- Voriconazole 200 mg vial
- Water for injection

Elaboration:

- Reconstitute the vial of voriconazole with 19 mL of water for injection (solution A).
- Withdraw 1 mL from solution A with a 20-mL syringe and complete with water for injection.
- Complete the syringe with water for injection. Close and shake (solution B).
- Transfer solution B in 2 sterile, empty vials with 10 mL each.
- Seal the vials and label as a sterile product.

Expiration time: 24 hours

Conservation: Store in the refrigerator.

Ophthalmic Suspensions

Amphotericin B Ophthalmic Suspension (2 mg/mL)

Components:

- Amphotericin B 50-mg vial
- Tears Naturale (Alcon Laboratories Inc, Fort Worth, TX) 10 mL
- Water for injection

Elaboration:

- Reconstitute amphotericin B 50 mg vial with 10 mL of water for injection (solution A).
- Remove and discard 4 mL from the vial of the artificial tears using a 25-gauge needle.
- Remove 4 mL from solution A with an insulin syringe and introduce the solution through the opening of the vial.
- Shake, close, and label.

Expiration time: 17 days

Conservation: Store protected away from the light and in the refrigerator.

References

1. Roth DB, Flynn HW Jr. Antibiotic selection in the treatment of endophthalmitis: the significance of drug combinations and synergy. *Surv Ophthalmol.* 1997;41(5):395-401.
2. Lalwani GA, Flynn HW Jr, Scott IU, et al. Acute-onset endophthalmitis after clear corneal cataract surgery (1996-2005). Clinical features, causative organisms, and visual acuity outcomes. *Ophthalmology.* 2008;115(3):473-476.
3. Krause L, Bechrakis NE, Heimann H, Kildal D, Foerster MH. Incidence and outcome of endophthalmitis over a 13-year period. *Can J Ophthalmol.* 2009;44(1):88-94.
4. Abreu JA, Cordovés L. Chronic or saccular endophthalmitis: diagnosis and management. *J Cataract Refract Surg.* 2001;27(5):650.
5. Williams A, Sloan FA, Lee PP. Longitudinal rates of cataract surgery. *Arch Ophthalmol.* 2006;124(9):1308-1314.
6. ESCRS Endophthalmitis Study Group. Prophylaxis of postoperative endophthalmitis following cataract surgery: results of the ESCRS multicenter study and identification of risk factors. *J Cataract Refract Surg.* 2007;33(6):978-988.
7. Bohigian GM. A retrospective study of the incidence of culture-positive endophthalmitis after cataract surgery and the use of preoperative antibiotics. *Ophthalmic Surg Lasers Imaging.* 2007;38(2):103-106.
8. Taban M, Behrens A, Newcomb RL, et al. Acute endophthalmitis following cataract surgery: a systematic review of the literature. *Arch Ophthalmol.* 2005;123(5):613-620.
9. Miller JJ, Scott IU, Flynn HW Jr, et al. Acute-onset endophthalmitis after cataract surgery (2000-2004): incidence, clinical settings, and visual acuity outcomes after treatment. *Am J Ophthalmol.* 2005;139(6):983-987.
10. Hatch WV, Cernat G, Wong D, et al. Risk factors for acute endophthalmitis after cataract surgery: a population-based study. *Ophthalmology.* 2009;116(3):425-430.
11. Bhagat N, Nagori S, Zarbin M. Post-traumatic Infectious Endophthalmitis. *Surv Ophthalmology.* 2011;56(3):214-251.
12. Duncan A, Mark L, Swejal A, et al. Bacterial susceptibility in trauma associated endophthalmitis. Invest. *Ophthalmol. Vis. Sci.* 2012;53:1675.
13. Andrew A, Phillip J, Harry W, et al. Endophthalmitis after intravitreal vascular endothelial growth factor antagonist: a seven year experience at a University Referral Center. Invest. *Ophthalmol. Vis. Sci.* 2012;53:1693.
14. Karsten U, Yazmin Y, Fabian S, et al. Spectrum of isolated microorganisms and their antibiotic resistance pattern in postoperative endophthalmitis. Invest. *Ophthalmol. Vis. Sci.* 2012;53:6193.

Financial Disclosures

Dr. Athiya Agarwal has no financial or proprietary interest in the materials presented herein.

Dr. Jorge L. Alió has no financial or proprietary interest in the materials presented herein.

Dr. Stephen F. Brint has no financial or proprietary interest in the materials presented herein.

Dr. Lucio Buratto has not disclosed any relevant financial relationships.

Dr. Iva Dekaris has no financial or proprietary interest in the materials presented herein.

Dr. Nikica Gabric has no financial or proprietary interest in the materials presented herein.

Dr. Tsutomu Hara has no financial or proprietary interest in the materials presented herein.

Dr. Ozana Moraru has no financial or proprietary interest in the materials presented herein.

Dr. Mauricio A. Perez has no financial or proprietary interest in the materials presented herein.

Dr. Šárka Pitrová has no financial or proprietary interest in the materials presented herein.

Dr. Mario R. Romano has no financial or proprietary interest in the materials presented herein.

Dr. Michael E. Snyder has no financial or proprietary interest in the materials presented herein.

Dr. Felipe Soria has no financial or proprietary interest in the materials presented herein.

Dr. Roger F. Steinert is a consultant for Abbott Medical Optics.

Dr. Eva Vlková has no financial or proprietary interest in the materials presented herein.

Index

For Product Safety Concerns and Information please contact our EU
representative GPSR@taylorandfrancis.com
Taylor & Francis Verlag GmbH, Kaufingerstraße 24, 80331 München, Germany

www.ingramcontent.com/pod-product-compliance
Ingram Content Group UK Ltd.
Pitfield, Milton Keynes, MK11 3LW, UK
UKHW052223190926
475702UK00006B/1181
* 9 7 8 1 6 1 7 1 1 6 0 8 7 *